W9-BIE-213

Second Edition *Manual of*

BASIC NEUROPATHOLOGY

by **RAYMOND ESCOUROLLE, M.D.**

Professor, University of Paris VI
School of Medicine
Chief of the Neuropathology Service
Charles Foix Laboratory
Hôpital de la Salpêtrière
Paris, France

JACQUES POIRIER, M.D.

Associate Professor, University of Paris XII
School of Medicine
Section of Neuropathology
of the Department of Pathology
Hôpital Henri-Mondor
Créteil, France

translated by **LUCIEN J. RUBINSTEIN, M.D.**

Professor of Pathology (Neuropathology)
Stanford University School of Medicine
Stanford, California

Negri
ε intracyto inclusions
ex, purkinje cell cerebellum.

W. B. SAUNDERS COMPANY

Philadelphia   London   Toronto
Mexico City   Rio de Janeiro   Sydney   Tokyo

W. B. Saunders Company: West Washington Square
                           Philadelphia, PA   19105

                           1 St. Anne's Road
                           Eastbourne, East Essex BN21 3UN, England

                           1 Goldthorne Avenue
                           Toronto, Ontario M8Z 5T9, Canada

                           Apartado 26370 — Cedro 512
                           Mexico 4, D.F., Mexico

                           Rua Coronel Cabrita, 8
                           Sao Cristovao Caixa Postal 21176
                           Rio de Janeiro, Brazil

                           9 Waltham Street
                           Artarmon, N.S.W. 2064, Australia

                           Ichibancho, Central Bldg., 22-1 Ichibancho
                           Chiyoda-Ku, Tokyo 102, Japan

Library of Congress Cataloging in Publication Data

Escourolle, Raymond, 1924–

Manual of basic neuropathology.

Translation of Manuel élémentaire de neuropathologie.

Bibliography: p.

Includes index.

1. Nervous system — Diseases.   I. Poirier, J., joint author.
   II. Title [DNLM: 1. Nervous system diseases —
   Pathology. WL100 E74m]

RC347.E8313 1978   616'8'04'7   77–80748

ISBN 0–7216–3406–0

Authorized translation. All rights reserved.

Title of the original French language edition:
Manuel Élémentaire de Neuropathologie
© 1971, Masson et Cie, Paris, France

English translation published 1978 by W. B. Saunders Company,
Philadelphia, London and Toronto.

Manual of Basic Neuropathology   ISBN   0-7216-3406-0

© 1978 by W. B. Saunders Company.   Copyright 1973 by W. B. Saunders Company.   Copyright
under the International Copyright Union.   All rights reserved.   This book is protected by copyright.   No part of it may be reproduced, stored in a retrieval system, or transmitted in any form
or by any means, electronic, mechanical, photocopying, recording or otherwise, without written
permission from the publisher.   Made in the United States of America.   Press of W. B. Saunders
Company.   Library of Congress catalog card number 77-080748.

Last digit is the print number: 9   8

PREFACE

The compilation of a basic work designed to familiarize students with such a highly specialized discipline as neuropathology entails two alternative risks: in attempting to compress the maximum information within the minimum of space, the text is liable to become unintelligible to beginners; if on the contrary one tries to maintain too elementary a level, the risk is that only the obvious will be stated. In presenting to the non-initiated reader neuropathological information that some may find too simple we have preferred the risk of the second pitfall.

This book is indeed designed not for neuropathologists, or even trained neurologists, but for medical students, particularly those with a special interest in neurology or neuropathology who have recently joined a neurology service or a neuropathology laboratory, and for students in anatomic pathology who wish to become familiar with the essential topics of the pathology of the nervous system. Those who do not plan a career in neurology or neuropathology need not extend their studies beyond the material covered herein; the others should regard this manual simply as an introduction to the textbooks and treatises listed in the bibliography. We have not added any other references, since to turn directly from this manual to the study of specialized articles would mean bypassing an essential intermediate stage of learning, namely an acquaintance with the well-recognized texts. The reader who wishes to specialize will find further references in these texts as well as in the volumes of journals devoted to neuropathology (*Acta Neuropathologica, Journal of Neuropathology and Experimental Neurology, Neuropathology and Applied Neurobiology*), to neurology (*Archives of Neurology, Brain, Brain Research, Journal of Comparative Neurology, Journal of Neurological Sciences, Journal of Neurology, Neurosurgery and Psychiatry, Neurology, Revue Neurologique*, etc.) and to anatomic pathology.

Names have purposely been avoided, with the exception of those traditionally associated with a particular disease. Discussion on the interpretation of lesions has been limited to the simplest observations. Many of the exceptionally rare diseases have been glossed over or mentioned only for the sake of completeness. Despite their interest, historical data have been omitted.

Among the recent contributions made by neuro- and histochemistry, electron microscopy, tissue culture, etc., only those well-accepted findings that have helped to clarify some of the more controversial aspects of the subject, especially in tumor pathology and in the dysmetabolic and degenerative disorders, have been retained. We have elected not to incorporate some of the recent data pertaining particularly to the basic cellular lesions in neuropathology, since we believe that they are still too fragmentary and in need of further study.

We express our grateful thanks to Miss Asselineau, Mrs. Fenoy, Miss Freytag, Mrs. Simonneau and Miss Vermeilley, our technicians of the Charles Foix Laboratory of Neuropathology, and to Mrs. Favolini, technician in the Anatomic Pathology Service of the Henri-Mondor Hospital, who performed the histological sections used in this text. We also thank Miss Tong for her gross and microscopic photographic work, and Mrs. Etchebehere and Mrs. Feyfant for typing the manuscript.

We are indebted to our several colleagues and friends who have given us the benefit of their criticisms and their suggestions. We are deeply grateful to our Chief, Dr. P. Castaigne, Dean of the Faculty of Medicine and Professor of Neurology at the Salpêtrière Hospital, for the constant support he has given to the development of our neuropathology laboratory and for the interest he has shown in this work, for which he wrote the introduction to the original edition. We warmly thank Dr. Fred Plum, of Cornell University School of Medicine, New York, for doing us the honor of introducing this English edition. Finally, we wish to express all our gratitude to Dr. Lucien J. Rubinstein for his kind interest in this manual and for his offer to translate it.

RAYMOND ESCOUROLLE, M.D.
JACQUES POIRIER, M.D.

TRANSLATOR'S FOREWORD

The publication, in 1971, of Escourolle and Poirier's *Manuel Élémentaire de Neuropathologie* met with immediate critical approval in European neurological journals. The clarity of its text, the selection and quality of its photographs and photomicrographs, and the simplicity of its drawings made it an obvious choice for translation for the benefit of English-speaking medical students and first-year residents in neurology, neurosurgery and pathology, for whom there had long been need of a basic primer in neuropathology that combines brevity with authority. The English version, which appeared in 1973, had a favorable reception and a revised updated edition of this work is now called for.

In this second edition, the text has undergone substantial changes. The chapters on nervous system tumors and on vascular pathology have been extensively reorganized, while those on infectious diseases and on genetic metabolic disorders due to enzyme defects have been virtually entirely rewritten. Those on the neuropathology of general pathological processes and on neuromuscular pathology have been updated and supplemented. The survey on neuropathological techniques which, in the earlier edition, constituted the introductory chapter has now been transferred as an appendix at the end of the manual and additional information on the special techniques applicable to muscle, nerve, and brain biopsy procedures has been incorporated. A number of photomicrographs, electron micrographs and diagrams have been added or replaced: approximately one-third of the illustrative material has been modified. Despite these fairly extensive revisions and additions, the authors have preserved the concision of the original format: the increase in size of this manual has been modest.

The authors of this text have medical backgrounds and qualifications which complement each other harmoniously. Both have had training in neurology. Professor Raymond Escourolle was for many years associated with the clinical service of the Salpêtrière Hospital in Paris, under Professor Alajouanine and later Professor Castaigne. Dr. Jacques Poirier's background and interests have been in histology and electron microscopy. Both are full-time neuropathologists, actively engaged in teaching and research. Their wide clinical and pathological experience is greatly strengthened by their having at their disposal the unrivaled neuropathological material of the Salpêtrière, where the French tradition of practice, teaching and research in clinical neurology and neuropathology is vigorously maintained.

A small number of minor changes have been made in the English text, usually to conform to taxonomic usages with which English-speaking medical readers may be more familiar. These changes have been made with the full approval of the authors. Where a divergence exists in the views held by the authors and those generally accepted by English-speaking neuropathologists—and these have been exceptionally few—a footnote has been added qualified as a "translator's note."

The translator is most grateful to the authors for their suggestions and for their concern in ensuring the authoritative character of the translation. He is indebted to Professor Dorothy S. Russell for her critical and helpful review of the English text of the first edition. He thanks Mrs. Melinda Callahan for typographical and secretarial help. Finally, he wishes to record his appreciation to Mr. John J. Hanley and Mr. Herbert J. Powell, Jr., W. B. Saunders Company, Philadelphia, for their assistance in the publication of the English edition of this manual.

Lucien J. Rubinstein, M.D.

INTRODUCTION TO
THE ENGLISH EDITION

As fields grow in the depth and scope of their knowledge, so do their textbooks tend to grow in size. This expansion has been notably true in anatomic neuropathology which, during recent years, has seen less and less of its important contributions incorporated into textbooks of general pathology and ever longer and more detailed volumes devoted exclusively to its varying aspects and their individual complexities. However, this necessary and fortunate effort of neuropathologists to bring us much needed details of their advances has left unfilled the parallel need for a modern, accurate, yet brief, exposition of the field. Surely, from the standpoint of teaching and patient care such statements are as needed as are the longer works. Undergraduate medical students for their first reading in a subject need a treatise that is, above all, accurate, clearly written, well-illustrated, and at least partly diagrammatic. Postgraduate students in neurology, neurosurgery, psychiatry and pathology require a comprehensive review of neuropathology that remains digestible in size, and these same specialists need an equally manageable volume later in their lives when they refresh their knowledge of a subject no longer in daily use.

Happily, this manual by Drs. Escourolle and Poirier fulfills all these needs. Originally published in France, the volume has had a deserved success on the Continent because of its combination of lucid prose, accurate description, clear photography, and generous use of clarifying line drawings and tables. All of this has been achieved within a size that permits almost any reader to survey its contents in a few hours. Now, with Dr. Rubinstein's felicitous translation, the manual is available to English-speaking audiences, for whom it will meet a need not presently fulfilled by any contemporary work. Drs. Escourolle and Poirier bring to their manual of neuropathology the special gifts of experienced pathologists who are thoroughly versed with the bedside nuances of clinical neurology. The result is an introductory and review text which is bound to serve a needed and important teaching function in its field.

FRED PLUM, M.D.

TABLE OF CONTENTS

Chapter 1

BASIC PATHOLOGY OF THE CENTRAL NERVOUS SYSTEM 1

Morphological analysis of central nervous system lesions 1
  Basic cellular lesions.. 1
    Neuronal lesions.. 1
    Astrocytic lesions 7
    Oligodendroglial lesions.. 10
    Microglial lesions 10
  Tissue lesions.. 12
  Appearances due to artifacts 15
    Gross artifacts 15
    Microscopic artifacts... 15
  Topographical analysis of central nervous system lesions 16
  Integration of morphological and topographical findings.............. 17

Chapter 2

TUMORS OF THE CENTRAL NERVOUS SYSTEM 18

Classification.. 18
Primary neoplasms 23
  Astrocytomas 23
  Glioblastomas... 25
  Oligodendrogliomas.. 26
  Ependymomas 28
  Choroid plexus papillomas 29
  Colloid cysts of the third ventricle................................. 30
  Medulloblastomas 31
  Ganglioneuromas and gangliogliomas............................... 31
  Pineal tumors... 31
  Schwannomas 33
  Neurofibromas.. 35
  Meningiomas 36
  Melanomas 41
  Sarcomas... 42
  Glomus jugulare tumors 44
  Pituitary adenomas 44

   Craniopharyngiomas 45
   Cholesteatomas 45
   Chordomas 48
   Lipomas 49
   Teratomas 49
   Hemangioblastomas 49
  Secondary tumors 51
  Bone tumors 54
  Structural changes resulting from expanding intracranial
  space-occupying lesions 54
   Focal changes 54
   Regional changes 54
   Recurrences, extracranial extensions, metastases 58

Chapter 3

TRAUMATIC LESIONS OF THE CENTRAL NERVOUS SYSTEM 60

  Craniocerebral injuries 60
   Closed craniocerebral injuries 60
    Primary traumatic lesions 60
    General and/or special consequences of primary traumatic
    lesions 64
    Summary 64
   Open craniocerebral injuries 65
  Injuries to the spinal cord and nerve roots 66

Chapter 4

VASCULAR PATHOLOGY 67

  Cerebral and/or meningeal hemorrhage 67
   Hypertensive hemorrhage 67
   Hemorrhage resulting from vascular malformations 72
   Hemorrhages due to blood dyscrasias 81
  Ischemic vascular pathology of arterial origin: infarctions 82
   General features 82
   Pathophysiology and etiology 85
    Hemodynamic factors 85
    Etiological factors 87
   Topography 90
    Cerebral infarcts 90
    Spinal intramedullary infarcts 98
  Other cerebrovascular lesions of ischemic nature 101
  Vascular pathology of venous origin 103

Chapter 5

PATHOLOGY OF INFECTIOUS DISEASES 105

    Bacterial infections 105
        Pyogenic infections 105
        Tuberculosis 107
        Syphilis 110
        Brucellosis 111
    Mycoses 111
    Parasitic infections 112
    Rickettsial infections.. 113
    Viral diseases 113
        Nonspecific nervous system manifestations of viral infections 113
        Viral encephalitis... 114
        Transmissible "slow-virus" cerebral infections 120

Chapter 6

MULTIPLE SCLEROSIS AND DISEASES OF THE WHITE MATTER............. 121

    General considerations 121
    Multiple sclerosis and Schilder's disease 124
        Multiple sclerosis 124
        Schilder's disease 128
    The leukodystrophies... 129

Chapter 7

PATHOLOGY OF DEGENERATIVE DISEASES 132

    Pathology of degenerative cortical diseases 132
    Pathology of subcortical degenerative diseases................................ 137
    Pathology of cerebellar degenerative diseases.................................. 139
        Cerebellar atrophy with chiefly cortical involvement.................... 139
        Other forms of cerebellar atrophy... 141
    Pathology of spinal medullary degenerative diseases 144

Chapter 8

NEUROPATHOLOGY OF GENERAL PATHOLOGICAL PROCESSES............. 150

    Cerebral lesions of anoxic nature 150
    Pathology of deficiency diseases 153
    Encephalopathies of metabolic origin... 157

Toxic encephalopathies 157
Chronic alcoholism 158
Nervous system lesions due to malignant visceral disease in the
absence of tumor deposits 161
Hematological and lymphoreticular diseases: dysglobulinemias 162
Amyloidosis of the nervous system 164
Diabetes mellitus 164
Collagen diseases 164

Chapter 9

GENETIC METABOLIC DISEASES DUE TO AN ENZYME DEFECT 165

Disorders of lipid metabolism 165
    The sphingolipidoses 166
        The gangliosidoses 166
        The cerebrosidoses 168
        The sulfatidoses 169
        Niemann-Pick disease 171
        Fabry's disease 172
        Farber's lipogranulomatosis 172
    Refsum's disease 172
    Other neurolipidoses 172
    The lipoproteinoses 172
Disorders of mucopolysaccharide (glycosaminoglycan) metabolism 173
Disorders of carbohydrate metabolism 174
Disorders of amino acid metabolism 174
Disorders of metal metabolism 175
Disorders of pigment metabolism 175

Chapter 10

CONGENITAL MALFORMATIONS OF THE NERVOUS SYSTEM AND PERINATAL PATHOLOGY 176

Etiology of congenital malformations 176
Disturbances due to defective closure of the neural groove
(or dysraphic states) 176
Ageneses and dysgeneses 178
Cortical anomalies 181
Arachnoidal cysts 182
Hydrocephalus 183
Syringomyelia 185
Blastomatous dysplasias and phakomatoses 187
Perinatal pathology 188

Chapter 11

NEUROMUSCULAR PATHOLOGY 191

   Histological examination of muscle biopsies................................. 191
      Principal lesions 191
      Chief etiological processes... 195
      Conclusion 202
   Histological examination of peripheral nerve biopsies 203
      Principal lesions 203
      Chief etiological processes... 207
      Conclusion 208

Appendix

BRIEF SURVEY OF NEUROPATHOLOGICAL TECHNIQUES........................ 213

   Methods of removal... 213
      Autopsy 213
      Surgical specimens.. 215
      Biopsy procedures 215
   Fixation of tissues... 217
   Gross examination of the central nervous system......................... 217
      Inspection of the brain and spinal cord................................. 217
      Cutting of gross slices... 218
      Histological sampling 221
   Embedding, sectioning, and staining methods............................. 221
      Embedding and sectioning procedures................................. 221
      Staining procedures 224
   Special techniques... 224

BIBLIOGRAPHY 227

INDEX 231

Chapter 1

BASIC PATHOLOGY OF THE CENTRAL NERVOUS SYSTEM

Diagnosis in neuropathology is based on the gross and microscopic study of the brain, brainstem, cerebellum, and spinal cord. Three consecutive steps are involved and are, in fact, closely interrelated:

A morphological analysis of the lesions;

A topographical analysis of the lesions;

A critical integration of these findings and their subsequent confrontation with the clinical data and the general autopsy findings, thus permitting an etiological diagnosis to be made in most instances.

I. MORPHOLOGICAL ANALYSIS OF CENTRAL NERVOUS SYSTEM LESIONS

With the exception of tumors and malformations, most disorders of the central nervous system are characterized morphologically by the association of a number of lesions that are not diagnostic by themselves. Some of these lesions are revealed only on microscopic examination and involve the cellular elements of the nervous system (basic cellular lesions), whereas others, which correspond to more massive changes, are often recognizable grossly or with the help of a magnifying lens.

A. BASIC CELLULAR LESIONS

These lesions may involve the neurons, the astrocytes, the oligodendrocytes, and the microglia.

Although it is possible, for didactic purposes, to evaluate separately the changes demonstrable in the neurons, glia, fibrous connective tissue, and vascular structures, it is essential to emphasize the close functional interdependence of these various tissue elements and the concomitance of their reactions to the various pathological processes. This is particularly important in the case of nerve cell alterations, whose artifactual nature must be suspected if they are not accompanied by glial cell changes.

I. NEURONAL LESIONS[1]

a. Nerve cell loss ("neuronal depopulation"). Nerve cell loss is understood to

---

[1]In addition to these basic lesions, classical authors have described numerous nerve cell alterations, most of which are regarded today as related to preagonal terminal events. Among these, *Nissl's acute cell disease* (Spielmeyer's acute swelling), characterized by cell swelling and cytoplasmic basophilia, would seem to be due to hyperpyrexia and terminal hydroelectrolytic disturbances. Nissl's "severe cell disease," with its picture of cytoplasmic vacuolization and satellitosis, would constitute a later, terminal and nonregressive stage in the evolution of acute cell disease. It is seen rather infrequently, as is Spielmeyer's *granular degeneration*, which would seem to be a stabilized stage of the same regressive cell process.

occur when the number of cell bodies in a particular area is appreciably lower than normal. This is difficult to estimate when it involves less than 30 per cent of the normal cell population, and its assessment depends on the thickness of the section and on the normal cytoarchitectonics of the region examined. In practice, neuronal cell loss cannot easily be evaluated in the absence of astrocytic changes (gliosis).

Sooner or later, neuronal cell loss constitutes the end stage of all pathological processes that involve the nerve cells and are irreversible.

b. Simple neuronal atrophy (or "chronic nerve cell degeneration"). Simple neuronal atrophy is characterized by retraction of the cell body, with diffuse basophilia of the cytoplasm, and pyknosis and hyperchromasia of the nucleus. In addition, excessive lipofuscin pigment ("pigment atrophy") is often present. Simple neuronal atrophy is the result of numerous progressive degenerative processes.

c. "Ischemic" nerve cell change (or "acute necrosis") (Fig. 1). Ischemic nerve

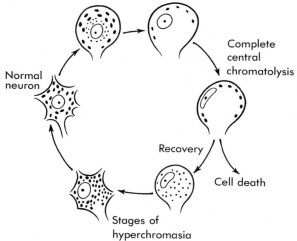

Figure 2. *Various nerve cell changes resulting from central chromatolysis.*

cell change is characterized by retraction of the cell body, with eosinophilia of the cytoplasm, disappearance of Nissl bodies, and pyknosis and hyperchromasia of the nucleus. Occasionally a few small basophilic masses are visible on the surface of the nerve cell; they correspond to degenerated terminal synaptic boutons.

Ischemic nerve cell change is linked to neuronal anoxia and results in total cell necrosis. It is seen in many acute processes.

d. Neuronophagia. In some processes that selectively affect the neurons, secondary phagocytosis of the cell body may occur. A collection of macrophages is then seen which surrounds debris from the cell body (see Fig. 141*A*).

e. Central chromatolysis (Fig. 2). Central chromatolysis is characterized morphologically by swelling of the cell body, disappearance of Nissl bodies—which persist only at the periphery of the cell—and flattening and displacement of the nucleus to the periphery (Fig. 3).[1]

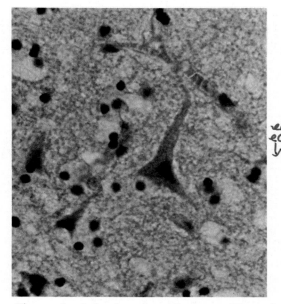

Figure 1. *Ischemic nerve cell change* (H. and E.). Cytoplasmic shrinkage and hyperchromatic nucleus.

---

[1]Neuronal chromatolysis may be so diagnosed only after comparison with the normal morphology of the appropriate nerve cell. Some nuclei (e.g., the mesencephalic tract of the fifth cranial nerve, Clarke's column) normally possess rounded neurons with marginated Nissl bodies, whose aspect may be misleading on cursory examination.

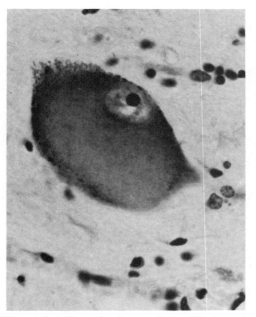

Figure 3. *Central chromatolysis* (Nissl stain). Note the cellular swelling, the eccentric displacement of the nucleus, and the margination of the Nissl bodies.

It is seen usually in lower motor neurons (anterior horns of the spinal cord, cranial nerve nuclei), where it represents a reaction of the cell body to a lesion of the axon ("axonal reaction" or "retrograde degeneration"). Subsequent recovery of normal cell morphology or, on the contrary, further progression to nerve cell degeneration depends on the reversibility of the axonal lesion.

Central chromatolysis may be seen in upper motor neurons, but is then more difficult to interpret. On the one hand, axonal lesions within the central nervous system either do not produce changes in cell body morphology or result in a simple type of atrophy ("Gudden's atrophy"); on the other, some disorders that do not *a priori* involve axonal lesions are accompanied by central chromatolysis (e.g., Wernicke's encephalopathy, pellagra encephalopathy) (see Figs. 180 and 184).

f. Peripheral chromatolysis (Fig. 4). Peripheral chromatolysis can be differentiated from central chromatolysis by the persistence of the Nissl bodies in the central portion, as opposed to the periphery, of the cell body. Peripheral chromatolysis is an exceptional occurrence and is usually considered to be a stage of recovery from central chromatolysis.

g. Fenestrated or vacuolated neurons (Fig. 5). Swelling with vacuolization of the cell body is an exceptional basic cellular lesion. In some cases it is thought to result from trans-synaptic degeneration,[1] e.g., in

---

[1]*Trans-synaptic degeneration* may also be found in other areas (e.g., in the lateral geniculate body following a lesion of the optic nerve). This process is also thought to occur in some of the systematic degenerative disorders that involve several neuronal systems (i.e., in olivopontocerebellar atrophy, in Friedreich's ataxia, and even in amyotrophic lateral sclerosis). *Retrograde trans-synaptic degeneration* is more exceptional. It is likewise assumed to occur in some of the cellular lesions associated with the Holmes type of cerebellar atrophy, in particular those involving the inferior olives. These various processes of trans-synaptic neuronal degeneration result in a simple type of neuronal atrophy. Only degeneration of the inferior olives produces a picture of nerve cell swelling with vacuolization.

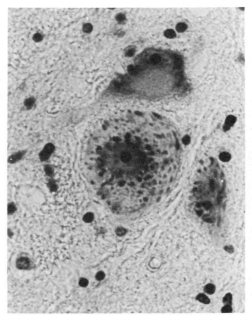

Figure 4. *Peripheral chromatolysis* (Nissl stain). Note: above the central cell is a small neuron showing central chromatolysis.

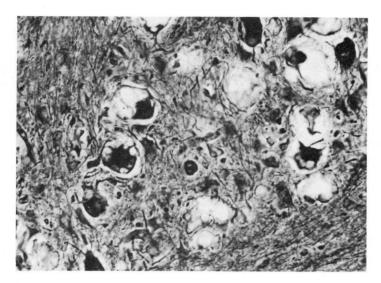

Figure 5. *Fenestrated neurons in a case of olivary hypertrophy* (Bielschowsky silver stain).

neurons of the inferior olives in olivary hypertrophy secondary to a lesion of the ipsilateral tegmental tract or of the contralateral dentate nucleus.

h. Mineralized (ferruginated) neurons (or "incrustated neurons") (Fig. 6). These lesions are caused by the deposition of iron and calcium salts in the cytoplasm of the cell body of some neurons at the edge of old hemorrhagic infarcts or of some traumatic scars.

i. Binucleated neurons. 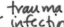 These lesions are seen rather infrequently, sometimes in the edges of old focal lesions. They are usually considered to be a form of neuronal reaction in response to adjacent tissue damage (i.e., traumatic, infectious).

Binucleated neurons may also be found in certain dysplastic processes characterized by the presence of monstrous neurons, as in tuberous sclerosis, for example.

j. Abnormal intraneuronal material. *1. The accumulation of lipofuscin* (Fig. 7) is an unremarkable aging change and, in the absence of other tissue alterations, cannot be considered to have pathological significance.

2. In *neurolipidosis* there is a diffuse accumulation of abnormal lipid products related to an intraneuronal enzymatic disorder. This results in swelling and distention of the cerebral cortical nerve cells (Fig. 8) as well as of the Purkinje cells of the cerebellum.

Histochemical stains are of help in deciding the nature of the stored material. Electron microscopy has demonstrated structural patterns that are fairly characteristic for each type (see Figs. 193, 194, and 196*B* and *C*).

3. Granulovacuolar degeneration (Fig. 9*A*) and *Alzheimer's neurofibrillary degeneration* (Fig. 9*B*) are chiefly the result of senile degenerative changes.

The former consists in the presence of small, clear vacuoles measuring 4 to 5 μm in diameter and containing an argyrophilic granule which is often also well stained with

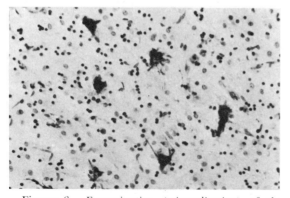

Figure 6. *Ferrugination (mineralization) of the neurons at the edge of an old hemorrhagic infarct.* Associated astrocytic gliosis (H. and E.).

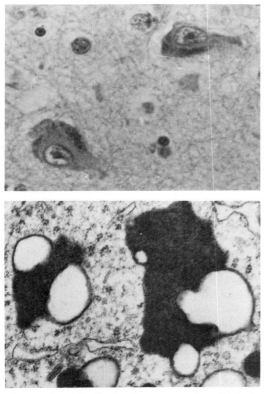

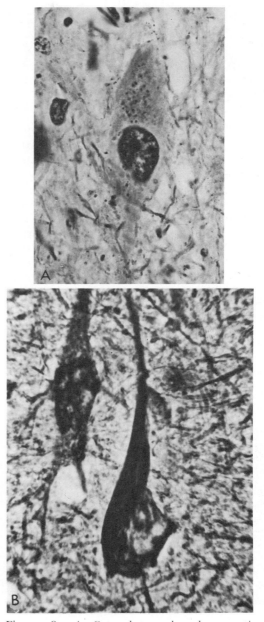

elongated, flame-shaped tufts in the cytoplasm. Other aspects consist of fine filaments entangled to form coils or more compact masses. Because of their twisted microtubular structure, as seen with the electron microscope, these changes are regarded as re-

Figure 7. *Lipofuscin in neuronal cell bodies.* Light microscopy above (periodic acid–Schiff), electron microscopy below.

hematoxylin. It is found mainly in Ammon's horn. Alzheimer's neurofibrillary degeneration has a more widespread distribution. Silver impregnations demonstrate thick,

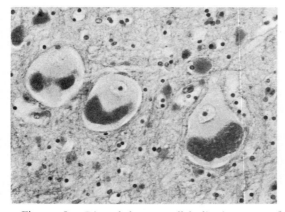

Figure 8. *Distended nerve cell bodies in a case of neurolipidosis* (combined luxol fast blue and Bodian stain).

Figure 9. *A, Granulovacuolar degeneration* (Bodian stain). *B, Neurofibrillary degeneration* (Bielschowsky silver stain).

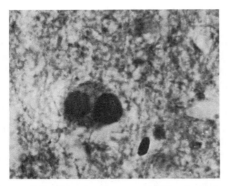

Figure 10. *Neuronal argyrophilic inclusion in Pick's disease.*

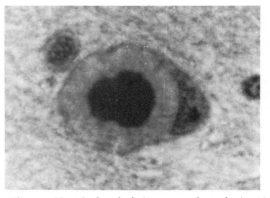

Figure 12. *Lafora body in a case of myoclonic epilepsy (dentate nucleus)* (periodic acid–Schiff).

sulting from a degeneration of the neurofilaments (see Fig. 161).[1]

Although these lesions are seen chiefly in senile dementia and in Alzheimer's disease, they are also one of the characteristic features of other degenerative processes (i.e., progressive supranuclear palsy of Steele, Richardson, and Olszewski; postencephalitic parkinsonism; and some forms of amyotrophic lateral sclerosis, such as the Guam type).

4. Round, homogeneous *neuronal argyrophilic inclusions* (Fig. 10) are characteristic of Pick's disease but are found in only one-third of the cases, mostly in the hippocampal cortex.

5. *Lewy bodies* (Fig. 11), which may be

---

[1]These structures are now believed to represent paired helical filaments. Their relationship to the normal neurofilaments is still uncertain (translator's note).

found in the pigmented nuclei such as the substantia nigra, locus coeruleus, and the dorsal motor nuclei of X, are characteristic of Parkinson's disease. These structures are rounded, rather crisply eosinophilic, are often surrounded by a paler halo, and are especially well seen in hematoxylin-eosin preparations.

6. *Lafora bodies* (Fig. 12) are rounded structures composed of mucopolysaccharides and are found chiefly in the dentate nuclei in myoclonic epilepsy.

7. *Viral inclusions.* The presence of eosinophilic *intranuclear inclusions* (see Fig. 145) which occupy a greater or lesser proportion of the nucleus and are surrounded by a clear halo is indicative of a viral infective process. These inclusions are associated with other inflammatory lesions (see below). They are seen chiefly in necrotizing encephalitis and in subacute sclerosing panencephalitis. Electron microscopy has demonstrated the presence of structures comparable to herpesvirus in the former (see Fig. 145) and to myxovirus in the latter (see Fig. 143). However, various other morphological forms that do not correspond to a viral structure are also frequently seen.

Intracytoplasmic inclusions are less often observed (e.g., Negri bodies in rabies).

k. Axonal alterations.[1] In axonal lesions, the distal part of the axon undergoes

---

[1]Recently electron microscopic studies have drawn attention to alterations in the terminal synaptic boutons which may be found in some forms of dementia.

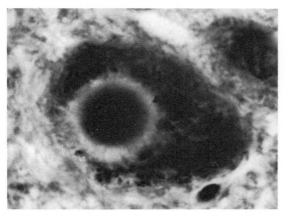

Figure 11. *Lewy body in a case of Parkinson's disease (substantia nigra)* (H. and E.).

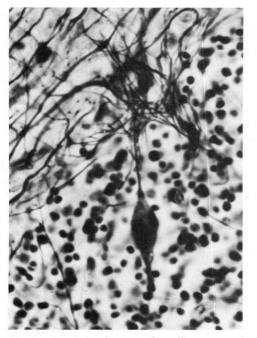

Figure 13. *Torpedo (axonal swelling) on a Purkinje cell axon in a case of olivopontocerebellar atrophy* (Bielschowsky silver stain).

various stages of wallerian degeneration (which will be described below in the context of the basic lesions affecting the peripheral nervous system).

In *simple neuronal atrophy* perikaryal lesions are associated with degeneration of the axon, which becomes moniliform and undergoes atrophy. In system degenerations the lesions appear to begin in the distal extremity of the longest axons.

A special form of axonal damage involves the Purkinje cells of the cerebellum and consists of *fusiform swellings*, with the formation of *torpedoes*. These are well seen in silver impregnations and are found to occur in the initial portion of the axis cylinder before the origin of the collateral branches (Fig. 13).

Massive rounded and globular *axonal swellings* are sometimes seen in certain forms of vitamin E deficiency. They also form part of the picture of *neuroaxonal dystrophy*.

II. ASTROCYTIC LESIONS

1. Gliosis. Gliosis is the most frequent change. It must be regarded as a *reaction* on the part of astrocytes to adjacent tissue damage. This type of reaction involves the proliferation of astrocytes (hyperplasia) and morphological changes that implicate the astrocytic nuclei and cytoplasmic organelles, especially glial filaments (hypertrophy).

Glial multiplication or proliferation (Fig. 14) is as a rule a relatively slow process in which it has been difficult, by the usual techniques, to document a mechanism of mitotic division. This is mainly due to the absence of identifiable mitoses in ordinary preparations, an observation that has in the past led some workers to postulate a mechanism of amitotic division or to envisage a process of differentiation and mobilization of undifferentiated precursor cell elements stimulated by the pathological process. However, recent work has shown that mitotic figures are readily demonstrable in astrocytes if the tissues are fixed by perfusion.

Hypertrophic *morphological changes* result in the classic picture of *fibrillary gliosis* and of *protoplasmic gliosis*.

Astrocytic hypertrophy involves the cell body and its processes. It is accompanied, although not invariably, by the production of glial filaments. These changes are secondary and follow degeneration of the nerve cells and myelin sheaths. Depending on the localization and nature of the primary degenerative process, they assume one of the following two forms: fibrillary or protoplasmic.

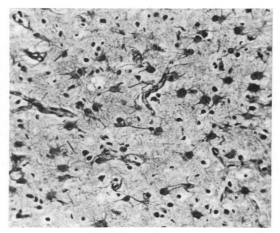

Figure 14. *Astrocytic glial proliferation* (Hortega's lithium silver carbonate impregnation).

Glial reaction at an early stage is characterized by hypertrophy of the nucleus, which is
often hyperchromatic and may demonstrate
inclusions (*nuclear bodies*), while the cytoplasm
and cell processes become visible and are
found to contain glycogen.

Ultimately, and typically *in slowly degenerative processes*, astrocytes regain their small size,
and their cytoplasm, cell processes, and glial
fibrils can be appreciated only with the help
of special stains (e.g., Holzer, Mallory's
phosphotungstic acid–hematoxylin). This is
the aspect of *fibrillary gliosis* (Fig. 15*C* and *D*).
In degenerative processes that affect the
nerve tracts, glial fibers and astrocytes orient
themselves in a direction parallel to the
degenerated nerve fibers, resulting in the
picture of *isomorphous gliosis*.

Destructive lesions of the central nervous

system, especially traumatic, provide the best
conditions for the proliferation and hypertrophy of glial cell elements. In cerebral
infarcts, astrocytes proliferate along the edge
of the focus of necrosis. Ballooning and cell
division are visible from the fourth to the
fifth day and develop in the course of the
following days. The hypertrophy chiefly involves the cytoplasm, which is homogenized
and eosinophilic, leading to the picture of
protoplasmic gliosis (Fig. 15*A*). Sometimes the
cytoplasmic hypertrophy is massive, with the
formation of *gemistocytic astrocytes* (Fig. 15*B*).
The frequent disposition of these cells in
pairs, with the formation of mirror images
on the part of the cellular elements, has long
suggested a process of amitotic division (but
see remarks above). Astrocytic gliosis, which
is often arranged in a disorderly pattern,

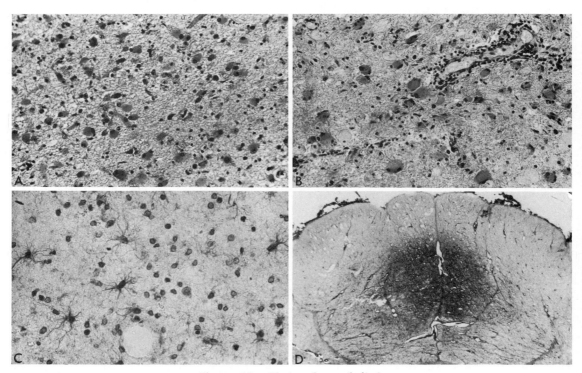

Figure 15. *Various forms of gliosis.*

A, Protoplasmic astrocytic gliosis (H. and E.).

B, Gemistocytic astrocytes in a case of Schilder's disease; note the associated perivascular lymphocytic
infiltrate (H. and E.).

C, Fibrous astrocytes (Holzer stain).

D, Fibrillary gliosis in posterior columns of the spinal cord (Holzer stain).

then assumes the aspect of *anisomorphous gliosis,* which differs markedly from the type of gliosis that accompanies degenerative processes involving the nerve tracts.

In the course of time, fiber formation progressively dominates the picture. Astrocytic cell processes and glial fibers are stouter and more numerous, whereas the cell bodies appear relatively reduced in size.

These progressive changes are seen also in a number of disorders affecting the white matter: these disorders include multiple sclerosis, Schilder's disease, leukodystrophies, and some inflammatory processes such as subacute sclerosing panencephalitis.

The precise conditions that determine these changes are still poorly understood. In some cases they may result in the monstrous giant cell forms with massive eosinophilic cytoplasm and short cell processes that represent the picture of *Alzheimer glia type I.* Multinucleated cell types are often noted. The presence of monstrous astrocytes is especially a feature of progressive multifocal leukoencephalopathy.

2. Alzheimer glia type II (Fig. 16). These changes essentially involve the astrocytic nuclei. These become massive, reaching 15 to 20 μm in diameter, and become lobated and often multilobulated. Their stain is pale because of the disappearance of chromatin granules. One or two dense spheroid bodies resembling nucleoli are often seen next to the nuclear membrane, which is always crisp

and well defined. The cell bodies are usually invisible in conventional stains, but in Nissl stains a few greenish granules are sometimes seen around the nuclei.

This lesion, which is characteristic of hepatolenticular degeneration, or Wilson's disease, is seen also in severe liver insufficiency associated with hepatic coma. It is always particularly well marked in the deep gray nuclei, especially the pallidum, the dentate nuclei, and to a lesser extent, the cerebral cortex.

"Naked nuclei gliosis," a term sometimes used to indicate the presence of rather voluminous, pale, and rounded astrocytic nuclei seen in certain forms of hepatic encephalopathy, especially associated with liver cirrhosis, may be related to the astrocytic lesion seen in Wilson's disease.

3. Glial necrosis. In ischemic and anoxic processes, the astrocytes, although less vulnerable than the neurons, may undergo degeneration. The cell bodies become ballooned and the cell processes undergo disintegration, with the picture of clasmatodendrosis, while the nuclei ultimately become pyknotic. The swollen aspect and irregular contour of these cells, which are seen in the course of a number of slowly evolving processes, correspond to the so-called "ameboid glia" of Alzheimer.

Viral infections may be the source of some instances of glial necrosis and may then lead to the presence of intranuclear inclusions, as in herpes simplex.

4. Storage material. *Lipofuscin* is frequently noted with age. The presence of large amounts of this material in certain degenerative disorders indicates a pathophysiological process that is still poorly understood.

In *neurolipidoses,* lipid glial storage may accompany neuronal storage. This is the case in Tay-Sachs disease and in some forms of mucopolysaccharidosis.

Corpora amylacea are rounded, basophilic, PAS-positive structures which measure 10 to 50 μm in diameter and are frequently noted, in the absence of pathological significance, in the subpial regions, especially near the temporal horns, and in the posterior columns of

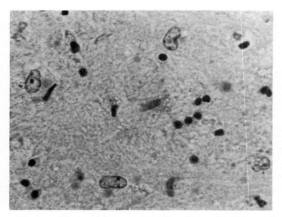

Figure 16. *Alzheimer type II glial cells* (H. and E.).

the spinal cord. By electron microscopy they are seen to arise within glial cell processes. They are found chiefly in elderly subjects and probably indicate a degenerative change in these glial processes.

III. OLIGODENDROGLIAL LESIONS

Most of the oligodendroglial cell changes noted in pathology are of doubtful significance.

a. This is the case with morphological changes corresponding to *oligodendroglial swelling* or *tumefaction.* This feature corresponds to an exaggeration of the clear perinuclear halos which are characteristic of oligodendroglia in light microscopy. It must be regarded as devoid of pathological significance and corresponds to an agonal or a postmortem artifact.

Mucicarminophilic perinuclear products are seen in the classic form of *mucoid degeneration* of the oligodendroglia. They have been noted in certain demyelinating diseases, but their significance is doubtful since they have also been found in other pathological conditions, notably in some oligodendrogliomas.

b. *The clustering of oligodendrocytes around neurons (satellitosis)* (Fig. 17) is likewise without obvious significance. This appearance is normal in some of the deep cortical layers and should, in any event, be clearly differentiated from the picture of neuronophagia that accompanies neuronal disintegration.

c. On the other hand, *loss of oligodendro-*

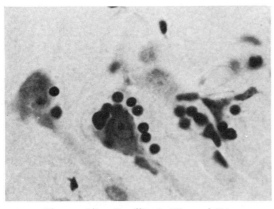

Figure 17. *Satellitosis* (H. and E.).

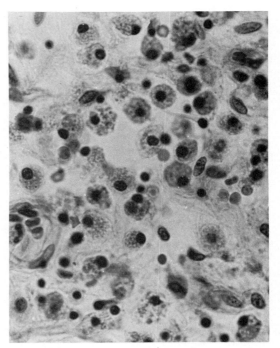

Figure 18. *Compound granular corpuscles (foam cells) or macrophages* (H. and E.). Note small blood vessel in lower left.

cytes in some of the demyelinating processes (i.e., multiple sclerosis and Schilder's disease) may be of significance.

d. Like neurons and astrocytes, oligodendrocytes may be the seat of

Intranuclear viral inclusions (especially in subacute sclerosing panencephalitis)

Lipid storage material (especially in metachromatic leukodystrophy)

e. Characteristic morphological changes have been described in progressive multifocal leukoencephalopathy.

IV. MICROGLIAL LESIONS

In *pathology* microglia play a part in three basic cell processes.

a. Proliferation of compound granular corpuscles (foam cells) or macrophages (Fig. 18) is very frequent. It is associated with demyelinating processes or with traumatic or vascular tissue destruction and assumes a fundamental phagocytic role. This cellular reaction rapidly makes its appear-

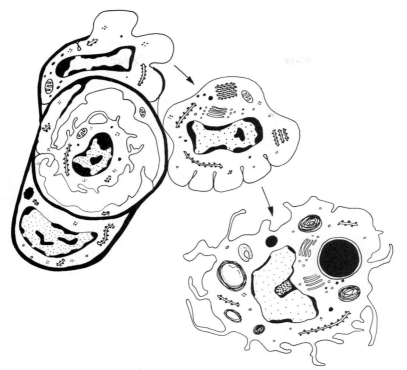

Figure 19. *Schematic drawing of macrophage formation, derived from a monocyte.* Monocytes from the blood leave the vascular lumen, become perivascular, then migrate into the cerebral parenchyma and are finally converted into macrophages. Pericytes do not participate in this process. (After Kitamura et al., J. Neuropathol. Exp. Neurol., *31*:502–518, 1972.)

macrophages

ance within 48 hours, with the development of rounded, frequently voluminous cell forms which measure 20 to 30 μm in diameter, have small, darkly staining and eccentric nuclei, and a clear granular cytoplasm that contains sudanophilic lipid or iron pigment originating from hemoglobin. The reaction increases in the course of subsequent days and weeks and may be observed after several months.

It is traditionally believed that these compound granular corpuscles are derived from microglial cells. However, experimental findings based on autoradiographic studies after tritiated thymidine labeling have now led to the belief that, in small rodents at least, the macrophages of the nervous system are, like those in the rest of the body, derived from monocytes in the circulating blood (Fig. 19).

b. Rod-shaped glial cell proliferation (Fig. 20) is usually regarded as a form of

microglial alteration characteristic of encephalitis (see Fig. 141C) and of subacute cerebral damage. Silver carbonate impregnations demonstrate the elongated nuclei and their

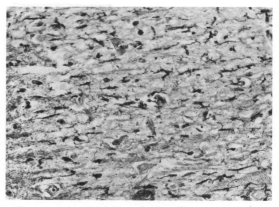

Figure 20. *Rod-shaped microglia in a case of general paralysis of the insane* (silver carbonate impregnation).

bipolar cell processes often better than conventional stains. The presence of iron in these cell processes is regarded as a characteristic feature of microglial proliferation in syphilitic general paralysis.

c. Nodules of neuronophagia are associated with acute nerve cell destruction, especially in viral encephalitis (see Fig. 141A). They are characterized by the accumulation, at the site of the damaged neuron, of rounded nuclei which somewhat resemble those of lymphocytes and are generally regarded as microglial, of round cells with nuclei that are often more voluminous, and sometimes of a few polymorphonuclear leukocytes with phagocytic features.

Occasionally in encephalitis, collections of darkly staining nuclei ("microglial nodules") may be found without the obvious picture of neuronophagia.

B. TISSUE LESIONS

The basic cellular lesions which have just been described, and which are closely interrelated, cause various changes in the neural structures. They may also be associated with meningeal, connective tissue, and vascular alterations which may result from the same pathological process. Moreover, they may bring about more massive tissue lesions, which are then often visible to the naked eye.

1. Cerebral atrophy. Cerebral atrophy is characterized by a narrowing of the gyri and a widening of the sulci and fissures over the cerebral convexity. On section the cortical ribbon is thinned, and ventricular dilatation is often present.

The histological substratum consists of a variable loss of neurons associated with gliosis and occasionally with lesions that are etiologically specific.

2. Ventricular dilatation. This lesion is difficult to evaluate when present to a mild degree and, in that case, only its focal distribution will give it practical significance.

On the other hand, it is easy to recognize when severe. It may then be due to various causes:

It may be associated with cortical and subcortical cerebral atrophy.

It may be secondary to obstruction of the cerebrospinal fluid circulation (see section on Hydrocephalus). In that case, the cerebral cortex is normal, at least in the early stages of the process.

3. Hemorrhages. Hemorrhages may be of highly variable etiology and may show different gross and microscopic features.

When only small, fresh subpial or even intracerebral hemorrhagic extravasations are present, they may be of limited significance and the result of agonal respiratory and circulatory disturbances.

4. Necrosis. This process consists essentially in destruction of the neural tissue. It may result from various etiological factors. It is obvious in old necrotizing processes that have culminated in the formation of intracerebral cavities of greater or lesser size. When recent, it is recognizable only by the softer consistency of the neural parenchyma. It is chiefly associated with edema. Microscopic changes include the disappearance of normal neural structures, the proliferation of compound granular corpuscles, and the contingent lesions that are specific for the etiological process.

5. Cerebral edema. Cerebral edema may occur as a result of various etiological factors. When severe, it is characterized by swelling of the cerebral hemispheres, flattening of the convolutions and of the ventricular cavities, and occasionally by internal herniations which are visible grossly. When unilateral, it causes displacement and compression of the midline structures, of the basal ganglia, and of the third ventricle.

Under light microscopy, myelin stains demonstrate pallor of the white matter. The cerebral tissue presents a loose appearance and is split by bullous formations of variable size. Glial cells are swollen, and perivascular spaces are dilated.

These gross and microscopic features correspond to electron microscopic appearances which vary according to the etiological

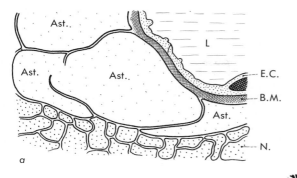

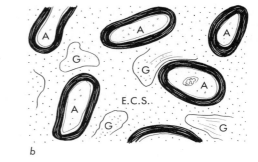

Figure 21. *Cerebral edema. Chief fine structural forms.*

a, Gray matter (traumatic and inflammatory edemas). Swelling of astrocytic cell processes, especially near capillaries. *Ast.*, astrocytic cell process; *E.C.*, capillary endothelial cell; *L.*, capillary lumen; *N.*, neuropil; *B.M.*, basement membrane.

b, White matter (traumatic and inflammatory edemas). Enlargement of extracellular spaces. *A.*, myelinated axon; *G.*, glial cell process; *E.C.S.*, extracellular space.

c, White matter (triethyltin edema). Splitting of myelin lamellae at the intraperiod line. *A.*, myelinated axon; *M.*, myelin; *V.*, vacuole.

and pathogenetic mechanism (Fig. 21); these appearances include

Astrocytic swelling

Dilatation of the perivascular and extracellular spaces

Splitting of the myelin lamellae

6. Spongiosis. Spongiosis is at present defined as a form of microcystic degeneration (see Fig. 147B) of the neural tissue. It may involve the gray or the white matter. In the former, it constitutes one of the chief features of some demential processes (see below) and corresponds to the presence of bullae and clear spaces in the astrocytes and occasionally in the neurons (see Fig. 147C).

It is seen also in some of the pathological processes that involve the white matter, such as subacute degeneration of the spinal cord (see Fig. 185) and spongy degeneration of the white matter in children (Canavan's disease).

7. Demyelination. Demyelination is defined as loss of tinctorial affinity on the part of myelin sheaths for the usual myelin stains. It may be of varying etiology (see Chapter 6).

8. Inflammatory lesions. These lesions consist of either disseminated or localized perivascular cuffings and inflammatory infiltrates of variable cell types depending on the etiology (i.e., lymphocytes, plasma cells, histiocytes, or polymorphonuclear leukocytes) (see Figs. 141B, 152A, and 155).

Their presence does not necessarily indicate an infectious etiology, since an inflammatory infiltrate of reactive, or symptomatic, character is well known to occur in other pathological processes, such as the presence of polymorphonuclear leukocytes in the early stages of cerebral infarction (see Fig. 107B) and lymphocytic infiltrations in some of the demyelinating diseases.

9.   *Connective tissue and vascular changes.*
a. Chapter 4 (Vascular Pathology) will deal with the arteriolar and arterial changes that may involve the superficial and deep vasculature as the result of various pathological processes.

b. Numerous basic neuropathological processes include among their chief lesions alterations of the vessel walls, especially of the capillaries.

Necrotizing processes, especially cerebral infarcts, very rapidly result in a capillary proliferation which, in association with the mobilization of macrophages, participates in the process of secondary phagocytosis (see Fig. 107*C*).

Some metabolic disorders such as Wernicke's encephalopathy show an association of neuronal and glial lesions with proliferation and swelling of the capillary endothelium, which is sometimes regarded as the main feature in the pathological process (see Fig. 180*A*).

Anoxic processes are accompanied by similar capillary changes (Fig. 22) which predominate in certain neural structures and in some of the cortical layers. A picture of capillary incrustation, especially in the globus pallidus, may be seen in carbon monoxide poisoning.

c. In encephalitic inflammatory processes, vascular changes characterized by perivascular lymphocytic cuffings are associated with neuronal and microglial alterations (see Fig. 141).

10.   *Meningeal and ependymal changes.*
a. The leptomeningeal tissue essentially participates in infectious processes and in vascular extravasations.

The ultimate formation of fibrous connective tissue scars and the development of adhesive arachnoiditis, which may impair the circulation and reabsorption of cerebrospinal fluid, constitute a further stage in the evolution of infective processes (see Fig. 135*C*).

Metastatic processes may likewise involve chiefly the subarachnoid meningeal spaces and present as a diffuse carcinomatous meningitis (see Chapter 2) (see Fig. 69).

b. The perivascular spaces of Virchow-Robin may pave the way for spread from the leptomeninges toward the cerebral tissue itself. In some neoplastic processes (e.g., in carcinomatous meningitis or in meningeal melanomatosis), it may thus form a pathway for the invasion of the underlying parenchyma (Fig. 23).

c. The formation of *ependymal granulations* is specific for certain meningeal infectious processes. The aggregation of subependymal histiocytes in tuberculous meningitis to form ependymal tubercles and the burgeoning proliferation of subependymal astrocytes in

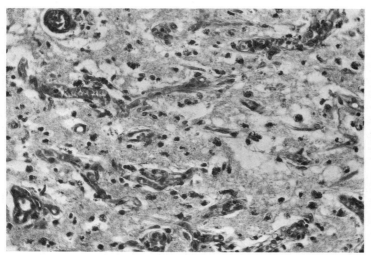

Figure 22.   *Capillary changes in anoxia.* Endothelial swelling; note the associated picture of edema.

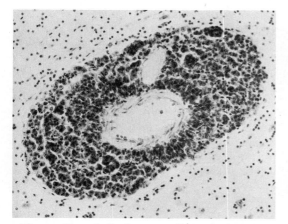

Figure 23. *Cuff of tumor cells in Virchow-Robin space in a case of carcinomatous meningitis.*

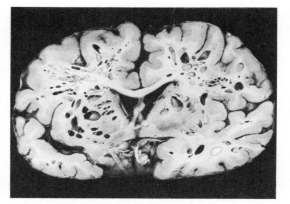

Figure 24. *Gas-forming bullae* ("Swiss-cheese brain") *due to inadequate fixation.*

general paralysis constitute a classic type of reaction on the part of the ependymal wall.

Proliferation of the *subependymal glia* often plays a part in the genesis of these ependymal changes. Thus, it may bring about a stenosis of the aqueduct of Sylvius, causing obstructive hydrocephalus in childhood.

C. APPEARANCES DUE TO ARTIFACTS

Because of its fragility, neural tissue may present appearances that are the result of a number of very different artifacts. These may be caused by terminal changes (i.e., terminal circulatory and asphyxial disturbances), the conditions of removal and fixation, or embedding, sectioning, and even staining procedures.

I. GROSS ARTIFACTS

Large bullous cavities with clear-cut edges ("Swiss-cheese brain"), visible to the naked eye, are the result of a phenomenon of postmortem putrefaction due to inadequate fixation (Fig. 24).

Inadequate fixation is likewise responsible for the pinkish appearance and soft consistency of the white matter (formalin solution of insufficient concentration). Conversely, fixation which is either excessive (because of

a formalin solution of excessive concentration) or unduly prolonged may be responsible for a yellowish, parchment-like appearance of the cortex. Both defects make the application of most histological techniques difficult, and sometimes even impossible.

The picture of congestion with vascular dilatation is most frequently the result of terminal asphyxial disturbances.

II. MICROSCOPIC ARTIFACTS

Multiple microscopic elongated cavities, often predominating in the cortex, are sometimes seen as the result of excessive freezing of the tissues (Fig. 25).

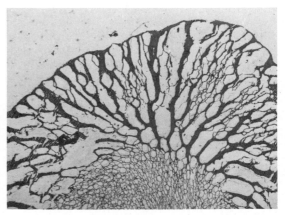

Figure 25. *Microscopic picture of multiple cavitations resulting from freezing artifact.*

A picture of nerve cell retraction, with the presence of clear pericellular spaces, is very frequently seen in paraffin-embedded tissues and is related to the temperature to which the paraffin has been heated. The same applies to the apparent dilatation of the perivascular spaces, which must therefore be differentiated from possible edema.

Dark neurons result from neuronal retraction with nuclear shrinkage and basophilia. They are frequently found in material removed by cerebral biopsy and are related to the traumatizing conditions of tissue removal or to over-rapid fixation. Their artifactual nature is obvious from the absence of alteration in the adjacent glial cell elements.

Pale ballooned *neurons* may be caused by excessive washing of the nervous tissue fragments with water before fixation or by other artifactual postmortem factors.

An artifact consisting of cellular pallor with conglutination of the neurons in the cerebellar granular layer ("état glacé of the cerebellum") is the result of a particular postmortem autolytic change. The absence of any associated glial cell alterations argues against the significance of this type of change.

II. TOPOGRAPHICAL ANALYSIS OF CENTRAL NERVOUS SYSTEM LESIONS

Topographical analysis of the lesions observed is just as important as study of their morphology. It constitutes a crucial step in the attempt to arrive at an etiological diagnosis. It necessitates a rigorous and systematic examination of all the neural structures and, by the same token, implies the need for multiple sampling at various levels and a technique of large sections that permits the synchronous study of the various areas of the central nervous system under the dissecting microscope.

1. Diffuse distribution. These lesions are produced chiefly by blood-borne infective processes. Some of the degenerative processes may, however, likewise be the cause of cerebral atrophy. It is nevertheless important to emphasize that, despite the diffuse character of these changes, lesions often show regional predominance, as in anoxic processes and in certain metabolic disorders.

2. Focal distribution. a. Lesions may be localized to an anatomically well-defined area (cerebral lobes, basal ganglia, brainstem), and certain preferential sites of involvement are linked to specific etiological entities (see, for example, cerebral tumors).

b. Lesions may be localized to a vascular territory. By definition, cerebral infarcts exemplify this type of focal lesion.

3. Disseminated distribution. This is seen essentially in multifocal processes, of which multiple sclerosis is the most characteristic example.

4. Systematized distribution. A number of nervous system disorders, especially degenerative diseases, cause changes that involve certain functionally related morphological systems, e.g., involvement of upper and lower motor neurons in amyotrophic lateral sclerosis, spinocerebellar involvement in Friedreich's ataxia.

III. INTEGRATION OF MORPHOLOGICAL AND TOPOGRAPHICAL FINDINGS

The two steps in neuropathological examination that have been somewhat artificially dissociated under the headings of morphological and topographical analysis must now be followed by a regrouping of the findings that will permit an etiological diagnosis of the lesions. As a matter of fact, these findings alone are not sufficient, and it is necessary to confront them with the clinical data, ancillary investigations, general autopsy findings, and possibly other investigative methods.

Thus, an understanding of cerebral infarcts, for example, is possible only after careful and complete postmortem examination of the vascular tree, heart, and lungs and after comparing the anatomical findings with information provided by the clinical picture, the chronology of the functional disturbances, and data from contingent arteriographic and computerized tomographic procedures.

Likewise, the study of the lipidoses cannot be based solely on neuropathological findings. It necessitates detailed alignment with data from the general postmortem examination and rigorous neurochemical analysis performed on unfixed material.

Chapter 2

TUMORS OF THE CENTRAL NERVOUS SYSTEM

Nervous system tumors are classified into two groups: those of the central nervous system and those of the peripheral nervous system.

Tumors of the peripheral nervous system, meaning broadly those situated outside the cranial and spinal cavities, essentially include tumors of the peripheral nerve trunks, sympathetic ganglia, adrenal medulla, and chemoreceptors. Generally speaking, the study of these tumors lies outside the context of traditional neuropathology.

Central nervous system tumors may be further divided into two groups: intracranial tumors (often erroneously labeled cerebral tumors) and tumors causing spinal root and cord compression (spinal and intraspinal tumors). The distinction has clinical significance. However, the same histological types are found in both groups, but with a different frequency. We shall chiefly be concerned with an understanding of these histological types.

I.   CLASSIFICATION

Both a *topographical* and a *histological classification* must serve as a basis for the pathological study of intracranial and intraspinal neoplasms.

1.   *Topographical Classification*

a.   Intracranial tumors (Figs. 26 and 27). Depending on whether they are situated above or below the tentorium cerebelli, intracranial tumors are either supratentorial or infratentorial (infratentorial tumors are also called posterior fossa tumors) (Fig. 28). In addition, there are intermediary sites, which include tumors of the tentorial notch (straddling the supra- and the infratentorial compartments) and foramen magnum tumors (straddling the posterior fossa and the spinal canal).

b.   Intraspinal tumors (Fig. 29). Tumors in this situation are either extradural (epi-

dural), in which case they originate from the spine or from within the spinal canal, or intradural (subdural), in which case they may be either extra- or intramedullary.

In addition, their segmental level of localization within the spinal canal (cervical, thoracic, lumbosacral, or cauda equina) is important.

2.   *Histological Classification*
(Fig. 30)

Three main groups of neoplasms are encountered: primary intracranial and/or intraspinal tumors; secondary intracranial and/or intraspinal tumors; and cranial and/or spinal bone tumors.

Those of the first group, the primary neoplasms, are classified according to the histological elements from which they are derived.

In practice, the various tumors must also

18

extradural (epidural)
subdural
intramedullary
extramedullary

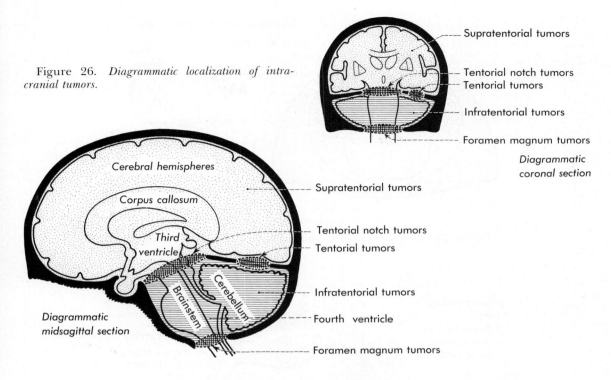

Figure 26. *Diagrammatic localization of intra-cranial tumors.*

		Supratentorial tumors
		Tentorial notch tumors
		Tentorial tumors
		Infratentorial tumors
		Foramen magnum tumors

Diagrammatic coronal section

Cerebral hemispheres

Corpus callosum

Third ventricle

Brainstem

Cerebellum

Supratentorial tumors

Tentorial notch tumors

Tentorial tumors

Infratentorial tumors

Fourth ventricle

Foramen magnum tumors

Diagrammatic midsagittal section

Supratentorial tumors	Cerebral lobe tumors	Frontal tumors Parietal tumors Temporal tumors Occipital tumors
	Deep hemispheric tumors	Lateral ventricle tumors Centrum ovale tumors Basal ganglia tumors
	Midline hemispheric tumors	Corpus callosum tumors Sella turcica tumors Third ventricle tumors Pineal tumors
Tumors straddling the supra- and infratentorial compartments: tentorial tumors, tentorial notch tumors.		
Infratentorial (posterior fossa) *tumors*	Midline tumors	Fourth ventricle tumors Vermis tumors
	Cerebellar lobe tumors	
	Brainstem tumors	
	Extraparenchymatous tumors	Cerebellopontine angle tumors Gasserian ganglion tumors Tumors of the base of the skull Anterior tumors (clivus tumors)
Tumors straddling the infratentorial and the cervical compartments: foramen magnum tumors.		

Figure 27. *Topographical classification of intracranial tumors.*

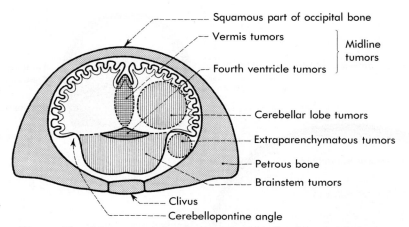

Figure 28. *Diagrammatic localization of principal infratentorial tumors.*

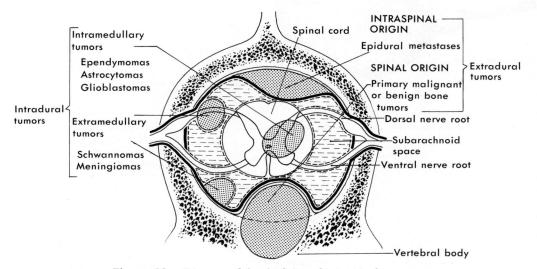

Figure 29. *Diagram of the chief sites of intraspinal tumors.*

be reclassified according to two further criteria that are most important from the prognostic point of view. Thus, intracranial neoplasms can be divided into *histologically benign tumors* (astrocytomas, oligodendrogliomas, ependymomas, pituitary adenomas, meningiomas, schwannomas, etc.) and those which are *histologically malignant* (glioblastomas, medulloblastomas, metastases, etc.) as well as into *parenchymatous tumors* (astrocytomas, glioblastomas, medulloblastomas, metastases, etc.) and those which are *extraparenchymatous* (pinealomas, schwannomas, meningiomas, pituitary adenomas, etc.).

3. Topographical and Histological Correlations
(Figs. 31 to 33)

It is important to be aware of the principal correlations that can be made between the topography of the tumors and their histological nature, and especially of the relationship that exists between the sites of election of the most frequent neoplastic types and their respective age incidence.

The neurologist and the neurosurgeon must be able to reconcile the data obtained

Primary tumors

Histological elements normally present within the cranial and/or spinal cavity

Cellular derivatives of the neural tube

Glial cells
- Astrocytes .... Astrocytomas / Glioblastomes } a
- Oligodendrocytes ... Oligodendrogliomas b
- Ependymocytes ...... Ependymomas / Choroid plexus papillomas / Colloid cysts

Neurons .... Medulloblastomas / Ganglioneuromas and / Gangliogliomas

Pinealocytes........................ Pineocytomas / Pineoblastomas

c

Cellular derivatives of the neural crest
- Schwann cells .... Schwannomas / Neurofibromas
- Arachnoidal cells .... Meningiomas
- Melanocytes .... Melanomas

Other cells
- Connective tissue cells .... Sarcomas
- Reticuloendothelial (? microglial) cells .... Reticulum-cell sarcomas– microgliomas
- Vascular cells (?) .... Hemangioblastomas
- Glomus jugulare cells............. Glomus jugulare tumors
- Adenohypophyseal cells .... Pituitary adenomas

Intracranial and/or intraspinal embryonal remnants
- Ectodermal derivatives... Craniopharyngiomas / Cholesteatomas
- Notochord.. Chordomas
- Adipose cells... Lipomas
- Germ cells.. Germinomas
- Derived from the three germ layers....................... Teratomas

Secondary tumors
(metastases)

Bone tumors
Primary or secondary, benign or malignant

Figure 30. *Simplified histological classification of intracranial and intraspinal tumors. a,* Gliomas in the usual sense; *b,* gliomas in the broad sense; *c,* gliomas in the broadest sense.

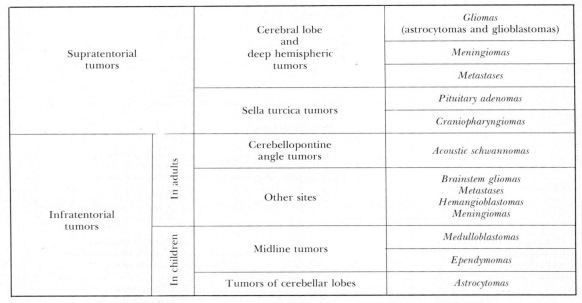

Supratentorial tumors		Cerebral lobe and deep hemispheric tumors	*Gliomas* (astrocytomas and glioblastomas)
			Meningiomas
			Metastases
		Sella turcica tumors	*Pituitary adenomas*
			Craniopharyngiomas
Infratentorial tumors	In adults	Cerebellopontine angle tumors	*Acoustic schwannomas*
		Other sites	*Brainstem gliomas Metastases Hemangioblastomas Meningiomas*
	In children	Midline tumors	*Medulloblastomas*
			Ependymomas
		Tumors of cerebellar lobes	*Astrocytomas*

Figure 31.   *Most frequent intracranial tumors and their sites of predilection.*

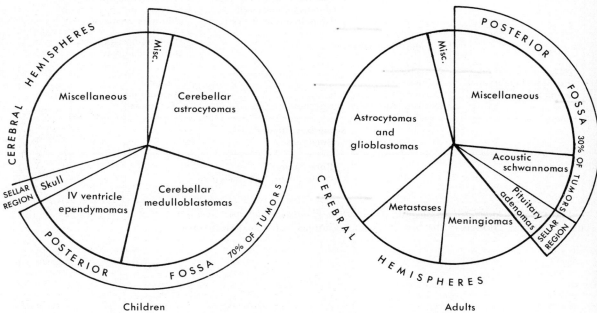

Children   Adults

Figure 32.   *Distribution and approximate incidence of the most frequent types of intracranial tumors in terms of their general topography and the age of the patient.*

Extradural tumors	Spinal	Vertebral metastases
		Primary malignant or benign tumors of bone
	Intraspinal	Epidural metastases
Intradural tumors	Extramedullary	Meningiomas
		Schwannomas and neurofibromas
	Intramedullary	Ependymomas
		Astrocytomas
		Glioblastomas

Figure 33.   *Most frequent tumors causing spinal root and cord compression and their sites of predilection.*

from both schemes of classification and recognize which of the two is the more important in each instance: the site of the tumor or its histological nature. In practice, both factors play a role in determining prognosis and therapeutic modalities, and each loses some of its significance when taken on its own.

II. PRIMARY NEOPLASMS

ASTROCYTOMAS

Astrocytomas are histologically benign astrocytic tumors which, in a fair number of cases and after a variable time interval, are susceptible of malignant change (see Glioblastomas). They account for 20 to 30 per cent of the tumors in the glioma group. Their gross, microscopic, and biological characteristics vary to a considerable degree according to their site. Thus, the following varieties are encountered.

1. Cerebral hemispheric astrocytomas.
These tumors are found chiefly in adults between the ages of 30 and 50. They diffusely infiltrate the hemispheric white matter (Fig. 34), cortex, and basal ganglia, and have no definite borders. They are usually of firm consistency.

Their *microscopic appearance* is very uniform: it is characterized by a rather sparse and fairly regular proliferation of astrocytes (more often fibrillary than protoplasmic or gemistocytic), without histological evidence of malignancy, mitotic figures or vascular endothelial proliferation, and without areas of necrosis or hemorrhage. However, microcystic areas, calcifications, and perivascular lymphocytic cuffings are fairly common (Fig. 35).

Malignant change after a variable lapse of time (often several years) occurs frequently.

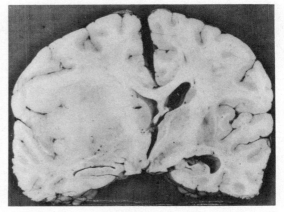

Figure 34.   *Astrocytoma of the left cerebral hemisphere.*

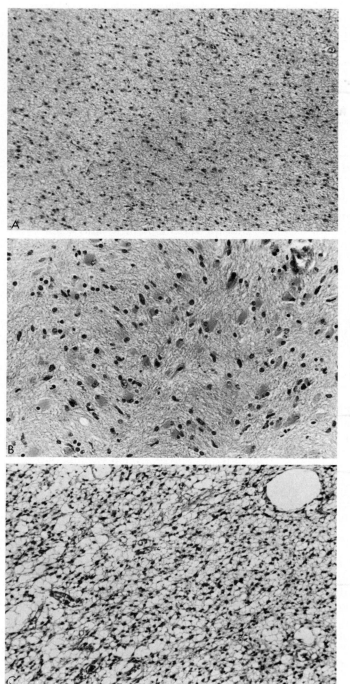

Figure 35. *Various microscopic features of cerebral astrocytomas.*

A, Grade 1 astrocytoma (increase of normal astrocytic density). *B*, Gemistocytic astrocytoma. *C*, Microcystic astrocytoma.

2. Astrocytomas of the floor of the third ventricle, chiasm, and optic nerves. These tumors, which are found mainly in children and adolescents, are grossly limited to any of the above regions, but often infiltrate all of them. The neoplastic astrocytes are elongated (pilocytic). Malignant change is exceptional. These tumors are sometimes encountered in von Recklinghausen's neurofibromatosis.

[handwritten: pilocytic < optic n / ii vent / chiasm   neuro fibromatosis]

3. Brainstem astrocytomas. These tumors, which are found most often in children or adolescents, present grossly as a diffuse, roughly symmetrical hypertrophy of the pons and medulla. Histologically, they closely resemble cerebral hemispheric astrocytomas except that their astrocytes are often elongated and bipolar (pilocytic), a morphological feature which results from the persistence of normal preexisting nerve fascicles along which the tumor cells align themselves. Malignant change occurs fairly frequently.

4. Cerebellar astrocytomas. These neoplasms are, likewise, essentially tumors of childhood and adolescence. They are usually well circumscribed, situated within a cerebellar hemisphere and/or the vermis, and often cystic. They are composed of protoplasmic and, more often, of fibrillary and pilocytic astrocytes. They frequently contain "Rosenthal fibers": these structures, which result from changes in the astrocytic cell processes, present by light microscopy as small, highly elongated bodies which are strongly eosinophilic and show a marked affinity for Mallory's phosphotungstic acid–hematoxylin. Malignant change is exceptional in cerebellar astrocytomas. Complete surgical excision may achieve definitive cure, but recurrences are possible.

5. Spinal cord astrocytomas. These tumors are most often found at the cervicothoracic level and then result in a fusiform swelling that is limited to that region (Fig. 36). Histologically, they closely resemble fibrillary cerebral hemispheric astrocytomas and, like those of the brainstem, have a tendency to be pilocytic. They may undergo malignant change.

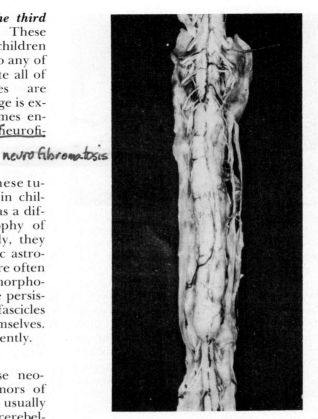

Figure 36. *Gross picture of an astrocytoma in the thoracic part of the spinal cord.*

GLIOBLASTOMAS

Glioblastomas are malignant, rapidly fatal, astrocytic neoplasms. Some result from a malignant change in a preexisting astrocytoma that may or may not have been clinically evident; the others presumably arise *de novo.* In either case, the gross and microscopic features are similar. Glioblastomas account for 50 per cent of the tumors of the glioma group; they may occur at any age, but show a maximal incidence between the ages of 45 and 55.

They may occur in any region of the central nervous system. However, the cerebral hemispheres, in particular the frontal lobes or temporal lobes, the basal ganglia, and the commissural pathways are sites of predilection. Multiple localization (multifocal gliomas) occurs in approximately 5 per cent of the cases.

[handwritten: • frontal / • temporal / • basal ganglia / • commissures]

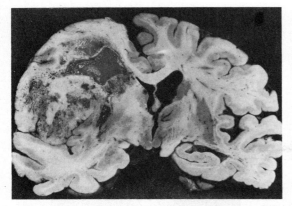

Figure 37. *Gross picture of a glioblastoma of the left cerebral hemisphere.* Note the variegated appearance, with zones of necrosis, hemorrhage, and cystic degeneration.

Grossly (Fig. 37), glioblastomas present as relatively well-defined tumors, but lack a capsule. Tumor tissue, which is grayish pink, soft and granular, often forms a thin peripheral rim, whereas in the center of the growth, creamy yellow areas of necrosis and/or fatty degeneration, reddish hemorrhagic zones, and occasionally one or more cysts containing clear yellow or brownish fluid account for its variegated pattern. At the periphery, dilated and sometimes thrombosed blood vessels are often observed.

Local extension is rapid and may be accompanied by meningeal invasion. Recurrence is the rule, even after apparently complete surgical removal. On the other hand, extraneural metastases are an exceptional rarity.

Microscopically (Fig. 38), the appearances vary greatly among cases and within the same case. The following features are found, though to a variable degree and randomly distributed: there are *more or less densely cellular areas* composed of neoplastic astrocytes of varying shape and size, corresponding both to classic protoplasmic, fibrillary, and gemistocytic astrocytes and to so-called "glioblasts," "spongioblasts," "astroblasts," and "giant cells." All these cells show considerable nucleocytoplasmic abnormalities and variable numbers of mitotic figures. There are also *necrotic zones*, around which the tumor cells are arranged in fairly character-

istic "pseudopalisades"; *hemorrhagic zones; cysts;* and finally, *vascular endothelial proliferation*, in which the picture consists of numerous, highly convoluted capillary blood vessels whose endothelial cells show evidence of active multiplication. In addition, a sometimes considerable *connective tissue reaction* is not infrequently observed; it may be due to invasion of the meningeal tissues by tumor, to the organization of zones of necrosis, or to a proliferation of collagen and reticulin fibers in the areas of vascular endothelial proliferation.

In a number of cases, the mesenchymal endothelial and/or perivascular fibroblastic proliferation is so severe and extensive that it acquires malignant neoplastic features, resulting in a picture of mixed glioma and sarcoma. Such tumors are sometimes referred to as *"gliosarcomas."* From the clinical and biological point of view, however, they behave essentially as glioblastomas.

A variant of the glioblastoma, the *giant-cell glioblastoma,* deserves separate mention. These tumors, which are often well circumscribed, are composed of giant, monstrous, and multinucleated cells whose astrocytic nature has been established by electron microscopy. They are often characterized by a considerable proliferation of connective tissue, which has led some authors to interpret them, erroneously, as giant-cell, or monstrocellular, sarcomas. Because of their relatively good demarcation, their prognosis is not necessarily as sinister as the microscopic picture might lead one to assume and, in some cases, several years' survival has been recorded after surgical excision.

OLIGODENDROGLIOMAS

Oligodendrogliomas (or oligodendrocytomas) account for approximately 5 per cent of the intracranial gliomas (Russell and Rubinstein). Their most frequent incidence is between *the ages of 30 and 50.*

They are most often found in *the cerebral hemispheres, where they usually involve the cortex and the white matter.* Intraspinal oligodendrogliomas are less common (accounting for 4.1 per cent of spinal intramedullary tumors,

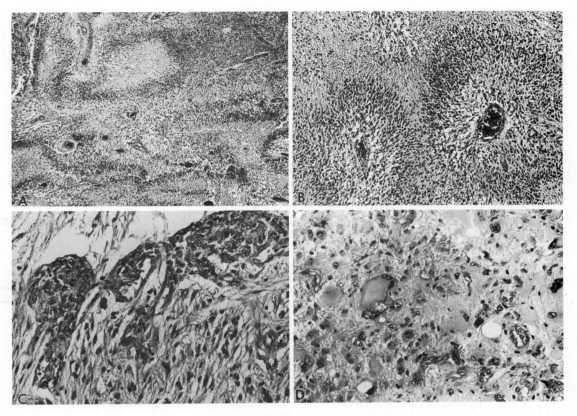

Figure 38. *Chief microscopic features in glioblastoma.*
A, Zones of necrosis with pseudopalisades.
B, Zone of necrosis, with tumor cells in perivascular pseudorosettes.
C, Capillary endothelial proliferation.
D, Giant astrocytes with monstrous nuclei.

according to Kernohan), and cerebellar examples are exceptional (only one case in Zülch's series of 4000 tumors).

Grossly, these neoplasms are usually well circumscribed and grayish pink, and often include areas of mucoid change, which may result in a gelatinous consistency; zones of necrosis and cystic degeneration; hemorrhagic areas; and calcifications.

Microscopically, they present a highly uniform appearance that is easily recognizable (Fig. 39). The oligodendrocytes, which are swollen and closely packed, exhibit small, round, darkly staining nuclei surrounded by a clear halo. This "honeycomb" aspect is

most characteristic. Mitotic figures are usually rare. The vascular connective tissue stroma is very discrete. In 20 per cent of the cases according to Zülch, calcifications are demonstrable either as isolated microscopic structures scattered amidst the tumor cells or as perivascular collections. The various mucoid, cystic, necrotic, and hemorrhagic changes that are sometimes already apparent to the naked eye are recapitulated under the microscope. Finally, astrocytes of diverse morphology are not uncommonly encountered as distinct areas admixed with the mainly oligodendrocytic cell population. This has led some observers to use the name "oligoastrocytoma" for such cases.

Traditionally the **prognosis** of oligoden-

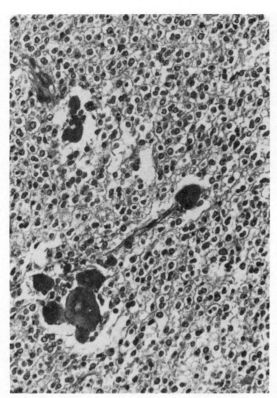

Figure 39.   *Oligodendroglioma* (H. and E). Note the presence of calcifications.

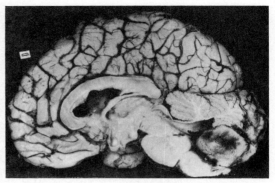

Figure 40.   *Fourth ventricle ependymoma.*

60% infratent.

rarer than infratentorial ones (approximately 60 per cent); the most frequent site therefore is the region of the *fourth ventricle* (Fig. 40). On the other hand, ependymomas account for approximately 60 per cent of the spinal cord gliomas and are then most often found in the *lumbosacral segments* and at the *filum terminale* ("ependymoma of the cauda equina").

Their **gross appearance,** which is reddish, nodular and lobulated, recalls that of the placenta. Although they are usually well circumscribed, they nevertheless grow by local extension and may spread in the cerebrospinal pathways so as to produce distant metastases in the central nervous system and even, exceptionally, outside it.

Microscopically (Fig. 41), the cellular density and histological architecture of ependymomas vary among cases and from area to area within the same case.

Most often, especially in the cerebral hemispheres and in the posterior fossa, the tumor is highly cellular and composed of closely grouped polygonal cells in the cytoplasm of which blepharoplasts can be visualized when stained with Mallory's phosphotungstic acid–hematoxylin. Two features, which are inconstant, are highly diagnostic: *ependymal tubules* (i.e., groupings of ependymal cells around true or potential circular cavities) and *perivascular pseudorosettes* (i.e., perivascular arrangements of ependymal cells into coronal structures in which the fibrillated cell processes form a clear halo between the central blood vessel and the more

drogliomas has been regarded as relatively favorable, but in practice it cannot be predicted, and no valid correlation has been established between the microscopic appearances of these tumors and their clinical evolution. Metastases through the cerebrospinal pathways as well as extensive postoperative recurrences may indeed occur. Moreover, they may undergo malignant change into a glioblastoma.

EPENDYMOMAS

Ependymomas account for approximately 6 per cent of the intracranial gliomas (Russell and Rubinstein). Although they are encountered at any age, they are *definitely more frequent in childhood and adolescence.*

They may occur at any level of the ventricular system. However, supratentorial tumors (approximately 40 per cent) are

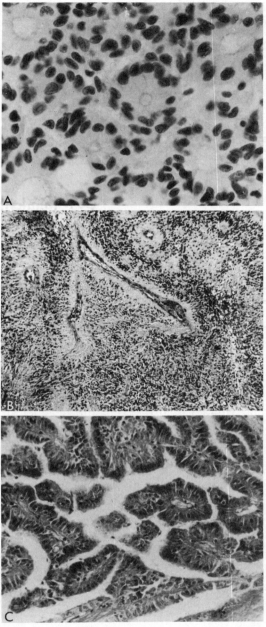

Figure 41. *Microscopic features in ependymomas.*
A, Ependymal tubules (H. and E.).
B, Perivascular pseudorosettes (H. and E.).
C, Papillary ependymoma (Masson trichrome).

peripherally situated corona of ependymal nuclei).

Occasionally, particularly in the spinal cord and at the filum terminale, the epen-

dymoma is *papillary*, in which case the cells are arranged as a simple epithelium that covers central cores composed of connective or gliovascular tissue. *Myxopapillary ependymomas*, in which the stroma is the seat of mucinous degeneration, are found only in the region of the filum terminale.

Although these neoplasms are usually well circumscribed and histologically benign, *malignant ependymomas* are known to exist. These tumors, which are difficult to distinguish grossly from glioblastomas, are highly invasive, and their histological picture is that of a highly undifferentiated tumor.

The existence of *ependymoblastomas* is under scrutiny. Rubinstein has recorded two cases in children in which the tumors were composed of highly primitive glial cells, but demonstrated ependymal tubules; he has suggested that these tumors might be true ependymoblastomas.[1]

Subependymomas (or subependymal gliomas) are ependymomas in which the subependymal glia plays a prominent role, resulting in the overall picture of a fibrillary glioma in which small groups of ependymocytes are scattered.

CHOROID PLEXUS PAPILLOMAS

Choroid plexus papillomas (Fig. 42) account for 0.5 per cent of intracranial tumors according to Zülch and for 2 per cent of the tumors of the glioma group according to Russell and Rubinstein. They are encountered most frequently *in the first decade of life.*

These neoplasms occupy the sites of the ventricular system in which choroid plexus is normally found. They occur, in order of decreasing frequency, in the *fourth ventricle*, the lateral ventricles (more so on the left), and in the third ventricle.

Their histological structure faithfully recapitulates that of the normal choroid plexus.

---

[1]A few more examples in very young subjects have since been noted (Russell and Rubinstein, 1977), thus confirming the delineation of this very rare form of malignant ependymoma (translator's note).

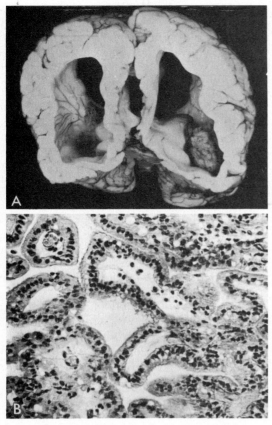

Figure 42.   *Choroid plexus papilloma.*
A, Gross picture of a papilloma of the right lateral ventricle in a child with marked hydrocephalus. *B,* Microscopic appearance (H. and E.).

It is therefore essentially papillary, i.e., characterized by an arrangement of vascular connective tissue cores lined by a simple columnar or cuboidal epithelium whose cells lack cilia and blepharoplasts and often contain granules and small vacuoles.

Although the tumors are histologically benign, leptomeningeal dissemination by the cerebrospinal pathways is observed fairly often. Moreover, oversecretion of cerebrospinal fluid by the papilloma is likely to produce hydrocephalus.

The existence of malignant choroid plexus papillomas has been established in a few cases, but these examples are so rare that the possibility of a metastasis from a visceral carcinoma to the choroid plexus must be rigorously eliminated before the diagnosis can be entertained.[1]

COLLOID CYSTS OF THE THIRD VENTRICLE

Colloid cysts of the third ventricle (Fig. 43) account for 2 per cent of the intracranial gliomas (Russell and Rubinstein) and are encountered chiefly in *young adults;* they are conspicuously rare in children.

They are always situated *at the anterior end of the third ventricle,* where they are suspended at the rostral end of the tela choroidea immediately against the foramen of Monro. The latter structure may be intermittently obstructed, resulting in episodes of acute hydrocephalus. When the cyst becomes large, it may distend the cavity of the third ventricle and sometimes may even extend caudally to the origin of the aqueduct.

The cyst wall consists of a fibrous capsule attached to the stroma of the choroid plexus and internally lined by cuboidal or columnar epithelial cells that contain mucous droplets and even cilia. Its contents are made up of amorphous PAS-positive material, which may contain lipid droplets and degenerated leukocytes.

---

[1] In practice, the only acceptable malignant choroid plexus papillomas that have so far been recorded have occurred within the first decade of life, i.e., at an age when visceral adenocarcinoma can be virtually excluded (translator's note).

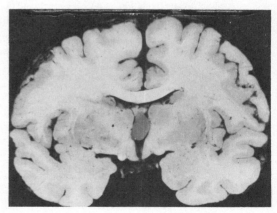

Figure 43.   *Colloid cyst of the third ventricle.*

Numerous theories have been advanced concerning the origin of colloid cysts of the third ventricle. A few could arise from persistent remnants of the paraphysis, a glandular structure that is found in the fetus and is derived from an invagination of the telencephalic vesicle immediately anterior to the diencephalo-telencephalic boundary. However, it seems that most colloid cysts are of ependymal origin.

MEDULLOBLASTOMAS

30% p fossa child

Medulloblastomas are malignant neoplasms which account for approximately one-third of the posterior fossa tumors in children.[1] They are quite radiosensitive.

Their site of predilection is the cerebellar vermis, especially its inferior portion; from this point the tumor tends to infiltrate the cerebellar hemispheres and invade the cavity of the fourth ventricle. Metastatic spread within the central neuraxis through the cerebrospinal pathways is frequent.

From the histological point of view (Fig. 44), medulloblastomas are highly cellular, homogeneous tumors. Their distinguishing

---

[1]There is evidence to suggest that medulloblastomas may originate from remnants of the superficial fetal granular layer of the cerebellum, which normally disappears by the twelfth month of postnatal life (translator's note).

feature is the presence of round or oval nuclei arranged in dense and diffuse sheets, in parallel rows or forming rosettes. Mitotic figures are numerous. Glial fibrils are absent as a rule, there are no reticulin fibers except when the leptomeninges are invaded, and blood vessels are scanty.

The nature and histogenesis of medulloblastomas present difficult problems of interpretation which are not yet resolved and are reflected in a diversity of ill-defined nosological tumor entities identified by different authors under the designations of neuroblastomas, so-called "circumscribed cerebellar sarcomas," malignant ependymomas, etc.

GANGLIONEUROMAS AND GANGLIOGLIOMAS

These extremely rare neoplasms are found predominantly in children and young adults. Their site of predilection is the floor of the third ventricle or the temporal lobe.

Grossly, the tumor, which is usually of small size, is well circumscribed, homogeneous, and finely granular on section.

Microscopically, gangliogliomas display two types of neoplastic cells—neuronal and astrocytic—whose proportions vary from case to case. In addition, a notable fibrous connective tissue stroma, an abundant vasculature, calcospherites, and small cystic cavities are encountered fairly often.

These neoplasms, in which a malformative element is likely, have a very slow clinical evolution, and the prognosis after surgical removal is usually favorable.

PINEAL TUMORS

The clinicopathological classification of pineal tumors has long been debated. Here we shall adhere to the classification of Russell and Rubinstein, which is the most widely used at this time.

Strictly speaking, the term "pinealoma" should be applied only to primary neoplasms originating from pineal parenchymal cells. Unfortunately, the term has been commonly (and often still is) used also to designate a

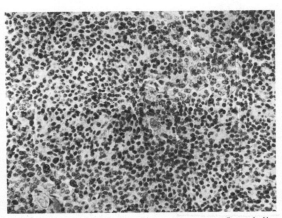

Figure 44. *Microscopic appearance of medulloblastoma* (H. and E.).

group of tumors that arise in the pineal region, but are in fact germinomas.

Germinomas (Figs. 45 and 46) indeed constitute the type of tumor most frequently found in that area (approximately 50 per cent) and, by the same token, the pineal region is the most common site of intracranial germinomas.[1] However, germinomas may also occur in the hypothalamic region; these tumors have traditionally been designated as "ectopic pinealomas."

Intracranial germinomas are encountered in subjects between the ages of 20 and 40 and occur predominantly in males.

The histological features are highly characteristic; two distinct cell populations are seen: areas of large polygonal or spheroidal cells with a frequently vacuolated cytoplasm and voluminous rounded nuclei containing a prominent nucleolus, separated by connective vascular trabeculae along which small round cells resembling lymphocytes are clustered. Tumors with this distinct "mosaic pattern" often contain calcifications.

Although these tumors are histologically malignant as well as invasive, the clinical

---

[1] As the name indicates, these tumors are thought to arise from germ cells, i.e., multipotential embryonal cells. Accordingly, they represent a form of teratoma, hence the name *atypical teratoma* that has often been given them in the literature (translator's note).

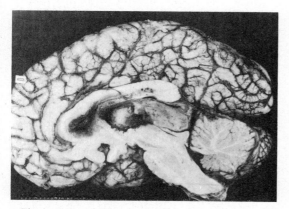

Figure 45. *Midsagittal section of the brain revealing a pinealoma.* Note the tumor between the splenium of the corpus callosum and the corpora quadrigemina.

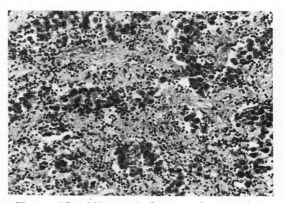

Figure 46. *Microscopic features of a pineal germinoma ("pinealoma"): "mosaic" appearance.*

course after radiotherapy may be more favorable than the microscopic picture might lead one to predict.

True pinealomas, i.e., those originating from pineal parenchymal cells, are divided into two groups.

Pineocytomas (or pinealocytomas) are circumscribed neoplasms of slow growth, with a microscopic appearance that recalls that of the normal pineal gland, i.e., small cells with eosinophilic cytoplasm extending their processes toward the blood vessels and grouped into lobules separated by vascular connective tissue trabeculae. The cells are sometimes arranged in rosettes around circular eosinophilic areas which demonstrate a fibrillary structure.

Pineoblastomas (or pinealoblastomas) are highly cellular neoplasms composed of small, poorly differentiated cells which are rich in chromatin and have an ill-defined cytoplasm. Microscopically, these tumors resemble medulloblastomas and share their degree of malignancy as well as their tendency to spread in the leptomeninges. In fact, some authors regard them as true medulloblastomas of the pineal gland.

Finally, it is important to remember that in addition to germinomas and to true pinealomas, the pineal region is a site of predilection for teratomas and may also be the site of origin of several other varieties of tumor (e.g., gliomas, meningiomas, cholesteatomas).

SCHWANNOMAS

Schwannomas (neurilemmomas or neurinomas) are benign tumors arising from Schwann cells.

Site. Schwannomas may originate wherever Schwann cells are present. They may therefore be found on cranial nerves, spinal nerve roots, peripheral nerve trunks, and even at nerve endings. We are, however, here chiefly concerned with the intracranial and spinal nerve roots.

Intracranial schwannomas. The most frequent intracranial schwannomas are the acoustic schwannomas (eighth cranial nerve) (Fig. 47), which are situated in the cerebellopontine angle. When they reach a certain size they cause changes in the neighboring structures that can easily be correlated with the clinical symptoms. These changes include the following: enlargement and erosion of the internal auditory meatus; stretching of the neighboring nerves, especially of the eighth cranial nerve, whose fibers are spread along the surface of the tumor and are later incorporated within its capsule, followed by stretching of the seventh and then the fifth cranial nerves, and eventually of the mixed cranial nerves; and cerebellar and brainstem compression.

Schwannomas of the fifth, ninth, and

Sens > mot.

tenth cranial nerves are considerably less common. Motor cranial nerves are involved only exceptionally.

Spinal schwannomas. These tumors are situated most frequently on the dorsal sensory nerve roots, but some have also been described on the ventral motor nerve roots (Fig. 48). The thoracic segments are most *D > V* often implicated, but cervical and lumbar schwannomas are not rare. They may also be situated in the cauda equina. The tumor is usually restricted to the subdural space, but may sometimes extend through the intervertebral foramen, resulting in an hourglass appearance.

Gross features. Schwannomas are firm, well-circumscribed, encapsulated tumors of variable size. When small, they are spherical, of elastic consistency, and whitish or slightly translucent. When larger, they are irregularly lobulated and may become cystic. On section, some may show hemorrhages and yellowish foci. These tumors displace and do not invade the nerves from which they originate.

As a rule, schwannomas are single solitary tumors. However, in von Recklinghausen's neurofibromatosis, multiple schwannomas, especially bilateral acoustic schwannomas, may be found.

The clinical evolution of schwannomas is slow. In principle, these tumors remain histologically benign; they may, however, recur. Some authors have described malignant schwannomas—either malignant from the onset or benign schwannomas that have undergone malignant change—but these cases are rare and in some instances debatable.

Microscopic features. Microscopically (Fig. 49), the growth is surrounded by a connective tissue capsule. The tumor tissue may be of two types, which are often intermingled within the same example:

1. **Dense fibrillary type** (type A tissue). Here the narrow elongated bipolar cells show very little cytoplasm and contain rod-shaped or cylindrical nuclei. These nuclei are arranged in elongated drifts, whorls, or characteristic palisades. Fine re-

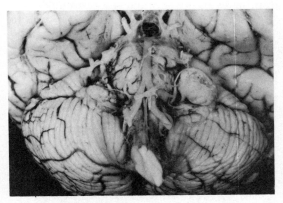

Figure 47. *Acoustic schwannoma arising in the left cerebellopontine angle.* Note the course of the facial nerve, which has been raised and stretched by the tumor.

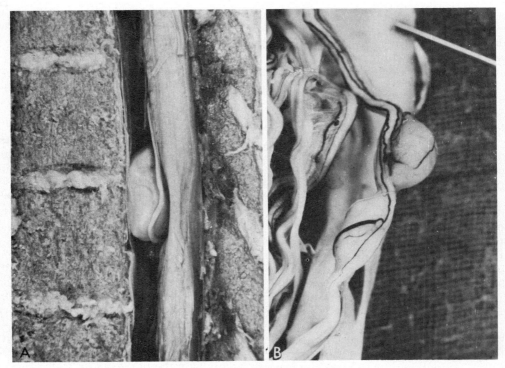

Figure 48.   *Gross features of spinal schwannomas.*
   A, Schwannoma of the thoracic region; note its relation to a dorsal nerve root and the lateral compression of the spinal cord. (Courtesy of Dr. L. Rouques.) *B*, Two small schwannomas of the cauda equina in a case of von Recklinghausen's disease.

ticulin fibers can be demonstrated with special stains.

2. Loose reticulated type (type B tissue). There is a lesser degree of cellular density in this tissue. Round and pyknotic nuclei are randomly arranged in a matrix that contains microcysts and vacuolated cells. The general appearance is finely honeycombed. Reticulin fibers are present. Type B tissue usually predominates in intracranial schwannomas.

Finally, we note the absence of mitotic

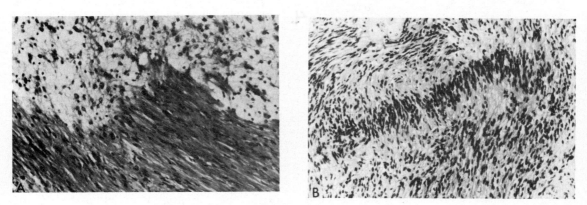

Figure 49.   *Microscopic features of schwannomas.*
   A, Antoni A type tissue in lower half: Antoni B type tissue in upper half. *B*, Nuclei arranged in palisades.

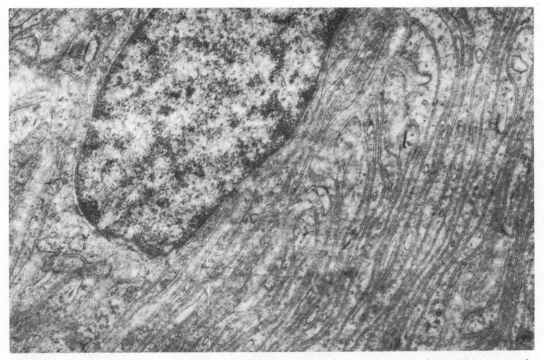

Figure 50. *Schwannoma*. Electron microscopic appearance of Antoni A type tissue. Numerous closely interwoven Schwann cells (× 17,500).

figures, the hyaline thickening of the tumor vessel walls, and the absence of nerve fibers within the growth. These are usually displaced, and incorporated in its capsule.

Whatever their appearance by light microscopy, schwannomas are found with the electron microscope to be formed by the sole proliferation of Schwann cells (Fig. 50), with a more or less conspicuous proliferation of collagen fibers.

NEUROFIBROMAS
(Figs. 51 and 52)

Neurofibromas form multiple tumors of nerve roots and peripheral nerves as part of the picture of von Recklinghausen's neurofibromatosis.

Although some authors have tended to confuse schwannomas and neurofibromas, we are unquestionably dealing with two different neoplastic processes. Neurofibromas can be differentiated from schwannomas by several features:

1. They almost always occur within the context of von Recklinghausen's disease.

2. They are almost always multiple.

3. With both light and electron microscopy they show the same constituents as normal nerves, i.e., myelinated and nonmyelinated nerve fibers, Schwann cells, fibroblasts, collagen fibers.

4. In contrast to schwannomas, which are true benign tumors arising from Schwann cells, neurofibromas may therefore represent a kind of hyperplasia of the schwannian and fibroblastic supporting elements of the nerve, the individual fibers of which appear to be dissociated by this benign proliferation.

The likelihood of a malignant change occurring in neurofibromas is just as conjectural as in the case of schwannomas.[1]

---

[1]Another view is that malignant change may occur in a neurofibroma, with the production of a neurofibrosarcoma, and that this event, although rare, is better documented than in malignant schwannomas (translator's note).

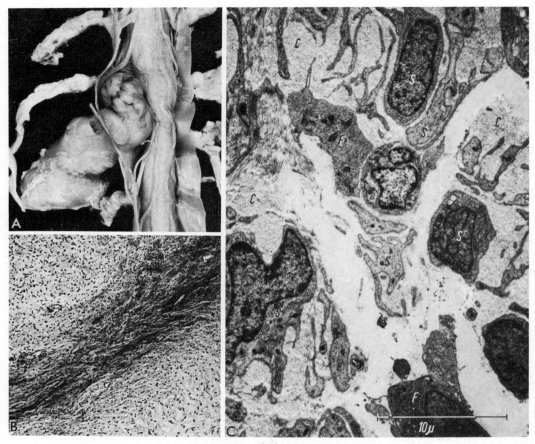

Figure 51.   *Spinal neurofibroma.*

A, Gross picture of a dumbbell neurofibroma. (Courtesy of Dr. L. Rouques.)

B, Microscopic features; myelinated axons and numerous collagen fibers are present in the center; laterally, more loosely textured areas contain Schwann cell and fibroblastic nuclei (Masson trichrome stain).

C, Electron microscopic features; Schwann cells *(S),* fibroblasts *(F),* and collagen fibers *(C).*

MENINGIOMAS

Meningiomas are benign tumors originating from arachnoidal cells.

They account for 13 to 18 per cent of primary intracranial tumors and approximately 25 per cent of intraspinal tumors. Most meningiomas occur in adults between the ages of 20 and 60, with a maximal incidence around 45. They are predominantly found in females.

Site. They are ubiquitous and may arise wherever arachnoidal cells are present (Fig. 53).

Intracranial meningiomas (Figs. 53 and 54). Sites of predilection are as follows:

1. Convexity meningiomas (parasagittal meningiomas, meningiomas of the falx, meningiomas of the lateral convexity) are the most frequent (approximately 50 per cent).

2. Basal meningiomas (olfactory groove meningiomas, meningiomas of the lesser wing of the sphenoid, meningiomas of the

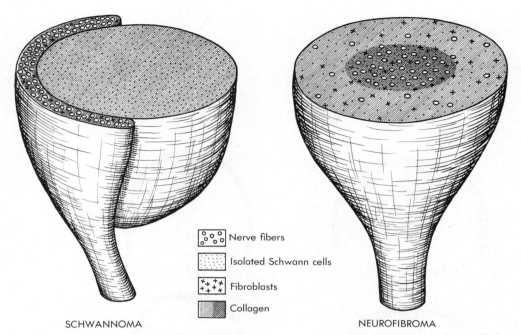

Nerve fibers

Isolated Schwann cells

Fibroblasts

Collagen

SCHWANNOMA   NEUROFIBROMA

Figure 52. *Comparative diagram showing the respective structures of schwannoma and neurofibroma.*

pterion, suprasellar meningiomas) are next in frequency (approximately 40 per cent of cases).

3. Posterior fossa meningiomas and meningiomas of the foramen magnum, as well as intraventricular meningiomas, are considerably less common (approximately 10 per cent of cases).

Spinal meningiomas (Fig. 55). They are most frequently situated in the thoracic segments and are usually located in the lateral compartment of the subdural space.

Gross features. Meningiomas are grossly spherical (Fig. 54) or lobulated, well circumscribed, and firmly attached to the inner surface of the dura. They displace the underlying neural parenchyma without invading it. Meningiomas *en plaque* spread along the deeper surface of the dura and tend to invade the overlying bone; as a result, hyperostosis may follow.

Meningiomas are usually single, but multiple tumors may occur. In some cases the condition consists in a diffuse meningiomatosis that may involve the entire leptomeningeal space.

in neurofibromatosis

Their clinical evolution is very slow. Surgical removal, even when apparently complete, is sometimes followed by recurrence.

Microscopic appearance. By light microscopy meningiomas present several aspects (Fig. 56).

1 **Endotheliomatous type.** The tumor is composed of polygonal epithelial-like cells, with ill-defined cell borders, a pale cytoplasm, and a relatively voluminous spherical nucleus containing a conspicuous nucleolus and occasionally showing a pseudoinclusion in the shape of a clear, well-defined intranuclear vacuole.

The distribution of the cells is fairly uniform, being diffuse and arranged in elongated sheets or in islands separated by scanty vascular connective tissue trabeculae. A characteristic and diagnostic cellular grouping is almost always present to a greater or lesser extent: it consists in a whorling pattern in which cells are closely wrapped around one another. These whorls show fairly frequently a hyalinized and calcified center and are then termed "psammoma bodies."

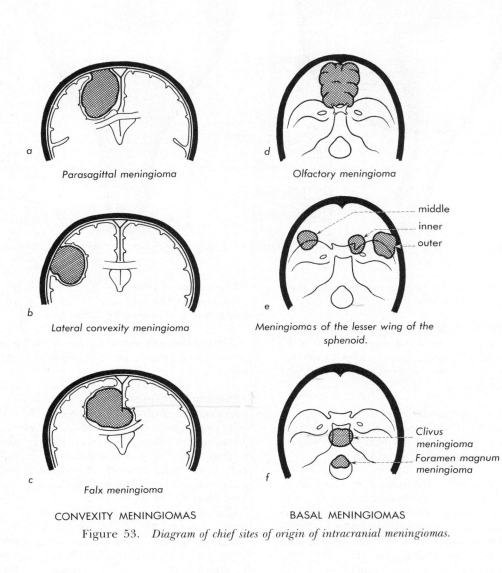

CONVEXITY MENINGIOMAS   BASAL MENINGIOMAS

Figure 53.   *Diagram of chief sites of origin of intracranial meningiomas.*

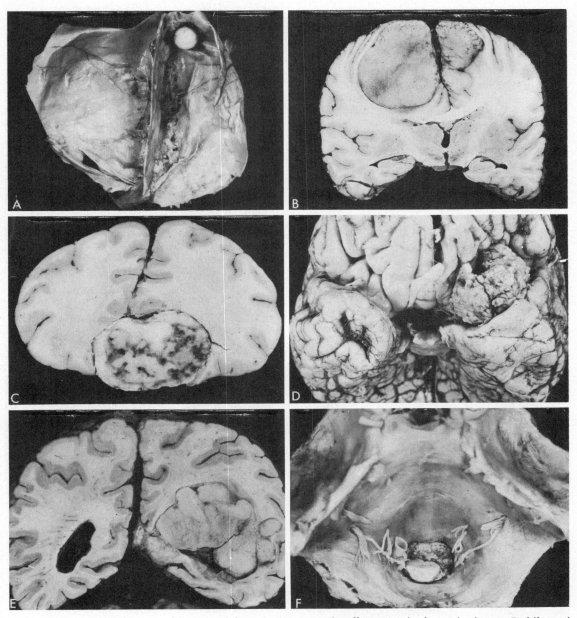

Figure 54. *Gross features of intracranial meningiomas.* *A*, Small parasagittal meningioma; *B*, bilateral falx meningioma; *C*, olfactory meningioma; *D*, sphenoidal wing meningioma; *E*, intraventricular meningioma; *F*, foramen magnum meningioma.

2. **Fibroblastic type.** The tumor is composed of elongated fusiform cells, arranged in wavy interlacing fascicles. A fairly well developed network of collagen and reticulin fibers is found between the individual cells. Whorls and occasionally psammoma bodies are also found in these cases.

Special features. Whether they are of endotheliomatous or fibroblastic type, meningiomas may be the seat of various histological changes or "degenerations." Thus, the following alterations may be seen:

Xanthomatous changes, with the presence of fat-filled cells;

Myxomatous changes, characterized by an

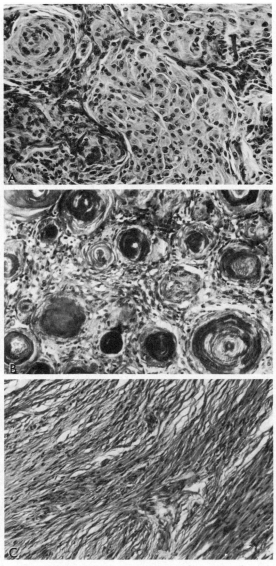

Figure 56. *Chief microscopic features of meningiomas.*

A, Endotheliomatous type; note here the unusually well-defined cellular outlines and the presence of whorls.

B, Calcified psammoma bodies (hematoxylin-phloxine-saffranin).

C, Fibrous type.

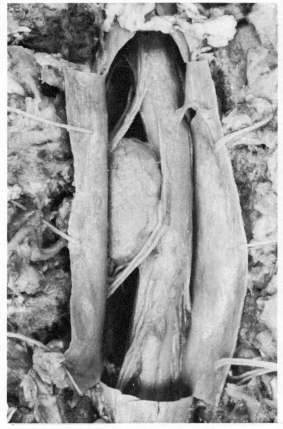

Figure 55. *Spinal thoracic meningioma.* Note the intradural localization of the tumor and the lateral compression of the spinal cord parenchyma between the two nerve roots. (Courtesy of Dr. L. Rouques.)

abundant homogeneous stroma separating the individual cells;

Areas of cartilage or bone within the tumor;

Foci of melanin pigment in the connective tissue trabeculae ("pigmented meningiomas");

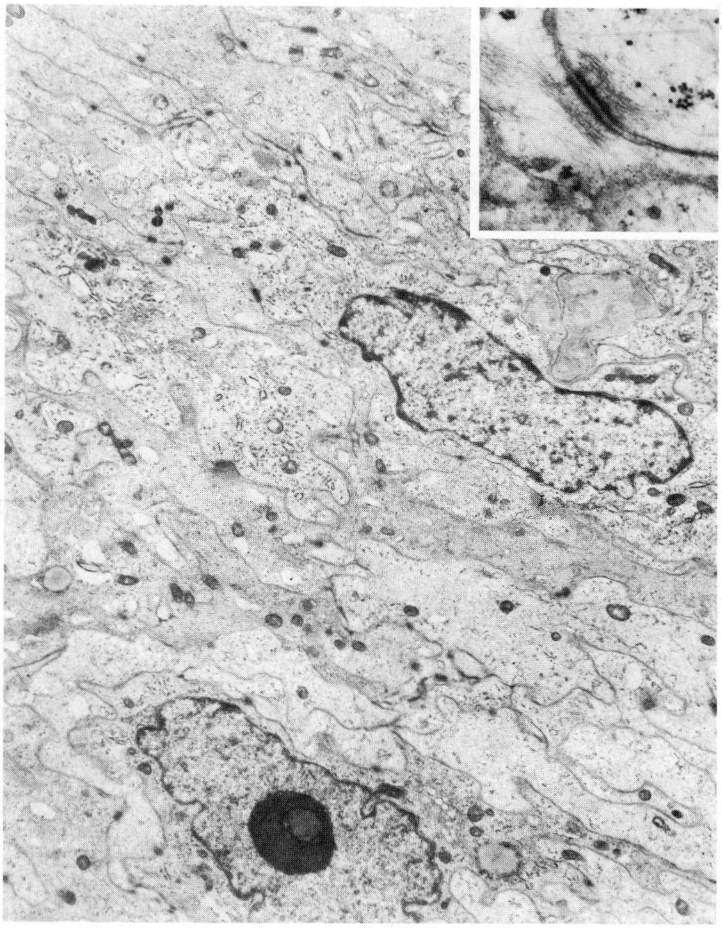

Figure 57. *Electron microscopic features of a meningioma.* Overall view, showing closely adjacent cells, tonofilaments, and desmosomes (× 6250). *Inset:* desmosome under high magnification (× 57,000).

Nuclear abnormalities and occasional *mitotic figures*, which have sometimes suggested "malignant transformation," but do not probably by themselves have a sinister significance;

A *very rich degree of vascularization* — so-called "angiomatous" meningiomas.

Despite the variation in appearance as seen by light microscopy, the unitary character of meningiomas should be emphasized: whereas various histological aspects may be found within the same tumor by light microscopy, the electron microscopic appearance (Fig. 57) is always similar and demonstrates arachnoidal cells — with tonofilaments and desmosomes — and a greater or lesser number of collagen fibers. Moreover, no correlation exists between these histological variants, the topographical distribution, and the clinical course of meningiomas as a whole.

MELANOMAS

A wide variety of disorders ranging from a simple increase in normal leptomeningeal pigmentation to highly malignant melanomas may be encountered. However, whether benign or malignant, primary melanomas of the nervous system are extremely rare. Before the diagnosis can be entertained, it is essential to exclude rigorously the possibility of a small occult primary cutaneous or ocular melanoma. In addition, other tumors, in particular meningiomas, may sometimes contain melanin pigment, and this may render their diagnosis from a true melanoma a matter of considerable difficulty.

SARCOMAS

Intracranial sarcomas are very rare neoplasms whose nature is often debated. They are estimated to account for 1 to 3 per cent of all intracranial tumors. Two main types can generally be recognized.

1. Fibrosarcomas (or fibroblastic sarcomas) are derived from fibroblasts, which may be situated in the dura, the leptomeninges, the perivascular spaces, the tela choroidea, or the stroma of the choroid plexuses. Fibrosarcomas are most frequently attached to the meninges, but may sometimes be entirely parenchymatous. Otherwise, they have no particular site of predilection.

Grossly, they are well circumscribed but nonencapsulated, of firm consistency, and with fairly homogeneous grayish cut surfaces. In some cases, the neoplasm is not a well-defined mass, but consists of a diffuse infiltration of the meninges (meningeal sarcomatosis).

Their *microscopic appearance* is identical with that of fibrosarcomas arising elsewhere in the body and presents the same range of cellular differentiation. The better differentiated examples are characterized by interlacing bundles of elongated fibroblastic cells of which only the nuclei are clearly visualized, separated by a rich network of reticulin fibers. Nuclear abnormalities are usually rare, but mitotic figures are common as a rule.

These sarcomas will to a greater or lesser extent invade the adjacent neural parenchyma in the shape of irregular neoplastic infiltrates.

2. Reticulum-cell sarcomas (Fig. 58) (sometimes erroneously identified as "granulomatous encephalitis" or "malignant reticulohistiocytic encephalitis") are of controversial origin. Some authors regard them as arising from reticulum cells, which are thought to be normally present in the meningeal and perivascular spaces (perithelial sarcomas). Others, in particular Russell and Rubinstein, are of the view that microglial cells participate in the neoplastic process and, hence, designate these tumors by the term **microglioma**. Whatever their origin, these neoplasms, which are not rare, are most frequently encountered in subjects between the ages of 50 and 70.

Reticulum-cell sarcomas–microgliomas are considerably more invasive and less well circumscribed than fibrosarcomas. They most often involve the cerebral hemispheres and show a certain predilection for the temporobasal regions and for the midline structures of the brainstem. The proliferation is sometimes multifocal or extremely diffuse, and the meninges may be infiltrated.

Microscopically, the appearances are fairly characteristic and consist of a proliferation of reticulum cells of varying size and shape, and of numerous small cells with darkly staining round nuclei that resemble lymphocytes. These small cells are often arranged to form perivascular cuffings. In addition, silver impregnations demonstrate a considerable increase of reticulin fibers, both perivascularly and within the substance of the tumor. Finally, mitotic figures are common.

3. Nosological problems. Except for the two main types of tumor described in the preceding paragraphs, we believe that the other kinds of sarcoma that have been isolated by a number of workers do not constitute proper entities and correspond in fact to other types of neoplasm. Thus, the "*circumscribed cerebellar sarcomas*" (or "arachnoidal sarcomas") are a variant of medulloblastoma; the "*monstrocellular sarcomas*" are in reality giant-cell glioblastomas;[1] the "*hemangioperi-*

---

[1]The term "monstrocellular sarcoma" has also apparently been used to designate examples of mixed glioblastomas and sarcomas (see above, p. 26) and perhaps exceptional cases of fibrous xanthomas and xanthosarcomas that may originate in the central nervous system (translator's note).

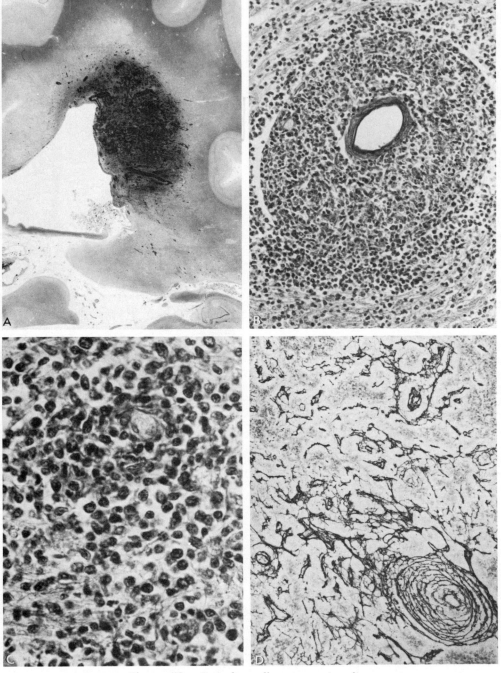

Figure 58. *Reticulum-cell sarcoma–microglioma.*

A, Right cerebral hemisphere (H. and E.). Tumor proliferation near right lateral ventricle, dorsal to pulvinar.

B, Tumor (H. and E., ×200). Tumor proliferation cuffing a blood vessel.

C, Tumor, cellular detail (H. and E., ×500).

D, Tumor (Gordon-Sweets' silver method for reticulin, ×180). Perivascular and intraparenchymatous reticulin fiber network.

cytomas" (included by Kernohan within the group of sarcomas) are difficult to distinguish from hemangioblastomas;[1] and "*sarcomatous meningiomas*" are in fact fibrosarcomas and not meningiomas.

Other varieties, such as myxosarcomas, chondrosarcomas, mesenchymal chondrosarcomas, and rhabdomyosarcomas, are exceptional rarities.

GLOMUS JUGULARE TUMORS
(or chemodectomas of the glomus jugulare)

These neoplasms, which are rare, originate from the cells of the glomus jugulare, or jugular body, which is situated in the adventitia of the jugular bulb. The tumor proliferates in the middle ear and may present in the external auditory meatus. However, in approximately 40 per cent of the cases the growth reaches the posterior fossa, in particular the region of the cerebellopontine angle.

present in CP angle or p.fossa

The histological appearance is identical with that of tumors of the carotid body: it consists of large clear polygonal cells grouped in lobules that are separated by a delicate connective tissue stroma rich in capillary blood vessels. By electron microscopy, dense-core vesicles may be demonstrated in the cytoplasm of the tumor cells, and biochemical studies have established that these cells secrete serotonin.

PITUITARY ADENOMAS

Adenomas are by far the most common neoplasms of the pituitary gland. Carcinomas of the adenohypophysis are an extreme rarity and are difficult to distinguish from pituitary metastases originating from visceral carcinoma.

Pituitary adenomas are of varying size and

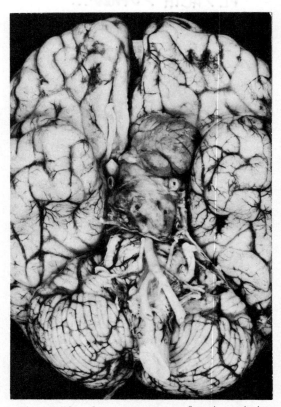

Figure 59. *Gross appearance of a giant pituitary adenoma.*

may range from a growth limited entirely to within the substance of the adenohypophysis to a giant mass (Fig. 59) that extends beyond the sella turcica and compresses the base of the brain. The tumors may be divided into two main groups.

1. Functionally inactive adenomas (true chromophobe adenomas). These adenomas are composed of cells of variable size, without definite tinctorial affinity, arranged either as diffuse masses or in trabeculae, or even in palisading or papillary formations.

2. Hormone-secreting adenomas. These tumors are identified by special staining techniques (e.g., Herlant's tetrachrome stain) and represent several varieties that are functionally dependent on the cell type from which they are derived. Thus, somatotropic adenomas are encountered in acromegaly; prolactin-secreting adenomas in the amen-

---

[1]A slightly different view on this controversial question is that craniospinal hemangiopericytomas are to be regarded as identical with a relatively malignant variant of angioblastic meningioma and that they differ both cytologically and biologically from the considerably more benign hemangioblastoma (Russell and Rubinstein, 1977) (translator's note).

PL > ACTH > other...

orrhea-galactorrhea syndrome; corticotropic and melanotropic adenomas in certain forms of Cushing's disease; and thyrotropic adenomas usually as a lesion secondary to primary thyroid myxedema.

CRANIOPHARYNGIOMAS
(Figs. 60 and 61)

Craniopharyngiomas account for approximately 3 per cent of intracranial tumors. They are encapsulated, solid and/or cystic, and intimately related to the pituitary gland and stalk. Because of their epithelial structure and their situation, they are often thought to arise from Rathke's pouch (which is an ectodermally derived diverticulum originating from the roof of the stomatodeum); however, that derivation has never

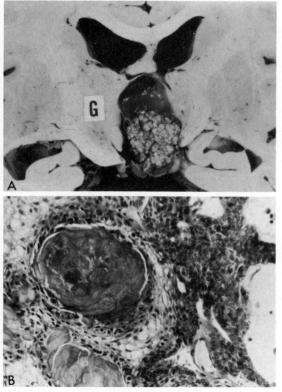

Figure 60. *Craniopharyngioma.*
A, Gross features; note cystic appearance and numerous foci of calcification. *B,* Microscopic appearance (H. and E.).

been established. They are encountered most often in children and adolescents, and are in fact the most common of the supratentorial tumors occurring in childhood. They form suprasellar masses that compress the chiasm anteriorly, the pituitary gland inferiorly, and the third ventricle superiorly. Although they are histologically benign, they often extend in various directions, which makes their complete surgical removal a matter of considerable technical difficulty.

Microscopically, the solid portions of the tumor are composed of cords or sheets of epithelial cells arranged in several layers: the periphery is formed by a basal layer of palisading cells beneath which several layers of stratified epithelial cells are found, resulting sometimes in the formation of "horny pearls" composed of keratinized cells. Amidst these epithelial areas, small cysts lined by palisading cells may be seen, as well as deposits of lamellar bone. These epithelial areas are separated by connective tissue trabeculae which are frequently narrow; the latter contain blood vessels and fairly often demonstrate a highly variegated appearance due to microcystic degeneration and to the presence of cholesterol crystals, macrophages, foreign body giant cells, and lymphocytic infiltrates.

The cystic portions of the tumor are lined by stratified squamous epithelium resting on a thin connective tissue layer. The cystic fluid contains numerous cholesterol crystals. Surrounding the tumor, a dense gliosis is often present, in the midst of which may be seen small epithelial islands that are apparently separate from the main tumor mass.

CHOLESTEATOMAS

Cholesteatomas (or "pearly tumors") are cystic neoplasms resulting from the inclusion of epiblastic elements in areas from which they are normally absent. Inclusion of these elements may take place in the fetal period,[1]

[1]Craniopharyngiomas have the same criteria, and some authors do not make a clear distinction between craniopharyngiomas and epidermoid cysts. However, craniopharyngiomas, though frequently and even occasionally entirely cystic, usually possess a solid portion, which is never found in cholesteatomas.

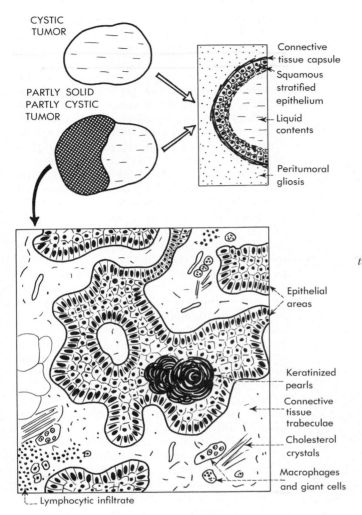

CYSTIC
TUMOR

PARTLY SOLID
PARTLY CYSTIC
TUMOR

Connective
tissue capsule

Squamous
stratified
epithelium

Liquid
contents

Peritumoral
gliosis

Epithelial
areas

Keratinized
pearls

Connective
tissue
trabeculae

Cholesterol
crystals

Macrophages
and giant cells

Lymphocytic infiltrate

Figure 61. *Diagram of structural features in craniopharyngiomas.*

or in later life as a result of mechanical trauma (repeated lumbar punctures, for example).

These tumors are very rare. Sites of predilection include the posterior fossa (especially the cerebellopontine angle), the intra- and suprasellar regions, and the lumbosacral spinal region.

Microscopically, two groups are distinguished, depending on their histological structure.

1. Epidermoid cysts (Fig. 62). These are cysts whose wall is composed of a thin connective tissue capsule upon which rests stratified squamous keratinized epithelium.

Their contents consist of more or less granular material, arranged in layers as in an onion bulb and rich in cholesterol crystals formed by the breakdown of keratin from desquamating epithelial cells.

2. Dermoid cysts (Fig. 63). In addition to epithelium of the epidermal type which is identical with that of epidermoid cysts, their structure includes an underlying layer comparable to the dermis; this may contain hair follicles, sweat glands, and sebaceous glands. In addition to desquamated keratinized cells, the cyst contents include glandular secretory products, among which hairs may be matted.

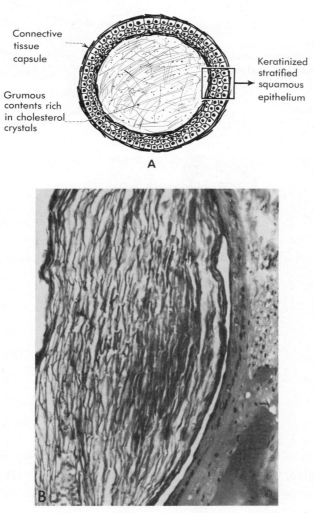

Figure 62. *Structure and microscopic appearance of epidermoid cysts.*

A, Diagram of overall structure. *B*, Microscopic appearance (hematoxylin-phloxine-saffranin).

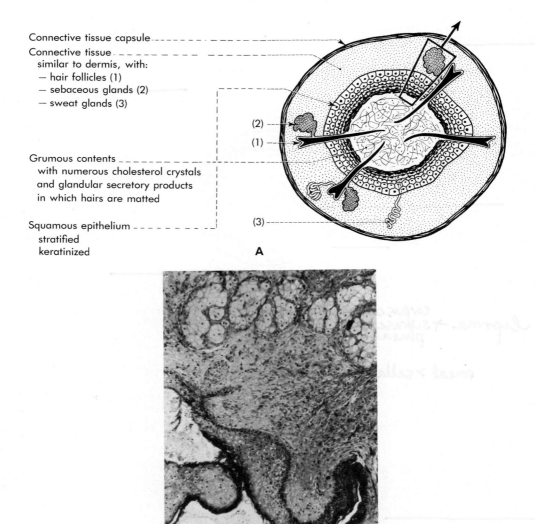

Connective tissue capsule

Connective tissue
   similar to dermis, with:
    — hair follicles (1)
    — sebaceous glands (2)
    — sweat glands (3)

                               (2)

                               (1)

Grumous contents
   with numerous cholesterol crystals
   and glandular secretory products
   in which hairs are matted

Squamous epithelium   (3)
   stratified
   keratinized

A

B

Figure 63.   *Structure and microscopic appearance of dermoid cysts.*
A, Diagram of overall structure. *B*, Microscopic appearance (H. and E.).

CHORDOMAS

Chordomas originate from intraosseous notochordal remnants. In the cranial cavity their site of election is at the level of the sella turcica and the clivus; in the spine they favor the sacrococcygeal region.

Microscopically, they consist of clear cells of variable size which demonstrate large PAS-positive vacuoles in their cytoplasm, hence the term "physaliphorous cells." The presence of connective tissue trabeculae, which are sometimes fairly dense, results in a conspicuous lobulation.

Rare malignant forms demonstrating mitotic figures exist, but, as a rule, chordomas are histologically benign and their rather unfavorable prognosis is attributable to their locally invasive character, which may result in bone destruction.

LIPOMAS

Lipomas are rare, benign growths. They tend to favor the corpus callosum, in which case they are often associated with partial or complete agenesis of that structure. Other sites are the suprasellar and the pineal regions. Within the spinal canal they are usually intradural and extramedullary, and are most often found at the thoracic level; in approximately one-third of the cases, they are associated with other congenital anomalies.

Microscopically, they are essentially composed of adipose cells in which connective tissue and vascular elements may coexist to a variable extent.

[handwritten: corpus callosum]
[handwritten: lipoma → suprasellar / pineal]

TERATOMAS

[handwritten: pineal > sella > p fossa]

Teratomas are extremely rare within the central nervous system, where they account for only 0.1 per cent of primary intracranial growths. They are found mostly within the first decade of life and tend to favor the midline. Their sites of predilection, in order of decreasing frequency, are the pineal region, the sellar and suprasellar regions, and the posterior fossa. With the exception of sacrococcygeal teratomas (which are relatively frequent), teratomas are even rarer in the spinal canal than within the cranial cavity; they are then often associated with spina bifida. The tumors are composed of various derivatives of the three primitive germ cell layers, i.e., epidermal, dermal, vascular, cartilaginous, glandular, muscular elements.

Intracranial teratomas are usually well circumscribed and encapsulated, and histologically benign. In some cases they display histological malignancy and are then sometimes designated as "teratoid tumors."

HEMANGIOBLASTOMAS

These growths account for approximately 1 to 2.5 per cent of all intracranial tumors.

They are encountered at any age, but are seen most frequently in young and middle-aged subjects.

Hemangioblastomas are most often situated in the *cerebellum* (Fig. 64). Indeed, they represent approximately 7 per cent of the primary tumors originating in the posterior fossa. In addition, they may be found within the parenchyma of the spinal cord, the medulla oblongata and, exceptionally, in the supratentorial compartment.

Although hemangioblastomas are often demonstrably or apparently solitary, they are also fairly frequently multiple and, in that case, they fall within the definition of **von Hippel–Lindau's disease** (see Fig. 66). The disease typically consists in the association of a retinal and a cerebellar hemangioblastoma with visceral lesions, in particular renal and/or pancreatic tumors or cysts; it is often familial. In fact, the disorder in its classic form represents but one variant of a larger, diversified nosological entity that is essentially characterized by the presence of one or more hemangioblastomas. For this reason, the overall entity deserves the name *hemangioblastomatosis*. It would therefore be desirable to replace the preceding three narrow criteria that originally defined von Hippel–Lindau's disease by three somewhat less rigid criteria: (1) the presence of one or more hemangioblastomas within the central nervous system, either at the same site (retina, cerebellum, spinal intramedullary) or at different sites (retina and cerebellum, retina and spinal intramedullary, cerebellum and spinal intramedullary), (2) the inconstant presence of visceral lesions, and (3) the frequent familial incidence (see Fig. 66).

Grossly (Fig. 64), hemangioblastomas are well circumscribed and very often cystic; they sometimes consist solely of a small mural nodule attached to the wall of a considerably larger cyst. The fairly characteristic yellow color is due to an abundant lipid contents. In addition, the tumor is usually vascularized and drained by well-developed vascular pedicles which in some cases may erroneously suggest the presence of an associated arteriovenous malformation. This rich vascularization accounts for the frequency of bleeding within the tumor.

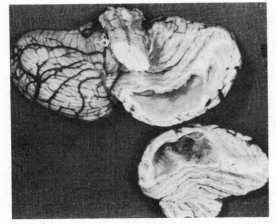

Figure 64.   *Gross features of cerebellar hemangioblastoma*. Note the presence of a mural tumor in the reflected lower portion of the cerebellar cyst.

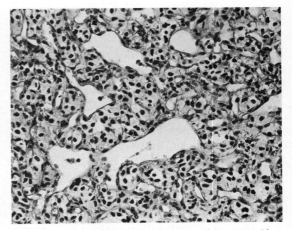

Figure 65.   *Microscopic features of hemangioblastoma* (Masson's trichrome).

Microscopically (Fig. 65), the appearances are highly characteristic. The histological picture is one of numerous capillary blood vessels of different sizes separated by trabeculae or sheets of varying dimensions composed of clear cells with round or elongated nuclei. These tumor cells, which lack all cytonuclear abnormality, often present a spongy appearance caused by an abundance of intracytoplasmic vacuoles that have been emptied of their lipid contents as a result of the embedding procedure. A fine network of

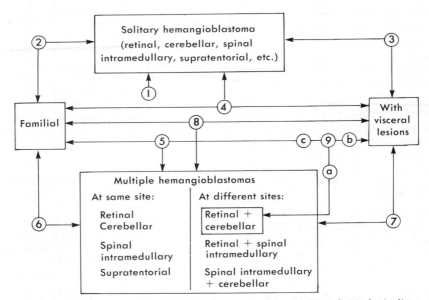

Figure 66.   *Diagram illustrating the nosological problems raised by von Hippel–Lindau's disease within the general context of the hemangioblastomas.*

1, Solitary hemangioblastoma (lowest grade of von Hippel–Lindau's disease).

2 to 8, Incomplete or atypical "formes frustes" of von Hippel–Lindau's disease.

9, Classical von Hippel–Lindau's disease (*a*, always; *b*, most often; *c*, often).

reticulin fibers surrounds the capillary blood vessels and the individual tumor cells. These cells have long been regarded as being derived from capillary endothelial cells, hence the classic view that these are "vascular tumors." In reality, their origin is still debated.[1]

Hemangioblastomas are histologically benign, but postoperative recurrences and, especially, the appearance of hemangioblastomas at other sites may darken the prognosis.

---

[1]The vascular endothelial origin of these tumors is generally accepted by most neuropathologists of the American and British schools (translator's note).

"Angioblastic meningiomas." The term "angioblastic meningioma" was applied by Bailey and Cushing to designate firm, largely supratentorial tumors that were microscopically similar to hemangioblastomas and were classified within the group of meningiomas on the basis of their meningeal attachment and on the hypothesis that meningioblastic cells were differentiating into angioblasts. In fact, this interpretation lacks supporting evidence, and electron microscopic studies have established that the so-called "angioblastic meningiomas" are simply hemangioblastomas and/or hemangiopericytomas.[1]

---

[1]See translator's note on p. 44.

III. SECONDARY TUMORS

Metastatic neoplasms from primary visceral cancer are among the most frequent histological types of intracranial and intraspinal tumor.

They may be situated in any region of the cranial cavity or spinal canal. They may involve the central neuraxis, e.g., cerebral hemispheres (Fig. 67), cerebellum, brainstem, or less often, the spinal cord; the spinal (Fig. 68) or cranial nerve roots; or the meningeal coverings, e.g., carcinomatous meningitis (Fig. 69), spinal epidural metastases, or dural metastases at the base of the skull or over the convexities. Their exact frequency is difficult to determine because statistical figures vary considerably according to the type of clinical material studied. Thus, in Cushing's series intracranial metastases were estimated to account for 3.2 per cent of all intracranial tumors, whereas in Kaufman's series they accounted for 36.8 per cent. As an average, a figure of 20 to 25 per cent is probably the most likely.

Metastases may be solitary, but are most often multiple. Their size ranges from that of a millet seed to that of a pigeon's egg. They generally present as well-circumscribed nodules, either firm or soft, the latter resulting from bleeding within the tumor, focal necrosis, or cystic degeneration. The two chief primary sites are **bronchopulmonary carcinoma** in the male and **mammary carcinoma** in the female. Next in frequency are malignant melanoma, renal carcinoma, and carcinoma of the alimentary tract (Fig. 70).

Microscopically, metastases essentially recapitulate the histological appearance of their primary source. However, highly atypical features are not rare and, if the primary site is not known clinically, its histological recognition in a metastatic deposit may be difficult in a fair number of cases and occasionally may be even impossible.

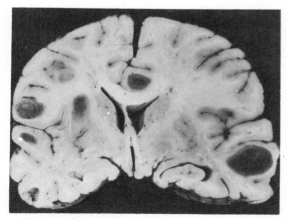

Figure 67. *Multiple hemispheric cerebral metastases.*

lung
breast
melanoma
renal
GI

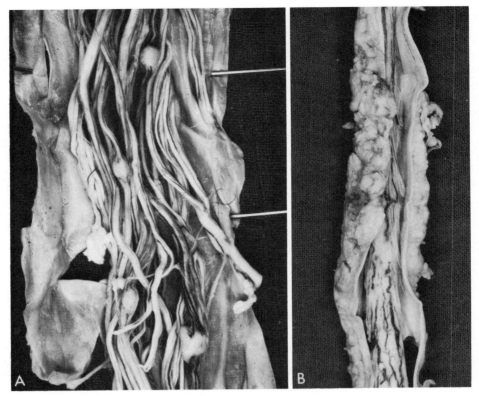

Figure 68.   *Intraspinal metastases.*

A, Nerve root metastases in the cauda equina. *B*, Epidural neoplastic infiltration.

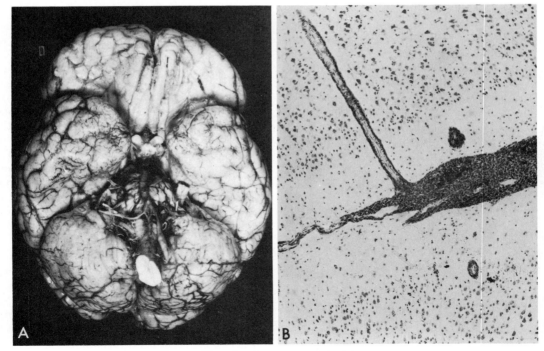

Figure 69.   *Carcinomatous meningitis.*

A, Gross features. *B*, Microscopic features. Note tumor infiltration along a perivascular space.

Metastatic neoplasms of the nervous system	Primary site																
	Lung	Breast	Kidney	Alimentary tract	Melanomas	Thyroid	Pancreas	Ear, nose, throat	Ovary	Uterus	Prostate	Testis	Sarcomas	Bladder	Biliary tract	Adrenal	Undetermined
Cerebral metastases (222)...........	97 (44%)	23 (10%)	16 (7%)	14 (6%)	7 (3%)	5 (2%)	4	4	3	3	2	2	3	2	1	1	35
Nerve root metastases (12) .... Isolated (6) .... Associated with other localizations (6)	3	1	1	1	0	0	0	0	0	0	1	0	1	0	0	0	4
Carcinomatous meningitis (39)........... Isolated (22) Associated with other localizations (17)	12	5	2	2	2	2	2	0	1	1	0	0	1	1	1	0	7
Total primary visceral malignancies	103 (41%)	25 (10%)	17 (7%)	17 (7%)	8 (3%)	6 (2%)	7 (3%)	4 (2%)	4 (2%)	4 (2%)	4 (2%)	2 (1%)	4 (2%)	2 (1%)	1	1	42 (16%)

Figure 70. *Sites of primary visceral malignancy in metastatic disease of the nervous system* (excluding epidural metastases). Data collected from 1951 to 1970 (Castaigne, Escourolle, and Hauw, 1972).

IV. BONE TUMORS

Bone tumors involving the skull and/or the spine may be benign (in which case they include osteomas, chondromas, aneurysmal bone cysts, cholesteatomas, etc.) or malignant. In the latter case, the malignancy may be primary (osteosarcoma, myeloma, etc.) or secondary (bony metastases from mammary, prostatic, renal, bronchial, or thyroid carcinoma, or the result of secondary bone invasion by an adjacent carcinoma). In any event, all these lesions fall more properly within the domain of bone pathology and therefore will not be further discussed in this chapter.

[handwritten margin note: 2° breast prostate renal lung thyroid .... 6I ...]

V. STRUCTURAL CHANGES RESULTING FROM EXPANDING INTRACRANIAL SPACE-OCCUPYING LESIONS

We shall consider here the effects of expanding intracranial space-occupying lesions in the broad sense of the term, therefore chiefly tumors, but including also abscesses, hematomas, large infarcts, parasitic cysts, etc.

FOCAL CHANGES

1. Changes within the tumor mass (Fig. 71). As a rule, these changes produce a more or less rapid increase in volume of the intracranial tumor mass. Such an increase in volume may result:

From local extension of the neoplastic process—of variable extent and rapidity.

Or, as a sudden event, from hemorrhage or cyst formation within the tumor.

2. Changes involving the adjacent neural parenchyma (Fig. 72). These changes are essentially of two kinds:

Compression and displacement of the neural parenchyma by an extraparenchymatous tumor, with the consequences of local damage (gliosis, necrosis, ischemia, etc.).

Destruction and invasion of the neural parenchyma by an infiltrating tumor.

The clinical consequences vary according to whether the process occurs in an "eloquent" or a "silent" region of the brain.

REGIONAL CHANGES

1. Cerebral edema. Increase in volume of the tumor is almost invariably accompan-

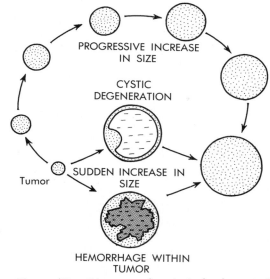

PROGRESSIVE INCREASE IN SIZE

CYSTIC DEGENERATION

Tumor

SUDDEN INCREASE IN SIZE

HEMORRHAGE WITHIN TUMOR

Figure 71. *Diagram of principal changes in tumor mass.*

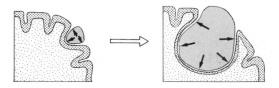

Compression and displacement of neural
parenchyma by an extraparenchymatous tumor

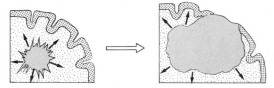

Destruction and invasion of neural
parenchyma by an infiltrating tumor

Figure 72. *Diagram of parenchymatous changes in intracranial tumors.*

ied by circulatory disturbances (e.g., venous stasis, arteriolar vasodilatation, increase of capillary permeability), which are responsible for the development of cerebral edema.

2. Disturbances of the cerebrospinal fluid circulation. Hydrocephalus may result either from disturbances in cerebrospinal fluid reabsorption or, more frequently, from obstruction to the flow of cerebrospinal fluid (Fig. 73) (foramen of Monro, aqueduct of Sylvius) due either to the location of the tumor mass or to cerebral edema which displaces the ventricular cavities and the paths of outflow of the cerebrospinal circulation.

3. Cerebral herniations (Figs. 74, 75, 76). Increase in volume of the tumor mass, cerebral edema, and ventricular dilatation resulting from hydrocephalus are all causes, either singly or in association, of *intracranial hypertension*.

Increase in volume of intracranial contents will lead to splaying of the still ununited cranial sutures in children, resulting in increase in size of the skull and in digital convolutional markings. In adults, however, in whom the bony skull can no longer enlarge because of union of the sutures, and after a certain age in children, the expanding cerebral mass will insinuate itself into the free residual openings that can accommodate it (cerebral herniations).

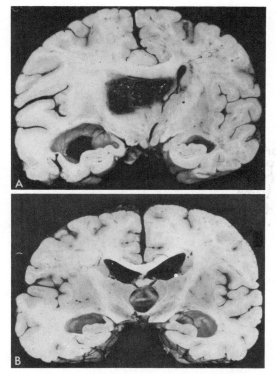

Figure 73. *Gross features of ventricular obstruction.*
A, Obstruction of the left foramen of Monro by a metastasis. *B,* Obstruction of the aqueduct of Sylvius, with hydrocephalus.

The problem differs according to whether the lesions are supra- or infratentorial (Fig. 74).

Cerebral Herniations in Supratentorial Lesions

a.   A unilateral lesion that increases the hemispheric volume is likely to cause a *herniation of the cerebral hemisphere through openings limited by the lower border of the falx and by the free edge of cerebellar tentorium on the same side.* Depending on the extent of the increase in size of the hemisphere and on the precise site of the expanding lesion, the thrust either will take place entirely through both these openings or will predominate in certain directions. As a result, several main topographical varieties of herniation, which are also

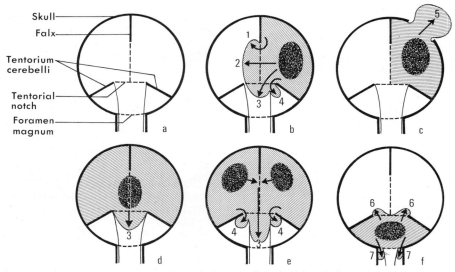

Figure 74. *Diagrammatic localization of the chief types of cerebral herniation.*

a, Normal aspect of rigid structures within the skull; *b*, unilateral hemispheric expanding lesion; *c*, herniation through bone flap; *d*, midline hemispheric expanding lesion; *e*, bilateral hemispheric expanding lesions; *f*, expanding infratentorial lesion.

1, Cingulate (subfalcine) herniation; *2*, lateral displacement of midline structures; *3*, central diencephalic herniation; *4*, temporal herniation; *5*, external herniation (through bone flap); *6*, superior cerebellar herniation (through tentorial opening); *7*, cerebellar tonsillar herniation (through foramen magnum).

likely to be associated with each other to a varying degree, may occur as follows:

Herniation of the supracallosal, or cingulate, gyrus under the falx (subfalcine herniation) will result in a lateral displacement of the anterior cerebral arteries, well visualized on arteriography.

Lateral displacement of the midline structures (i.e., the third ventricle, pineal gland, the vein of Galen) may occur.

Downward herniation of the diencephalon through the tentorial notch will cause downward displacement of the floor of the hypothalamus and of the mamillary bodies (central diencephalic herniation).

Herniation of the hippocampal gyrus in the tentorial notch between the brainstem and the free edge of the tentorium cerebelli may occur. In that case, the herniated temporal rim is likely to *compress the third and sixth cranial nerves, the cerebral peduncle* (with the likelihood of producing a lesion in the crus of the contralateral peduncle against the free

edge of the tentorium, thus giving rise to Kernohan's notch), and the *posterior cerebral artery* (with the likelihood of secondary infarction within its territory of supply). Finally, compression due to temporal herniation and the downward thrust of central diencephalic herniation may result in stretching of the blood vessels, especially venous, which may be responsible for *secondary brainstem hemorrhages*, particularly in the pontine tegmentum.

External cerebral herniation through the surgical bone flap occurs under special circumstances.

b. A bilateral lesion that increases the volume of both hemispheres will chiefly result in central diencephalic herniation and/or bilateral temporal lobe herniation.

c. A midline expanding lesion will largely result in central diencephalic herniation.

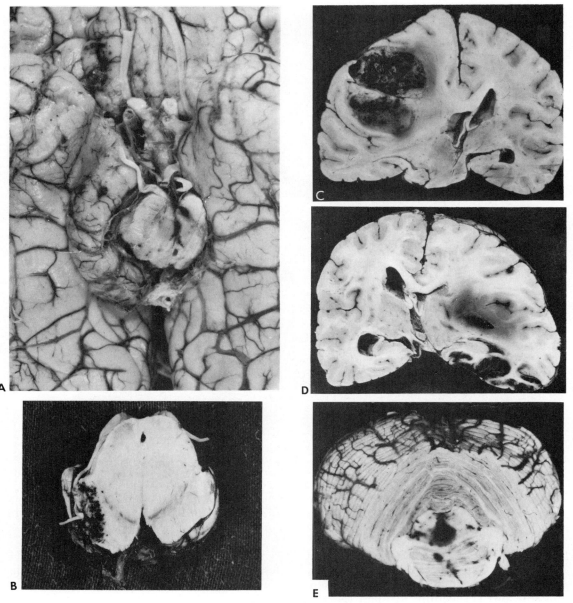

Figure 75. *Cerebral herniations.*

A, Inferior aspect of cerebral hemispheres; note the herniated rim of the right hippocampal gyrus compressing the oculomotor nerve and displacing the brainstem.

B, Cerebral peduncle; note hemorrhagic lesion in the crus of the peduncle contralateral to the temporal herniation (Kernohan's notch).

C, Cerebral metastases causing temporal herniation; note displacement of the midline structures and cingulate herniation.

D, Central diencephalic herniation and hemorrhagic infarction in the territory of the posterior cerebral artery (tumor of the right basal ganglia).

E, Pontine hemorrhage involving mostly the tegmentum, secondary to temporal herniation.

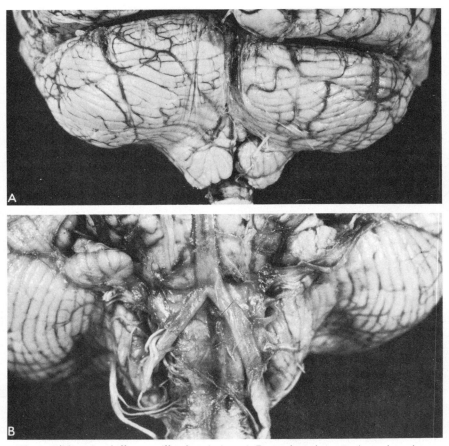

Figure 76. *Cerebellar tonsillar herniation. A*, Posterior view. *B*, Anterior view.

Cerebellar Herniations in Infratentorial Lesions

Two types of herniations exist:

a. Upward herniation of the mesencephalon and cerebellum through the tentorial notch. Direct mesencephalic lesions may result from this complication, as well as secondary lesions due to vascular compression.

b. Cerebellar tonsillar herniation through the foramen magnum is the most frequent and most dangerous complication of infratentorial expanding processes, regardless of their nature or degree of malignancy. As a result of increased intracranial pressure in the posterior fossa, the cerebellar tonsils are thrust downward through the foramen magnum, which they override, culminating in medullary compression and fatal lesions in the floor of the fourth ventricle (Fig. 76).

RECURRENCES, EXTRACRANIAL EXTENSIONS, METASTASES

1. Recurrences are generally found in malignant tumors (glioblastomas, metastases), but may also be seen in so-called benign tumors when removal has been incom-

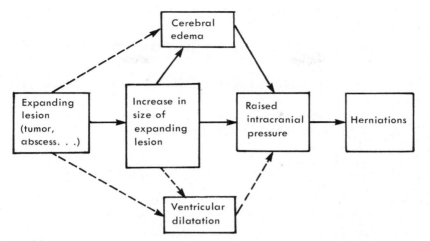

Figure 77. *Diagram of chief regional complications secondary to an intracranial tumor.*

plete—and sometimes even when removal has been complete.

2. *Extracranial tumor extensions* are rare and may occur as the result of local bone invasion (cranial vault or base of skull).

3. *Metastases.* *1.* Primary tumors of the central nervous system only exceptionally give rise to blood-borne metastases.

2. On the other hand, metastasis within the central nervous system resulting from meningeal dissemination is possible, especially with certain types of tumor (medulloblastomas, ependymomas, pinealomas).

Chapter 3

TRAUMATIC LESIONS OF THE CENTRAL NERVOUS SYSTEM

I. CRANIOCEREBRAL INJURIES

A. CLOSED CRANIOCEREBRAL INJURIES

I. PRIMARY TRAUMATIC LESIONS

Lesions due to head injury may involve the following anatomical planes of the cranial cavity:

The skull;

The extradural space (between the skull and the dura);

The subdural space (between the dura and the leptomeninges);

The subarachnoid space (strictly speaking, between the arachnoid and the pia, but actually formed by the leptomeningeal network);

The brain itself.

In practice, the pathological entities to be considered have their strict clinical counterparts only when trauma has caused a single and relatively simple lesion—a rare event, since most severe injuries lead to multiple lesions.

1. Within the bony plane: skull fractures. Skull fracture by itself is of no serious consequence, but it may be responsible for complications that result from vascular tear (extradural hematomas), meningeal tear (cerebrospinal fluid leaks), or brain contusion (depressed fractures).

a. Fractures of the cranial vault. The fracture line is usually linear and situated between the bony ridges (Fig. 78).

b. Fractures of the base of the skull. These fractures also include fractures of the vault in which the fracture lines have radiated toward the base. Three main locations are recognized: fractures radiating to the an-

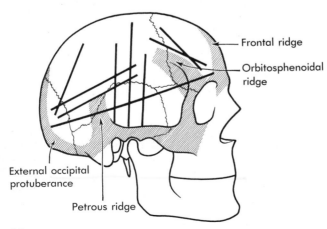

Figure 78. *Diagram of fracture lines along the cranial vault.* Note that the lines are usually found between the bony ridges of the skull (hatched).

Frontal ridge

Orbitosphenoidal ridge

External occipital protuberance

Petrous ridge

terior fossa, to the middle fossa, and to the posterior fossa.

All these fractures share a common proclivity to lead to a communication between septic cavities, such as the nasal fossae or the external auditory meatus, and the extradural or the subarachnoid space, hence the special risk of infection. Furthermore, cranial nerves may suffer mechanical damage at their sites of exit from the skull.

2. Extradural space: extradural hematoma

(Fig. 79). An extradural hematoma is an extravasation of blood between the dura and the inner table of the skull. It is composed of dense blood clot which tends to adhere early and firmly to the dura; its color is dark red, and it is jelly-like in consistency.

Bleeding is usually the result of injury to a blood vessel caused by skull fracture; it is most often due to rupture of the middle meningeal artery or one of its branches, but in some cases the trauma is venous (superior longitudinal sinus, lateral sinus, sphenoparietal sinus, etc.).

Extradural hematomas are usually situated in the temporal region, but fairly frequently extend beyond the confines of the temporal fossa, either rostrally, caudally, or inferiorly. There are, however, also atypical sites (i.e., frontal, subfrontal, subtemporal, occipital, and even posterior fossa hematomas).

In the absence of prompt surgical intervention, the extravasation of blood very rapidly increases in volume and results in cerebral compression and fatal internal herniation.

3. Subdural space: subdural hematoma

(Figs. 80 and 81). Subdural hematomas are collections of liquid composed of a variable mixture of blood and cerebrospinal fluid,[1] situated between the dura and the outer surface of the leptomeninges.

It is necessary to distinguish between early (or acute) subdural hematoma and late (or chronic) subdural hematoma.

---

[1]All intermediate forms exist between subdural hematomas composed of almost pure blood and subdural hygromas (or post-traumatic serous meningitides), which are composed of almost pure cerebrospinal fluid.

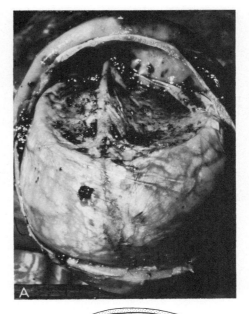

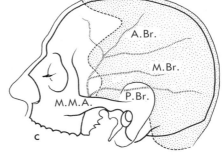

Figure 79. *Extradural hematomas.*
A, Gross appearance of a bifrontal extradural hematoma as seen in the cadaver. *B*, Diagram showing the surface projections of the middle meningeal artery (M.M.A.) and its branches (anterior, middle and posterior) on the vault of the skull (the hairline is outlined within the *stippled* area.).

a. Early subdural hematomas may be solitary lesions due to rupture of the cortical veins, but they are most often associated with an underlying cerebral contusion, i.e., a hemorrhagic contusion in which blood extends along the surface of the brain (hemorrhagic cerebral damage).

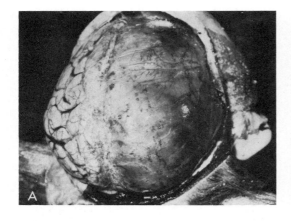 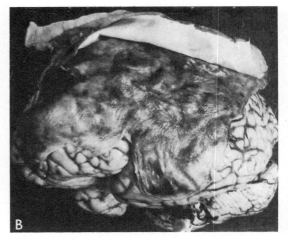

Figure 80.   *Subdural hematomas.*

A, Appearance on the cadaver before incision of the dura. *B,* Old organized subdural hematoma; gross appearance after removal of the dura.

b. Late subdural hematomas are seen several weeks or months after head injury and are solitary lesions. Their pathogenesis is obscure. There is no satisfactory theory that accounts for the delay in their appearance.

In contrast to extradural hematomas, subdural hematomas are composed of a sepia colored collection of fluid which resembles tincture of iodine and does not clot. They may be localized on any site of the convexity and extend for a variable distance both rostrally and caudally, but are always situated near the vertex, with a greater or lesser tendency to extend toward the base. Not uncommonly they are bilateral. Other rarer

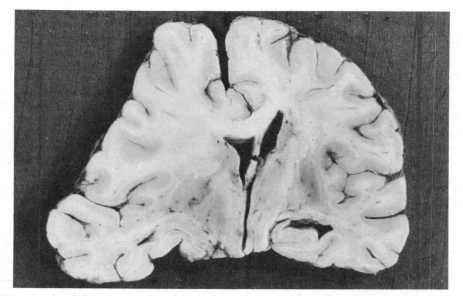

Figure 81.   *Subdural hematoma.* Note hemispheric compression, the contralateral displacement of midline structures, and the cingulate and hippocampal herniations.

sites include the subfrontal region, the interhemispheric fissure, and the posterior fossa. Chronic subdural hematomas may undergo organization and lead to fibrous tissue proliferation, resulting in the formation of a thick membrane between the dura and the leptomeninges.[1]

4. Subarachnoid space: subarachnoid hemorrhage. Meningeal subarachnoid hemorrhage is defined by the presence of blood in the subarachnoid spaces. Bleeding is due to rupture of a corticomeningeal blood vessel.

Most craniocerebral injuries of any severity are accompanied by some degree of subarachnoid hemorrhage. It is exceptional for severe traumatic subarachnoid hemorrhage

---

[1]In this group are included the classic "hemorrhagic pachymeningitides" found in chronic alcoholics and demented patients.

to be solitary; it is usually associated with the lesions of cerebral contusion.

5. Brain: cerebral lesions. a. Intracerebral hematoma. Isolated traumatic intracerebral hematomas are exceptional. They form circumscribed, well-limited collections of blood, without notable associated cerebral lesions.

b. Cerebral contusions (Fig. 82). From the strictly pathological point of view, cerebral contusions may range from a simple subpial hemorrhagic extravasation to an extensive laceration of the neural tissue accompanied by hemorrhages—subdural, subarachnoid, and intracerebral—of varying severity.

In practice, two main types are recognized:

Lesions of diffuse contusion are due to a contrecoup mechanism and are preferentially localized over areas of the brain which, at the time of injury, have impinged on bony

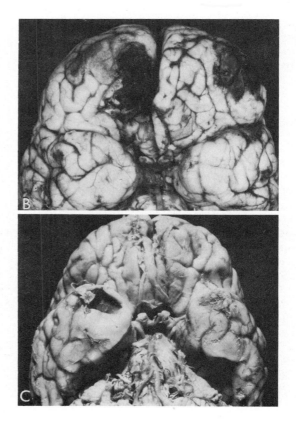

Figure 82. *Cerebral contusions.*

A, Diagram of sites of predilection.

B, Gross appearance of a recent fronto-orbital contusion.

C, Gross appearance of an older fronto-temporal contusion.

and meningeal surfaces or ridges: these areas include the tip of the temporal lobe, the orbital surface of the frontal lobe (Fig. 82B and C), the inner surface of the cerebral hemispheres, the brainstem, and the occipital pole.

Single (or chief) *foci of contusion.* In some cases, a single focus of contusion, which is often localized in the anterior part of the temporal lobe, may produce, as a result of intracerebral and subdural hemorrhage and subsequent edema, an acutely expanding lesion (hemorrhagic cerebral damage) that may necessitate neurosurgical intervention.

In cases in which the immediate course is favorable, the cerebral lesion undergoes organization, with the formation of a retractile connective tissue–glial scar, with meningeal adhesions and with demyelination of the underlying white matter. These cortico-meningeal scars may be the cause of some cases of post-traumatic epilepsy.

c. Cerebral edema. Cerebral edema is almost invariably found in severe head injury and is never solitary. It is always secondary either to a single lesion, as in intracerebral hematoma, or to multiple lesions, i.e., from multiple foci of contusion.

II. GENERAL AND/OR SPECIAL CONSEQUENCES OF PRIMARY TRAUMATIC LESIONS

a. Herniations. Whether they are due to an extradural or a subdural hematoma compressing the brain, or to edema resulting from single or multiple intracerebral lesions, cerebral herniations constitute a very serious and frequently fatal type of complication, especially temporal herniation as it compresses the rostral portion of the brainstem (see Chapter 2).

b. Acute hydrocephalus. Truly acute traumatic hydrocephalus may result from mechanical blockage of the pathway of flow of cerebrospinal fluid, either from herniation or from the presence of blood clot.

On the other hand, chronic, so-called "normal-pressure" hydrocephalus may be a sequel of post-traumatic meningeal hemorrhage, although it may also be observed after other scar-producing conditions, such as meningeal hemorrhage of various etiology or acute meningitis, when chronic arachnoiditis may result in impairment of cerebrospinal fluid resorption.

c. Infections. The complications of infection (meningitis, abscess, etc.) are generally found only in open craniocerebral injuries. A number of skull fractures (i.e., of the ethmoid sinus, of the frontal sinus, of the petrous bone) cause dural tears that are responsible for external leakage of the cerebrospinal fluid through the nose or ear. Infection is of course the major risk in these cases.

d. Prolonged coma. In these cases, the lesions of contusion as well as those due to secondary ischemia and anoxia are found.

III. SUMMARY

Most of the lesions that have been separately analyzed in the preceding paragraphs are seldom met in isolation and must be correlated with one another. A summary of the interaction of the chief lesions is shown in the diagram of Figure 83.

In any event, it is important to stress the difficulty of achieving an exact clinicopathological correlation in every case. It is well known that the same clinical picture may result from different types of lesion, and furthermore, the various lesions are often found together.

In addition, there are a number of cases with head injuries of variable severity that do not demonstrate any gross or even histological lesions in the brain: the term *commotio cerebri* (or "concussion") is then used in these instances. None of the pathogenetic theories proposed so far appear to provide a satisfactory explanation for this phenomenon.

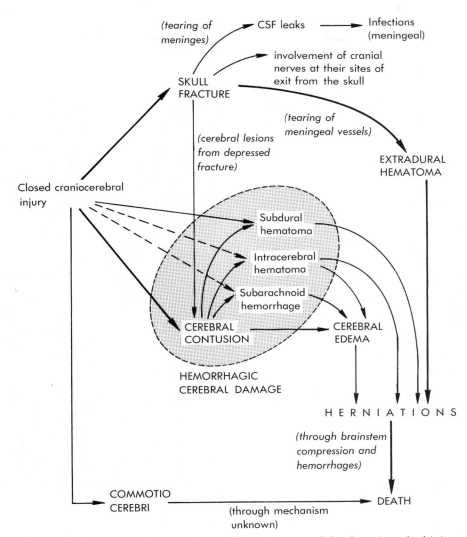

Figure 83. *Summary diagram of the chief complications of closed craniocerebral injury.*

B. OPEN CRANIOCEREBRAL INJURIES

Whatever its etiology (open fracture, missiles, etc.), the course of a *cerebral wound* may be summarily described as follows. Three stages of evolution are found:

A phase of damage, in which necrosis from direct destruction, associated with vascular phenomena (thromboses, hemorrhages), and edema are present.

A phase of clearing, in which compound granular corpuscles mixed with blood-borne polymorphonuclear leukocytes, lymphocytes, and plasma cells, clear the tissue debris and transport them toward the blood vessels.

A phase of repair, consisting of a proliferation of reactive astrocytes accompanied, in the adjacent meningeal zones, by a connective tissue proliferation of perivascular and meningeal origin. Thus, a retractile, mutilating, and ultimately definitive glial or gliomesenchymal scar is formed.

Naturally, the risk of infection is here at its highest.

II. INJURIES TO THE SPINAL CORD
AND NERVE ROOTS

Closed injuries of the spinal cord and nerve roots are due to forced movements or to fractures or subluxations of the spine.

The same basic traumatic lesions are found as in the skull:

Within the bony plane (Fig. 84): vertebral fractures or subluxations.

Extradural space: extradural hematoma.

Subdural space: subdural hematoma.

Subarachnoid space: spinal subarachnoid hemorrhage.

Spinal cord: various cord lesions (hematomyelia, spinal cord contusions, spinal cord edema).

Commotio cordae, without histological lesions, may also be found. Infarcts of ischemic origin (myelomalacia) resulting from vascular damage are a dangerous complication of spinal cord trauma and are met more frequently than in the case of cerebral trauma.

The stretched, bruised, or compressed nerve roots may also be the site of contusive, edematous, and hemorrhagic lesions.

In contrast to severe craniocerebral injuries, spinal cord injuries are seldom fatal.

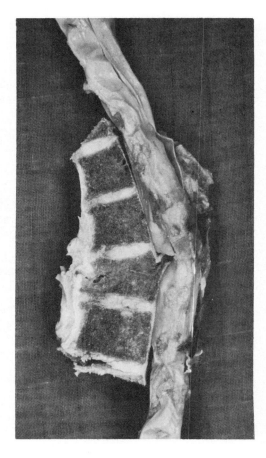

Figure 84. *Spinal vertebral fracture, with indenting of the spinal cord by bony fragment.*

VASCULAR PATHOLOGY   Chapter 4

I. CEREBRAL AND/OR MENINGEAL HEMORRHAGE

[handwritten: Causes: ↑BP, AVM, blood dyscrasias]

Any extravasation of blood within the brain and/or the leptomeninges, whatever its cause, constitutes a cerebral and/or meningeal (subarachnoid) hemorrhage.

Traumatic hemorrhages arise in a different context (see pp. 61–63) and will therefore be omitted from this chapter. Traditionally excluded also from present considerations are hemorrhagic infarcts (see p. 83), hemorrhages within neoplasms (see p. 54), and brainstem hemorrhages secondary to herniation (see p. 56). Likewise we shall exclude here those mild hemorrhagic suffusions which may sometimes be microscopic only and can occur in many disorders of various etiology, usually secondary to terminal events such as circulatory collapse or asphyxia.

Within the limits delineated above, therefore, the three main causes of cerebral and/or meningeal (subarachnoid) hemorrhage are *arterial hypertension*, rupture of a *vascular malformation*, and *blood dyscrasias* (see Fig. 104). In order to understand the pathophysiological mechanisms that underlie the development of these hemorrhages, it is necessary to have recourse to a few *definitions* (Fig. 85).

In *cerebral hemorrhage*, bleeding occurs primarily within the brain parenchyma. Such a hemorrhage may remain entirely cerebral, or it may irrupt into the ventricular cavities *(cerebral hemorrhage with ventricular rupture)* or, less often, into the leptomeningeal spaces *(cerebromeningeal hemorrhage)*; most frequently, irruption of the blood into the ventricles results in its passage into the leptomeningeal spaces and, notably, in the posterior fossa via the foramina of Lushka and Magendie, thus culminating in a cerebromeningeal hemorrhage secondary to *ventricular rupture*.

In *meningeal, or subarachnoid, hemorrhage* bleeding primarily takes place in the leptomeningeal spaces. It may remain purely subarachnoid, either diffuse or localized, and in the latter case may sometimes form a true *subarachnoid hematoma;* or it can extend into the brain by penetrating the cortex (meningocerebral hemorrhage) and in some cases ultimately burst into the ventricular cavity *(meningocerebral hemorrhage with ventricular rupture)*.

1. Hypertensive Hemorrhage

The major cause of *cerebral hemorrhage*, within the above definition, is arterial hypertension. It occurs mostly between the ages of 40 and 70.

a. Evolution. The bleeding, which is primarily intraparenchymatous, results in a collection of blood that is under tension,[1] contains little parenchymatous debris, and displaces the cerebral structures. Since the lesion is essentially infiltrative, its edges are irregular, and small petechial hemorrhages are visible along its borders in the gray matter and in the edematous and softened white matter.

---

[1]The term "intracerebral hematoma" is synonymous with cerebral hemorrhage.

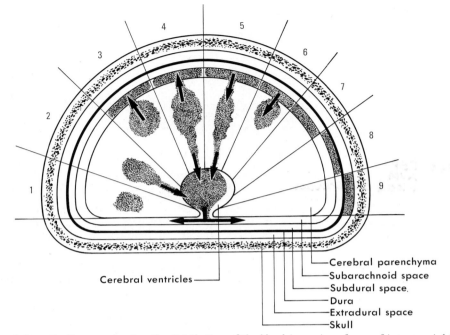

Cerebral ventricles

Cerebral parenchyma
Subarachnoid space
Subdural space
Dura
Extradural space
Skull

Figure 85. *Schematic diagram showing the distribution of the blood in various forms of intracranial hemorrhage.*

1. Pure cerebral hemorrhage (or cerebral hematoma) ⎫
2. Cerebral hemorrhage with ventricular rupture   ⎪
3. Cerebromeningeal hemorrhage   ⎬ Cerebral hemorrhages
4. Cerebromeningeal hemorrhage with ventricular rupture ⎭

5. Meningocerebral hemorrhage with ventricular rupture ⎫
6. Meningocerebral hemorrhage   ⎪
7. Pure meningeal (subarachnoid) hemorrhage   ⎬ Meningeal hemorrhages
8. Subdural hematoma   ⎭

9. Extradural hematoma

In severe cases, the hemorrhage presents as a rapidly expanding process that may result in cerebral herniation, with its own vital consequences (see pp. 55–58). It can also rupture into the ventricles, with the subsequent passage of blood into the subarachnoid space.

Less often, cerebromeningeal hemorrhage may be due to the direct irruption of intracerebral bleeding through the cortex into the leptomeninges.

Fairly frequently, a cerebral hemorrhage may remain relatively circumscribed; then the fatal evolution that is characteristic of a severe bleeding, described above, does not take place.

Phagocytic processes may follow the initial bleeding and its accompanying edema. The focal hemorrhage will be cleared by polymorphonuclear leukocytes and by macrophages derived from blood monocytes. A cicatricial cystic cavity with orange-yellow borders, surrounded by a reactive astrocytic gliosis, will then be formed. Old hemorrhagic scars of this type are often noted in the brains of hypertensive subjects.

b. Principal sites. 1. HEMISPHERIC

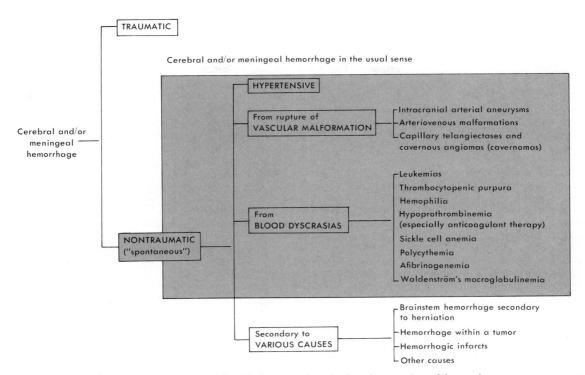

TRAUMATIC

Cerebral and/or meningeal hemorrhage in the usual sense

Cerebral and/or meningeal hemorrhage

HYPERTENSIVE

From rupture of VASCULAR MALFORMATION
- Intracranial arterial aneurysms
- Arteriovenous malformations
- Capillary telangiectases and cavernous angiomas (cavernomas)

From BLOOD DYSCRASIAS
- Leukemias
- Thrombocytopenic purpura
- Hemophilia
- Hypoprothrombinemia (especially anticoagulant therapy)
- Sickle cell anemia
- Polycythemia
- Afibrinogenemia
- Waldenström's macroglobulinemia

NONTRAUMATIC ("spontaneous")

Secondary to VARIOUS CAUSES
- Brainstem hemorrhage secondary to herniation
- Hemorrhage within a tumor
- Hemorrhagic infarcts
- Other causes

Figure 86. *Diagram of the chief causes of cerebral and/or meningeal hemorrhage.*

HEMORRHAGES. Approximately 80 per cent of hypertensive cerebral hemorrhages are situated in the cerebral hemispheres. Among these, most (about 80 per cent) are found in the basal ganglia. The others (about 20 per cent) are distributed throughout the white matter of the various cerebral lobes (intralobar hemorrhages).

Basal ganglia hemorrhages (Fig. 87). *Lateral* hemorrhages are the most frequent in this group: they involve the putamen and the external capsule (capsulolenticular hemorrhages). They may extend:

Superiorly and medially into the internal capsule and the lateral ventricle;

Inferiorly into the digital white matter of the superior temporal gyrus;

Medially, posteriorly, and inferiorly into the thalamus, the third ventricle, and the midbrain.

Medial hemorrhages, i.e., those situated in the thalamus, are rarer.

The preceding distinction between lateral and medial basal ganglia hemorrhages is, ad-

mittedly, somewhat arbitrary, since intermediary sites exist as well as massive lesions that may involve the entire region and then extend from the insula (island of Reil) laterally to the third ventricle medially.

Cerebral white matter hemorrhages (Fig. 88). Such a hemorrhage, of variable extent, may be situated in the frontal, temporal, parietal, or occipital lobe (intralobar hemorrhage) or in the white matter near the trigone of the lateral ventricle. Since the basal ganglia usually escape, the prognosis of such a hemorrhage is generally more favorable.

The brains of hypertensive patients frequently exhibit small, orange-yellow, cat-scratch–like slits, most often at the junction between cortex and white matter (Fig. 89), especially in the temporo-occipital lobes ("slit hemorrhages"). These represent the scars of old circumscribed hemorrhages.

2. INTRACEREBELLAR HEMORRHAGES (Fig. 90). Approximately 10 per cent of hyper-

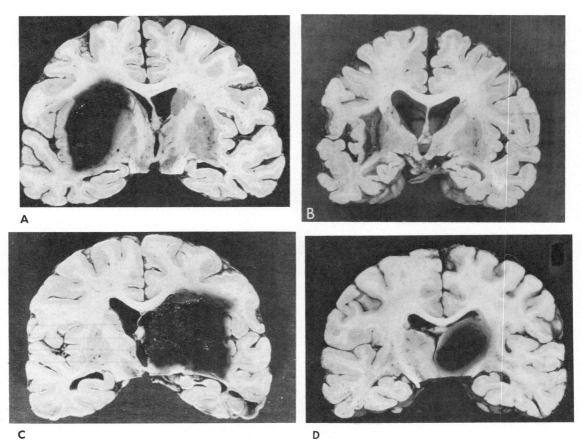

A

B

C

D

Figure 87.   *Basal ganglia hemorrhages.*

A, Lateral capsulolenticular hemorrhage.

B, Cystic scar of an old capsulolenticular hemorrhage.

C, Massive quadrilateral hemorrhage. Note scar from a hemorrhage in the ipsilateral inferior temporal gyrus.

D, Medial (thalamic) hemorrhage.

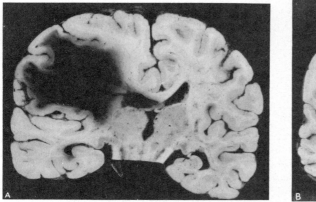

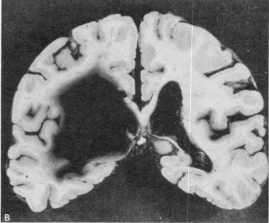

Figure 88.   *White matter hemorrhages.*

A, Left parietal hemorrhage. *B*, Hemorrhage involving the trigone of the lateral ventricle.

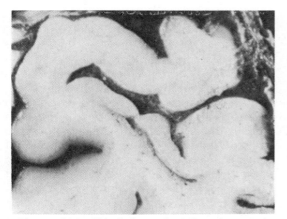

Figure 89. *Old slit-hemorrhage in a hypertensive subject.*

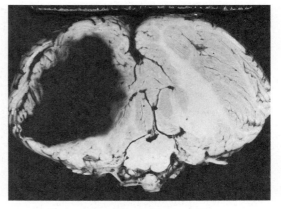

Figure 90. *Cerebellar hematoma.*

tensive cerebral hemorrhages occur in the cerebellum, most often in the central hemispheric white matter. Such a "cerebellar hematoma" behaves as a space-expanding mass in the posterior fossa, with the likely risk of herniation and medullary compression. It is also apt to rupture into the fourth ventricle.

3. BRAINSTEM HEMORRHAGES (Fig. 91). Approximately 10 per cent of hypertensive cerebral hemorrhages are situated in the brainstem, most often in the pontine tegmentum.

c. Mechanism. Hypertensive hemorrhages are due to the rupture of small intracerebral arteries, measuring 50 to 200 μm in diameter, whose walls are the seat of severe changes secondary to arterial hypertension. Indeed, arterial hypertension causes mechanical distention of these vessels, resulting in the formation of *microaneurysms* (Fig.

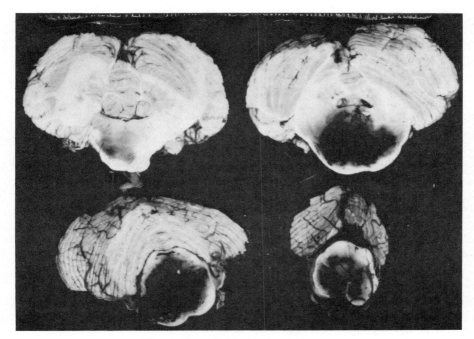

Figure 91. *Brainstem hemorrhages.*

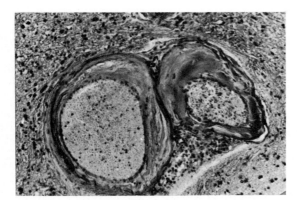

Figure 92. *Arteriolar hyalinosis in the putamen* (H. and E.).

ment of cerebral hemorrhage. This pathogenetic theory is supported by the good correlation that exists between the sites of predilection of arteriolar lesions and microaneurysms in hypertensive cerebral hemorrhage and the sites of election of the hemorrhages themselves.

The high frequency of microaneurysms and arteriolar lesions in the basal ganglia and, consequently, the greater frequency of hemorrhage in that region are attributed to the relatively higher arterial pressure that exists in the perforating blood vessels, which originate directly from the main trunk of the middle cerebral artery.

2. *Hemorrhage Resulting from Vascular Malformations*[1]

a. Intracranial arterial aneurysms. 1. SACCULAR ARTERIAL ANEURYSMS. Rupture from a saccular, so-called "congenital" arte-

93). First discovered by Charcot and Bouchard, these microaneurysms result in a total replacement of the normal endothelial, muscular, and elastic elements of the arteriolar wall by a thin layer of connective tissue. The destruction of the normal vessel wall architecture apparently favors its infiltration by blood plasma, with the consequent deposition of fibrin and lipid products (*arterial lipohyalinosis;* Fig. 92). This would then lead to increased fragility of the vessel wall and ultimately to its rupture and the develop-

---

[1]The term vascular "malformation" is sanctioned by usage. In the present context, however, it is not always appropriate, since vascular lesions of very different etiologies are included in this chapter and congenital malformative factors may constitute only one element, inconstant at that, in the genesis of these lesions.

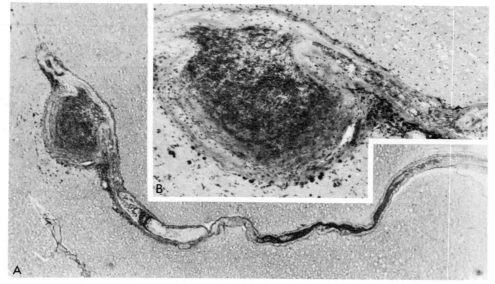

Figure 93. *Miliary aneurysm (Charcot and Bouchard) on a pontine arteriole.*

A, Low magnification. *B,* High magnification. Note alteration of arteriolar wall and the presence of peripheral iron blood pigment.

rial aneurysm is the main cause of nontraumatic *subarachnoid meningeal hemorrhage.*

The primary lesions consists in a localized saccular arterial dilatation. The aneurysmal sac is usually linked to the artery by a narrow segment, or neck. The wall of the sac is formed by fibrous connective tissue that is often extremely thin; the normal muscular and elastic elements of the arterial wall are entirely lacking.

The *pathogenesis* of these lesions is debated at this time. While the primary existence of congenital structural factors in the vessel wall, e.g., medial defects, must still be taken into account, greater stress is now being placed on the role of secondarily acquired factors, especially atherosclerosis, arterial hypertension, and hemodynamic disturbances attributable, among others, to the anatomy of the circle of Willis.

Their localization is characteristic (Figs. 94 and 95). They are situated chiefly on the vessels that form the circle of Willis, at the sites of arterial forking. Ten per cent of all aneurysms are found in the vertebrobasilar territory, especially at the termination of the basilar artery, and 90 per cent are situated in the carotid territory. The latter aneurysms show *three main sites of predilection,* for which the frequency differs according to various authors:

The termination of the internal carotid artery.[1] These aneurysms are often large and may compress the neighboring neural structures, such as the third cranial nerve. They may be situated either (1) in the angle formed by the internal carotid artery with the posterior communicating artery (*so-called posterior communicating aneurysms*) or (2) at the site of forking of the internal carotid artery into the anterior and middle cerebral arteries (*aneurysms of the carotid bifurcation*).

The anterior communicating artery and the adjacent segments of the anterior cerebral arteries.

The middle cerebral artery, approximately 2 to 3 cm from its origin, at the site of origin of its first main branches.

In about 10 to 20 per cent of cases, *multiple* aneurysms (seldom more than three) may be found: they are often bilateral and symmetrical.

Their evolution is determined by the risk of *rupture.* Because of their situation, rupture results in direct bleeding into the leptomeningeal compartment. Such a meningeal hemorrhage rapidly spreads to the entire subarachnoid space and will produce local changes in the underlying cortex as well as focal irritation of the cranial nerves and arteries situated in that space; arterial spasm may occur. A very extensive subarachnoid hemorrhage may result in rapidly increased intracranial pressure.

Most often, the hemorrhage undergoes *resorption*[1] within approximately three weeks. This takes place by way of the arachnoidal villi after the polymorphonuclear leukocytes and macrophages have begun their scavenging operations and become filled with hemosiderin. However, a very serious risk of *recurrent hemorrhage* exists between 10 and 15 days after the original bleeding.

This relapsing tendency accounts for the formation of loculations that may impede the circulation of cerebrospinal fluid and, particularly, limit the extension of the bleeding at the time of its recurrence, therefore resulting in a true *subarachnoid hematoma* that is apt to rupture into the adjacent cerebral parenchyma (meningocerebral hemorrhage). The localization and the extension of these subarachnoid hematomas, and the *intracere-*

---

[1]So-called "vestigial" aneurysms, which form finger-like extensions, may also be found at the termination of the internal carotid artery; they represent embryonal vascular remnants (Fig. 94*A*).

---

[1]An exceptional sequel of subarachnoid bleeding is characterized by the picture of subpial cerebral siderosis. This consists in iron pigment infiltration of the underlying neural tissue, along the vascular tree, and in necrosis of the crests of the cerebellar folia. These lesions are apparently determined by repeated episodes of insidious, smouldering subarachnoid hemorrhage.

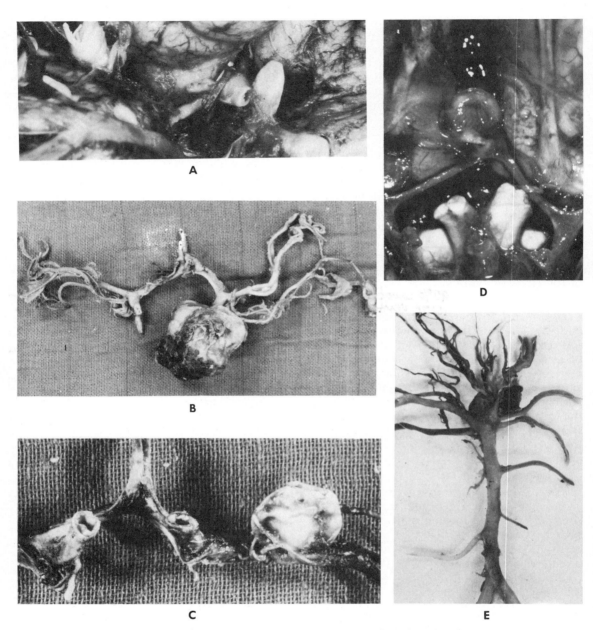

Figure 94.   *Main types of so-called "congenital" intracranial arterial aneurysm.*

A, Vestigial aneurysm at the termination of the internal carotid artery, obliterated by a clip.
B, Massive aneurysm at the termination of the internal carotid artery.
C, Middle cerebral artery aneurysm.
D, Aneurysm of the anterior communicating artery.
E, Aneurysm of the bifurcation of the basilar artery.

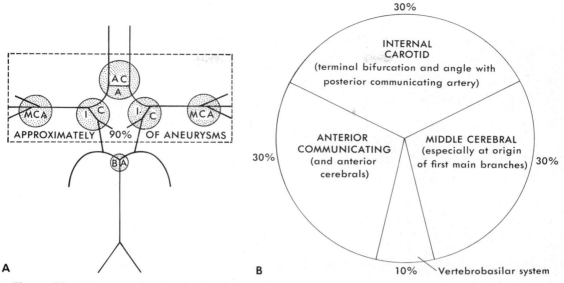

Figure 95. *Diagrams showing the distribution and frequency of arterial aneurysms.* ACA = anterior communicating artery. IC = internal carotid artery. MCA = middle cerebral artery. BA = basilar artery.

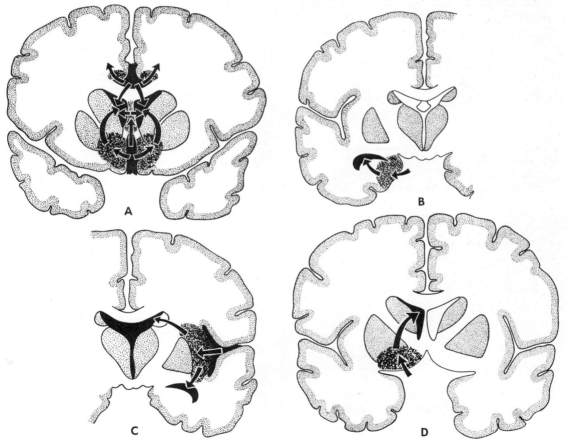

Figure 96. *Diagram showing the sites of hematomas secondary to rupture of an arterial aneurysm. A,* Aneurysm of the anterior communicating artery (and of the anterior cerebral artery). *B,* Aneurysm of the posterior communicating artery. *C,* Aneurysm of the middle cerebral artery. *D,* Aneurysm at the bifurcation of the internal carotid artery.

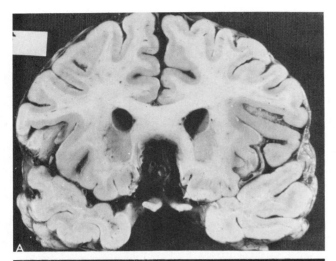

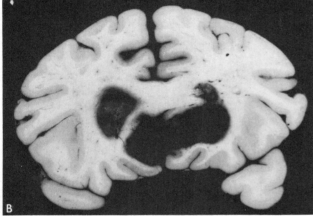

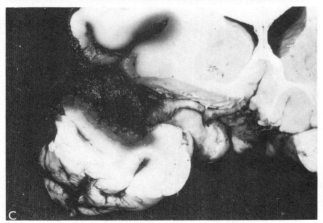

Figure 97. *Hematomas resulting from the rupture of an arterial aneurysm.*

A, Interhemispheric hematoma from rupture of an aneurysm of the anterior communicating artery.

B, Bifrontal hematoma with ventricular rupture, following rupture of an aneurysm of the anterior communicating artery.

C, Hematoma in the sylvian fissure, following rupture of an aneurysm of the middle cerebral artery.

bral hematomas that are thus produced, are determined by the site of origin of the aneurysm (Figs. 96 and 97). Such a meningocerebral hemorrhage naturally carries the risk of subsequent intraventricular rupture and/or cerebral herniation.

Although rupture is undoubtedly the main complication of intracranial aneurysms, it is not the only one (Fig. 98).

Cerebral infarcts are frequent, although their pathogenesis is uncertain. Favored theories include vascular compression resulting from a subarachnoid hematoma, thrombosis in the sac of the aneurysm and consequent embolization, and arterial spasm.

Finally, *compressive lesions* affecting structures adjacent to the aneurysmal sac — in particular, the cranial nerves — may occur, especially in relation to large aneurysms (some giant aneurysms may attain several centimeters in diameter).

2. OTHER TYPES OF INTRACRANIAL ARTERIAL ANEURYSM. These aneurysms are encountered much less frequently.

Fusiform atherosclerotic arterial aneurysms (Fig. 99) may develop to a considerable size, especially on the basilar artery. Their risk lies more in the compression of neighboring structures than in their ability to rupture.

Infectious arterial aneurysms (so-called "mycotic" aneurysms) are caused by infective lesions involving the arterial wall (Fig. 100). They may be due to *adjacent infection* (e.g., purulent meningitis, rarely chronic syphilitic meningitis) or to an *infected arterial embolus*, which most frequently occurs in subacute bacterial endocarditis. In the latter case the aneurysms, which are often multiple, are usually situated in the small corticomeningeal branches of the middle cerebral arteries, and their rupture may result in subarachnoid or meningocerebral hemorrhage.

Post-traumatic intracranial arterial aneurysms are rare.

b. Arteriovenous malformations (AVM), or angiomas (Fig. 101). These malformations consist of vascular clusters *that form direct arteriovenous shunts* without any intermediary capillary network. The arterial ped-

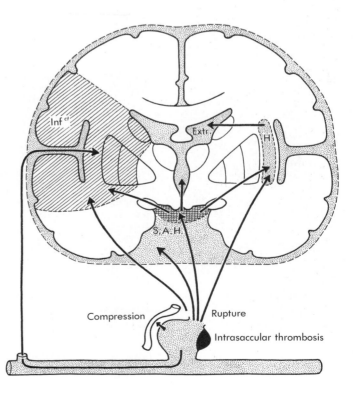

Figure 98. *Diagrammatic representation of the chief complications resulting from arterial intracranial aneurym. Inf^{ct}*, infarction; *Extr.*, ventricular extravasation; *H*, intracerebral hematoma; *S.A.H.*, subarachnoid hematoma.

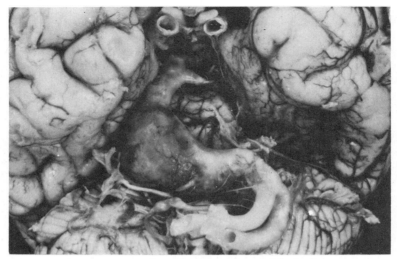

Figure 99. *Giant atherosclerotic aneurysm of the basilar artery.*

icles that feed the malformation are dilated and sinuous, and its draining veins are likewise tortuous and dilated, sometimes to a monstrous degree. The blood vessels which make up the malformation are highly variable in number, length, and caliber; their histological appearances are intermedi-

ary between those of arteries and veins, and they often exhibit secondary changes such as thrombosis, sclerohyalinosis, calcification, and even bone formation. Amidst the malformed vascular channels, interstitial tissue (which, according to the site of the AVM, may be either central nervous system

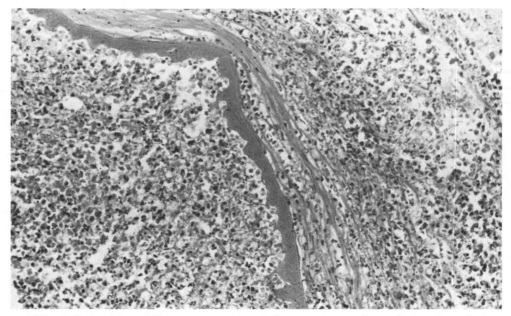

Figure 100. *Infective ("mycotic") aneurysm,* microscopic appearance. Note destruction of the arterial wall and the infiltration by altered polymorphonuclear leukocytes.

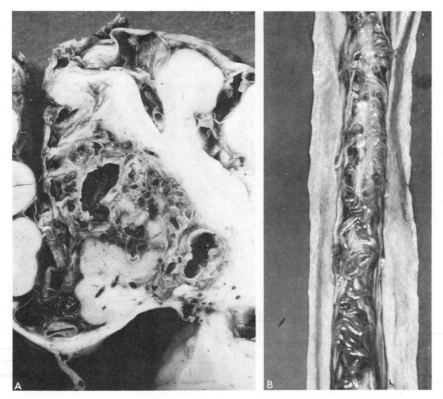

Figure 101. *Arteriovenous malformations. A,* Cerebral (medial frontal). *B,* Spinal medullary.

parenchyma or leptomeninges) is always present. This tissue is often the seat of ischemic changes and reactive gliosis.

Approximately 90 per cent of arteriovenous malformations are situated in the cerebral hemispheres (Fig. 101*A*), most often on the hemispheric surface (frontal, parietal, or temporal lobes especially), less often in their depths. The remaining 10 per cent are distributed in the brainstem, cerebellum, and spinal cord.

Rupture is the chief complication. Superficial AVM's largely give rise to subarachnoid hemorrhage, whereas deep AVM's may cause intracerebral hemorrhage, which may result in a cerebromeningeal hemorrhage consequent to intraventricular rupture.

Vascular malformations situated in the spinal cord (Fig. 101*B*) result in hematomyelia and/or spinal subarachnoid hemorrhage; also, they are apparently responsible for the condition of "subacute necrotic myelitis" of Foix and Alajouanine (Fig. 102*A*), which is characterized by progressive secondary necrotic lesions in the lower spinal cord.

Finally, two special forms of AVM occur:

Caroticocavernous fistulae, which may or may not be of traumatic origin;

Aneurysms, or "*varices,*" of the vein of Galen (Fig. 103), which are in fact arteriovenous aneurysms that drain into the vein of Galen, which undergoes extreme dilatation as a result.

c. Telangiectases and cavernous angiomas. These small vascular malformations may be encountered either in isolation or in association with each other. Although they often are incidental neuropathological findings, they may also be at the origin of cerebral and/or subarachnoid hemorrhage, but their demonstration amidst the vascular extravasation is often very difficult.

Capillary telangiectases are formed by collections of dilated capillary blood vessels that are separated from each other by nervous

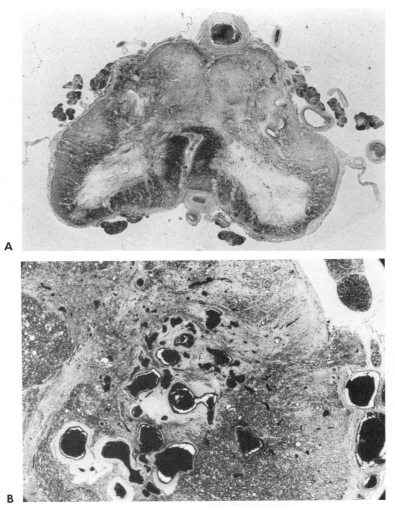

Figure 102. *Spinal medullary arteriovenous malformation.*

A, Low-power view. Subacute necrotic myelitis of Foix and Alajouanine. (First published case. Lumbosacral cord. Weigert myelin stain. Courtesy of, and legend endorsed by, Prof. Alajouanine.) Arteriovenous malformation composed of numerous large perimedullary vessels showing thickened altered walls, and of intramedullary vascular lumens; necrosis chiefly affecting anterior horns, suggesting the presence of arteriovenous shunting. Secondary ascending degeneration of posterior columns.

B, Microscopic appearance of intramedullary abnormalities in case illustrated in Figure 101B.

tissue parenchyma. They may be situated in the cerebral hemispheres, the cerebellum, or the spinal cord, but they tend to predominate in the brainstem, especially in the pons.

Cavernous angiomas (or *cavernomas*) form well-circumscribed nodules composed of wide-open vascular cavities surrounded by entirely fibrous walls. The cavities are closely packed together, without intervening nervous tissue parenchyma. These vascular lesions are often situated in the cortex of the cerebral hemispheres or cerebellum, but the basal ganglia or the brainstem may also be affected.

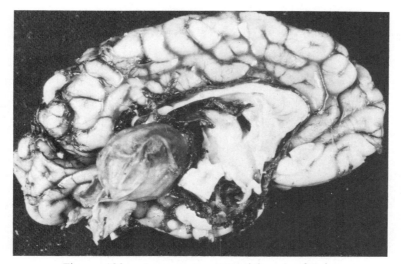

Figure 103. *Aneurysm ("varix") of the vein of Galen.*

3. *Hemorrhages due to Blood Dyscrasias*

Numerous blood diseases may cause cerebral and/or subarachnoid hemorrhage (see Fig. 86) as well as subdural or spinal (usually epidural) hematomas.

In *acute leukemia* (especially myeloblastic) (Fig. 104) and in *chronic myeloid leukemia*, about 20 per cent of the cases may develop intracranial hemorrhages, which may be of variable size and are often multifocal.

Among the neurological hemorrhagic complications that may follow *anticoagulant therapy*, subdural hematomas, cerebral and/or subarachnoid hemorrhage, spinal epidural hemorrhage, and intramuscular hematomas (e.g., bleeding into the sheath of the psoas muscle with consequent compression of the femoral nerve) are especially notable.

Some of these hemorrhagic episodes may be caused by incidental trauma that has escaped clinical notice.

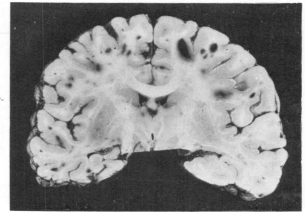

Figure 104. *Cerebral hemorrhages in acute leukemia.*

II. ISCHEMIC VASCULAR
PATHOLOGY OF ARTERIAL ORIGIN:
INFARCTIONS

The terms *cerebral infarct,* cerebral softening, and encephalomalacia are used to denote an area of tissue necrosis localized to a particular territory of vascular supply and secondary to occlusion, at a variable level, of the feeding arterial tree.

A. GENERAL FEATURES

Arterial occlusion of sufficient duration produces ischemic necrosis, in which the gross and microscopic appearances undergo a series of sequential changes that are identical regardless of the distribution of the affected territory.

Two main types of infarction are generally recognized[1]:

Anemic, or pale, infarcts, in which the lesions of ischemic necrosis remain relatively unaltered;

Hemorrhagic infarcts, in which the lesions are associated with hemorrhagic phenomena that selectively involve the cortical ribbon and the basal ganglia implicated in the ischemic process.

1. Anemic Infarction
(Fig. 105)

a. In the initial phase the lesions are difficult to delimit.

During the first six hours no visible alteration can be demonstrated, although the neural tissue is already irreparably damaged.

8-48°

From 8 to 48 hours, the damaged zone becomes pale, and the demarcation between the white and gray matter becomes indistinct. Edematous swelling is apparent and is sometimes accompanied by a certain degree of vascular congestion which is more marked in the cortex. At this stage, the softer consistency of the involved area is the only feature that permits the infarct to be recognized after proper formalin fixation.

Microscopically (Fig. 107), the neurons within the infarcted territory demonstrate the features of ischemic cell change, as described in Chapter 1 (see Fig. 1). These alterations are evident after six hours, while the glial cells undergo comparable changes.

In the cortex and white matter, the capillary blood vessels show endothelial swelling accompanied by exudation of edematous fluid and by extravasation of red blood cells, even in anemic infarction. From eight hours onward the myelin structures lose their usual tinctorial affinity (Fig. 118*A*).

Phagocytic activity rapidly makes its ap-

---

[1]Traditionally, a third type of infarct—the "*edematous infarct*" (Fig. 105)—is also described. Admittedly, all forms of infarction are associated with edematous lesions in their early stage of development. These lesions are naturally of the greatest importance in massive infarction in view of the extent of the ischemic territory, and will cause increased intracranial pressure with consequent cerebral herniation. The term *massive infarct* is therefore preferable to "edematous infarct."

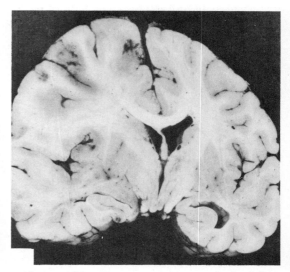

Figure 105. *Recent massive cerebral infarct.* Gross appearance.

pearance. Between 24 and 48 hours this is evidenced by an exudation of <u>neutrophil</u> leukocytes which is often very severe and may even simulate an inflammatory process (Fig. 107*B*).

>48° macrophage

b. During the first few days *2-10 d* the phago-cytic process will increase while the edematous reaction remains.

From 2 to 10 days, the swelling and water-logging persist, but to a decreasing extent, while the softened tissue becomes more <u>fria</u>-ble and the boundaries of the infarcted terri-tory become better defined.

After 48 hours the leukocytic infiltration is rapidly replaced by foamy compound granu-lar corpuscles, or <u>macrophages</u> (Fig. 107*C*). These cells, which are laden with sudanophi-lic breakdown products originating from myelin disintegration, group themselves around the swollen walls of the capillary blood vessels, which increase in number. The macrophage proliferation becomes con-siderably more marked after <u>five</u> days.

c. After 10 days *>10 d* <u>liquefaction</u> begins, and from the third week onward the process of <u>cavitation</u> becomes more evident. From then on, the area of necrosis is replaced by yel-lowish-gray tissue, which causes depression of the cortical surface. The macrophage pro-liferation becomes more marked in this zone and persists, although to a decreasing de-gree, during the subsequent months (Fig. 107*D*).

d. After a few months a <u>cystic cavity</u> is organized in the softened area. This cavity has ragged outlines, is intersected by vascu-lar connective tissue strands, and is covered on its outer border by a thin meningeal membrane which is visible on the cortical surface (Fig. 106).

During the phase of cicatrization, the residual cystic cavity becomes surrounded by a glial proliferation which is at first protoplasmic, then fibrillary, while a few foamy compound granular corpuscles remain demonstrable along the numerous vascular connective tis-sue strands that run across the cavity (Fig. 107*E*).

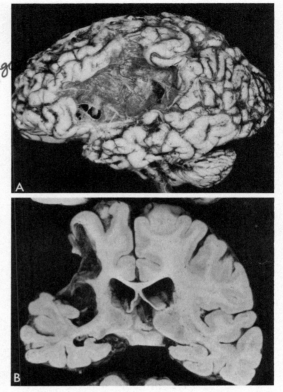

Figure 106. *Old cystic infarct in the territory of the middle cerebral artery.*

A, Left lateral aspect. *B,* Coronal section; note the involvement of a large part of the superficial territory of the middle cerebral artery, sparing, however, the temporal lobe.

2. *Hemorrhagic Infarction*
(Fig. 108)

This type of infarction is classically regarded as distinct from anemic infarction, although microscopic hemorrhagic extrava-sations are frequently found in the latter. On the contrary, it has frankly hemorrhagic fea-tures, which consist of petechial zones that are sometimes confluent and are situated in the cortex. These <u>hemorrhagic areas</u> may in-volve the entire zone of infarction, but tend most often to predominate along <u>boundary</u> zones supplied by meningeal arterial anas-tomoses or, in the case of middle cerebral in-farcts, in the <u>basal ganglia.</u>

The role of venous stasis has been can-vassed in determining the character of these

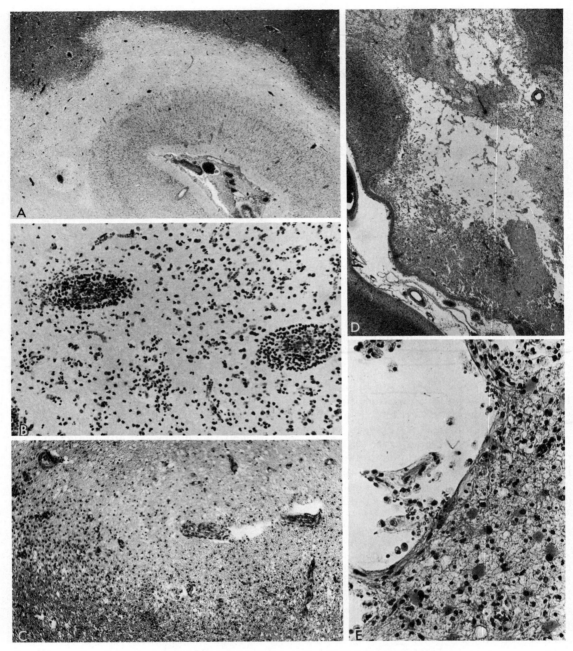

Figure 107. *Microscopic features of cerebral infarcts* (H. and E.).

A, 36-hour-old infarct; cortical and subcortical myelin pallor, with edematous border.

B, Diffusely scattered and perivascular groups of polymorphonuclear leukocytes after 36 hours.

C, On the fifth day the periphery of the infarct is invaded by compound granular corpuscles, and there is capillary proliferation.

D, Old infarct in the third month; note the sparing of the superficial layer, and the cortical and subcortical disintegration with preservation of the vascular and connective tissue network.

E, Astrocytic gliosis (gemistocytic astrocytes) around an infarct of several months' duration; note the presence of a few residual compound granular corpuscles.

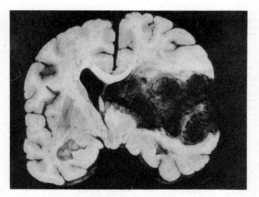

Figure 108. *Hemorrhagic infarct.*

hemorrhagic infarcts, but this mechanism seems negligible when compared with the secondary cortical reirrigation which takes place in capillary blood vessels that have been damaged by the initial anoxia and, especially, when compared with the sudden irruption of blood after lysis or secondary mobilization of the thrombus (Fig. 110*f*) This type of infarction is found particularly to accompany cerebral emboli.

B. PATHOPHYSIOLOGY AND ETIOLOGY (Fig. 109)

Cerebral infarction caused by prolonged ischemia localized to a particular vascular territory is always secondary to arterial occlusion. The latter may be due to:

Thrombosis, most often supervening on atherosclerotic lesions;

An *embolus,* in most cases of cardiac origin.

However, in a fairly large number of cerebral infarcts, careful examination of the arterial tree fails to disclose any definite occlusion. The pathogenesis of these cases has been envisaged in the following manner:

Present-day opinion tends to exclude arterial spasm as an etiological factor;

The factor of a hypotensive episode could be invoked, but only if it was severe or prolonged, or if it supervened in a case with severe, extensive, or multiple atheromatous stenosis of the arteries;

Most authors interpret these infarcts in which arterial occlusion cannot be demonstrated on the basis of emboli that have undergone secondary lysis.

The appearance and extent of the cerebral lesions depend on a number of hemodynamic and etiological factors (Figs. 109 and 110).

I. HEMODYNAMIC FACTORS

a. Presence and efficacy of anastomotic substitution pathways of vascular supply. In the course of arterial occlusion the ische-

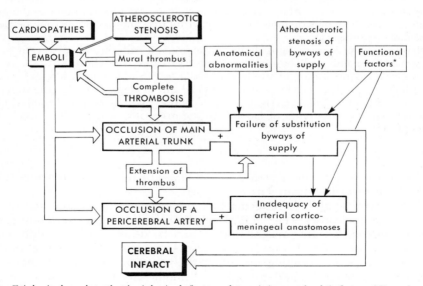

Figure 109. *Etiological and pathophysiological factors determining crebral infarcts. *Functional factors:* decrease in caliber of ischemic arteries; drop in blood pressure; loss of autoregulation of arterial caliber.

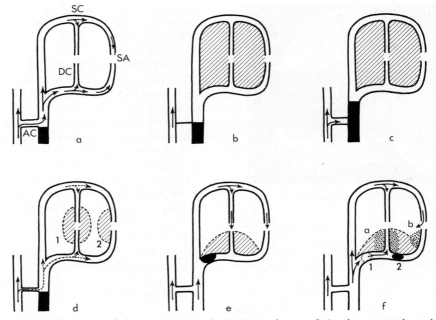

Figure 110. *Respective roles of the anastomotic substitution pathways of circulatory supply and of the type of vascular occlusion in determining the occurrence and extent of cerebral lesions (AC, anastomotic vascular network; SC, superficial arterial circulation; DC, deep vascular territory; SA, superficial meningeal anastomoses).*

a, Arterial occlusion, but with effective and adequate anastomotic substitution network of supply: no infarction.

b, Arterial occlusion without anatomically effective anastomotic network of supply (*AC*): massive infarction of the corresponding cerebral territory.

c, Arterial occlusion extending beyond the origin of the anastomotic network of supply. No anastomotic substitution byway of vascular supply: massive infarction.

d, Occlusion proximal to the anastomotic network of supply. Insufficient anastomotic substitution byway of arterial supply. Anemic infarct of variable extent in territory (2) distal to the junction of two vascular territories (last field of irrigation or watershed infarct) and in border zone between superficial and deep vascular territories (1).

e, Proximal occlusion of one dividing branch; anastomotic substitution byway of vascular supply provided by superficial meningeal anastomoses: limited proximal infarction.

f, Embolic occlusion. Mobilization of thrombus from 1 to 2. Sudden occlusion in 1, resulting in total ischemia of both deep and superficial vascular territories and in hemorrhages in the superficial territory when border zones are undergoing reirrigation (*b*); secondary mobilization of thrombus in 2, with hemorrhages due to secondary irruption of blood into the originally ischemic deep vascular territory (*a*) (hemorrhagic infarct).

mic cerebral territory is partially reirrigated by arteries at the base of the brain (circle of Willis, ophthalmic artery) and by superficial corticomeningeal anastomoses (Fig. 110*a*). This potential reirrigation by anastomotic substitution byways of arterial supply explains why in most cases the resulting area of cerebral softening remains limited to only part of the vascular territory that is normally served by the occluded artery (Fig. 110*d* and *e*).

However, this anastomotic arrangement of the vascular tree varies from case to case. It may be developmentally different in various subjects, and all anatomical deviations from the norm are possible. Moreover, these anastomotic substitution byways of arterial supply may be occluded either by atherosclerotic lesions or as the result of extension from the thrombus. In these cases it is easy to see why the territory of softening may reach its maximal extent (Fig. 110b and c).

b. Site of occlusion. Proximal occlusion of a blood vessel such as the internal carotid artery may, as the result of anastomotic substitution irrigation from the contralateral arterial network of supply and from the ophthalmic artery, produce a limited lesion only. Reirrigation is in general adequate in the proximal territory, and the lesions will then predominate in the distal regions ("last fields of irrigation") or at the junction of two vascular territories ("watershed or boundary zone infarct") (Figs. 110d and 119).

Should the arterial substitution network of supply be anatomically absent or occluded as the result of extension from the thrombus, the infarct will then be massive and will involve the entire arterial territory (Fig. 110c).

In distal arterial occlusion, i.e., involving an end-artery, such as the middle cerebral artery, the only possibility of reirrigation will depend on the presence of a superficial anastomotic network. The latter is often precarious and, as a result, the infarct proximal to the superficial anastomotic network will usually be extensive (Fig. 110e).

c. Type of occlusion. In general, *thrombosis* leading to gradual occlusion will permit the adaptation of an anastomotic substitution network of supply. The resulting infarct is then usually pale and of relatively limited extent.

By contrast, *emboli* produce massive and sudden occlusion, following which reirrigation is inadequate. Hence, the resulting infarct is usually extensive. In addition, the frequency of cortical hemorrhages in the marginal territories is explained by the occurrence of reirrigation through blood vessels that were initially damaged by sudden ischemia. On the other hand, migration or secondary fragmentation of the embolus accounts for hemorrhages observed in the proximal part of the ischemic territory in the course of sudden reentry of arterial blood (e.g., deep territory of the middle cerebral artery and territory of the superior temporal

artery in the course of embolization in the middle cerebral artery) (Fig. 110f).

II. ETIOLOGICAL FACTORS

1. Atherosclerosis

a. General features. Atherosclerosis is the chief etiological factor in the production of cerebral infarction. The structural features and general course of atherosclerosis in the brain are comparable to those of atherosclerosis in other organs.

In the brain, atherosclerosis affects chiefly

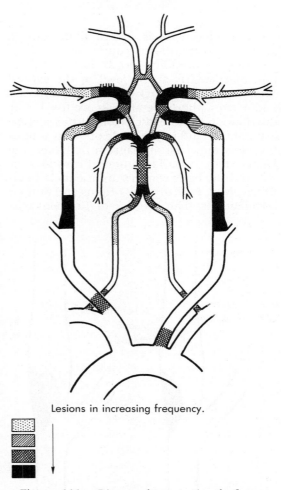

Lesions in increasing frequency.

Figure 111. *Diagram demonstrating the frequency and severity of atherosclerotic lesions in the arterial cervicocerebral tree.*

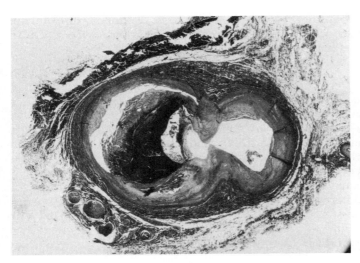

Figure 112. *Carotid bifurcation, transverse section* (H. and E.). Stenosing atherosclerotic lesions of the external carotid (right) and of the internal carotid (left). Voluminous mural thrombus in the internal carotid artery.

the large blood vessels, first of all the carotid arteries in their cervical course and the basilar artery. It predominates at sites of bifurcation (particularly at the level of the carotid sinus), at sites of curvature of the arteries, and in sites where the arteries are fixed. The distribution of atherosclerosis in the cervical arterial tree and in the circle of Willis is illustrated in the classical diagram by Baker and Fisher (Fig. 111). The internal carotid arteries and the basilar artery are the most heavily involved, both at their origins and at their terminations. The arteries of the convexity

are less severely affected than the vessels of the base, and they are only exceptionally involved in isolation.

Increase in size of the plaque and local changes—intramural hemorrhage, calcification, mural thrombosis—lead to increasing arterial stenosis (Fig. 112). It is generally believed that the latter must involve more than 75 per cent of the original lumen of the artery in order to cause a significant decrease of blood flow.

The course of arterial stenosis is variable (Fig. 113). The main danger lies in the de-

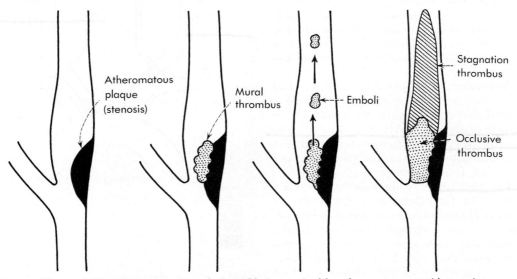

Figure 113. *Diagrammatic evolution of lesions caused by atheromatous carotid stenosis.*

velopment of arterial thrombosis secondary to local changes whose precise mechanism is still unclear. Thrombosis may occlude the arterial lumen completely and, as a result, a new event may take place, namely anterograde extension of a so-called "stagnation thrombus," usually up to the first sizable collateral branch. The thrombus is ultimately replaced by loose-textured connective tissue in which new vessels of variable permeability are often seen.

It seems equally possible that the mural thrombus, in many cases, can fragment and in doing so may give rise to arterial emboli. These emboli have been held to account for a number of cerebrovascular accidents from which recovery may to some extent be possible when ischemia is of short duration or which may be permanent when disintegration of the thrombus has not been sufficiently rapid. Finally, incorporation of the thrombus within the vessel wall has also been invoked to account for certain instances of underlying arterial stenosis.

b. Special features. ATHEROSCLEROTIC THROMBOSIS. *1. Internal carotid thrombosis* tends to supervene on stenosing atheromatous lesions. These lesions are most often observed at the carotid bifurcation or at the level of the carotid sinus (see Fig. 112). A stagnation thrombus (see Fig. 113) is formed and usually extends rostrally to the ostium of the first collateral branch, namely the ophthalmic artery, which later ensures, through the external carotid artery, a more or less adequate reirrigation of the proximal hemispheric territory. The zone of infarction is then limited to the distal portion of the middle cerebral territory and, to an incidental extent, of the anterior cerebral territory. Anterograde extension of the thrombus beyond the ophthalmic artery, as well as beyond the origin of the posterior communicating and the anterior cerebral arteries, will then cause massive infarction.

Less often, thrombosis takes place at the level of the carotid syphon, i.e., at the termination of the internal carotid artery. Occlusion, which supervenes upon atheromatous lesions in this terminal portion of the artery, is usually accompanied by retrograde extension of the thrombus into the carotid sinus.

It may be difficult in an old, organized lesion to decide whether thrombosis of the carotid artery originally took place at its distal or at its proximal end.

2. Isolated middle or anterior cerebral thrombosis is much less common than internal carotid thrombosis. It usually follows extension of a carotid thrombus beyond the termination of the internal carotid artery.

3. Vertebral artery thrombosis may be clinically and/or pathologically silent, or it may cause discrete lesions, provided the thrombosis does not reach the ostium of the posterior inferior cerebellar artery and provided it is unilateral.

4. Basilar artery thrombosis supervenes on atherosclerotic lesions, which are frequently present at that site. It may also result from ascending extension of a vertebral artery thrombosis. It may cause infarcts in the cerebral peduncles or in the pons.

5. Thrombosis of the posterior cerebral artery is seldom an isolated event. It usually occurs as the result of anterograde extension of thrombosis in the basilar artery. When the posterior cerebral artery is a tributary of the internal carotid artery, its occlusion may be secondary to extension from carotid thrombosis. As a result, the lesions frequently form part of the picture of massive hemispheric infarction.

6. Subclavian artery thrombosis may result in ischemic lesions in the vertebrobasilar territory following diversion of the arterial flow (so-called "subclavian steal syndrome").

EMBOLI OF ATHEROSCLEROTIC ORIGIN. According to current statistics, these emboli apparently play a very important role in the development of cerebral infarcts.

1. Platelet emboli. These emboli are of small size, having been detached from a white thrombus, and may cause transient cerebral accidents or occlude terminal arterial branches.

2. Fibrin emboli. Fibrin emboli originate

from a mural thrombus or from fragmentation of a stagnation thrombus. They often produce occlusion in the branches of larger arteries (middle, anterior, or posterior cerebral), secondary to carotid or vertebrobasilar thrombosis.

3. Purely atherosclerotic emboli. These emboli, which are seen less frequently, either may be detached spontaneously from ulcerated plaques or may be the result of arteriographic puncture.

2. Cardiac Emboli[1]
(Fig. 114)

Cardiac emboli are an extremely frequent cause of arterial occlusion, whether they originate from an atrial thrombus in mitral stenosis, from a mural thrombus in the course of a myocardial infarction or various forms of endocarditis (e.g., bacterial endocarditis, nonbacterial thrombotic endocarditis of malignant disease), or from a cardiac prosthesis, etc.

---

[1]Emboli of other than cardiac origin are less frequent; they may originate from a thrombus in the pulmonary veins in certain chronic lung diseases, or they may be fat emboli.

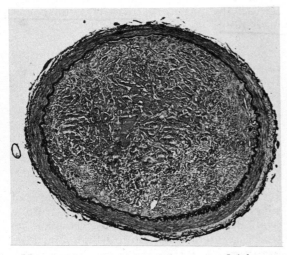

Figure 114. *Arterial embolus* (superficial temporal artery). Note the normal appearance of the arterial wall (H. and E.).

3. Other Causes

syphilis
tuberculusm
parasitm
polyant. n-
om (child)

a. Arteritis. Arteritis is a rare cause of cerebral infarction. Syphilitic arteritis, which affects especially the basal arteries, is seen only exceptionally today. Tuberculous meningitis and meningitides caused by parasitic organisms can produce occlusive arteritic lesions which may account for cerebral and spinal infarcts.

Collagen diseases, especially polyarteritis nodosa, may sometimes affect a few small superficial arterioles and, more exceptionally, the deep intracerebral or spinal intramedullary vessels; parenchymatous lesions thus produced consist of limited and more or less disseminated foci of softening.

In children, otitis media and rhinopharyngitis can occasionally be the cause of internal carotid occlusion, which may result in cerebral infarction.

b. Trauma. *Injuries* to the neck or in the mouth may occasionally give rise to internal carotid occlusion.

c. Vascular malformations. Finally, among the *vascular malformations,* arterial aneurysms may sometimes be associated with cerebral infarcts, but it is rarely possible to demonstrate that intrasaccular thrombosis is the cause.

C. TOPOGRAPHY

Regardless of the particular cerebral or spinal territory that may be involved by an infarct, the extent of the infarct will follow the general rules outlined above. Within the limitations already expressed, its localization will correspond to a greater or lesser portion of the relevant vascular territory.

I. CEREBRAL INFARCTS

Cerebral infarcts can be explained fully only after complete anatomical study of both vascular carotid axes and of the vertebrobasilar system, from the aortic arch up to their

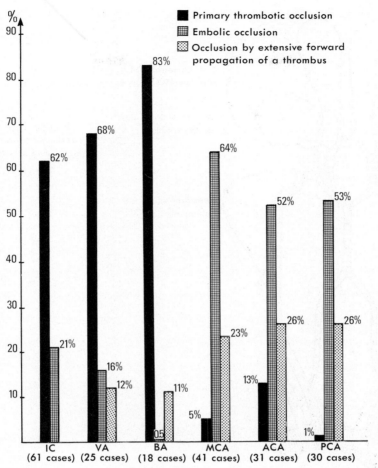

Figure 115. *Diagram showing the respective frequencies of the chief causes of cervicocerebral arterial occlusion.* IC = internal carotid artery. VA = vertebral artery. BA = basilar artery. MCA = middle cerebral artery. ACA = anterior cerebral artery. PCA = posterior cerebral artery. (Statistics from the Charles-Foix Laboratory of Neuropathology, Hôpital de La Salpêtrière, Paris.)

cerebral branches (Fig. 116).[1] The study must be completed by a meticulous examination of the heart cavities, heart valves, and myocardium.

1. Infarcts of the Carotid Territory

Infarction may involve either the whole or only part of each of the territories of the

---

[1]Only the removal *en bloc* of the cervical vertebral column and of the base of the skull at the time of autopsy will permit rigorous study of the cervicoencephalic vascular supply. This study must be done on sequential sections after decalcification.

branches of the internal carotid artery (Fig. 117).

A single infarct may be found, but it is important to emphasize the frequency of multiple infarcts. These may be of variable extent, either concomitant or consecutive. This qualification applies equally well to infarcts resulting from internal carotid thrombosis and those secondary to cardiac emboli.

a. Infarct of the anterior cerebral artery territory (Fig. 118E). This area consists of the superior frontal gyrus, inferior and medial surfaces of the frontal lobe back to

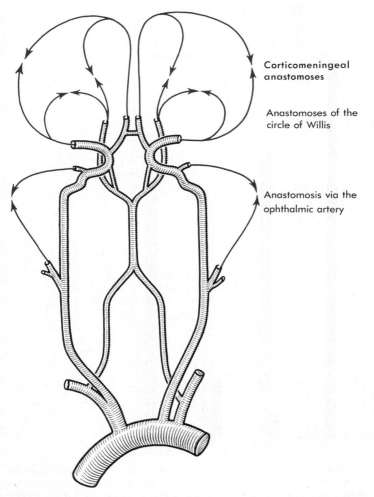

Corticomeningeal
anastomoses

Anastomoses of the
circle of Willis

Anastomosis via the
ophthalmic artery

Figure 116. *Diagram of the caroticovertebral vascular tree and of its chief anastomotic pathways.*

the level of the precuneus, corpus callosum, and anterior portion of the basal ganglia supplied by the recurrent artery of Heubner. Because of the potential substitution byways of supply provided by the contralateral artery and by the anterior communicating artery, infarcts of the anterior cerebral territory are less common than those of the middle cerebral territory.

ACA

The existence of anomalies in the circle of Willis, i.e., a single anterior cerebral artery, may account for bilateral infarction in some cases.

Such an infarct is rarely single and is usually found in association with an infarct of the middle cerebral territory as a result of internal carotid thrombosis.

b. Infarct of the middle cerebral artery territory. This area includes the lateral surface of the frontal and parietal lobes, insula, superior and middle temporal gyri, and deep striatal territory.

Occlusion of the proximal part of the middle cerebral artery results in total middle cerebral infarction (Fig. 118C), since the superficial collateral circulation is able to assume only a slight margin of arterial substitution. The occlusion is more often the result of embolization than of primary intravascular thrombosis (Fig. 115).

Isolated superficial middle cerebral infarction (Fig. 118B) results from occlusion distal to the origin of the perforating branches, whereas occlusion of the ostia of the latter by

Figure 117. *Cerebral vascular territories. a,* Outer surface; *b,* inner surface; *c,* lower surface; *d, e, f, g, h, i, j,* and *k,* coronal slices from before back.

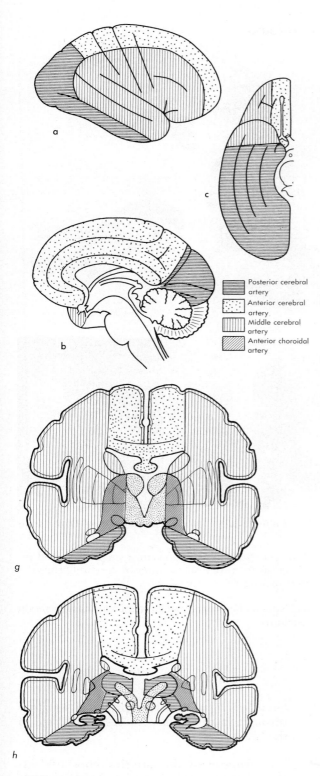

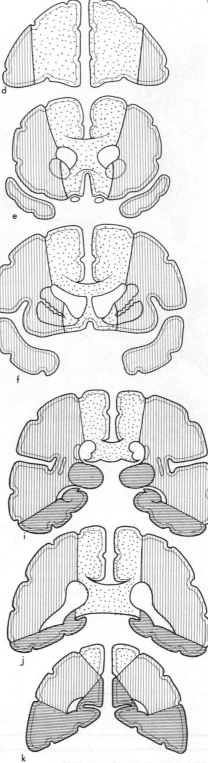

Posterior cerebral artery

Anterior cerebral artery

Middle cerebral artery

Anterior choroidal artery

g, anterior communicating artery; h, thalamic perforating arteries

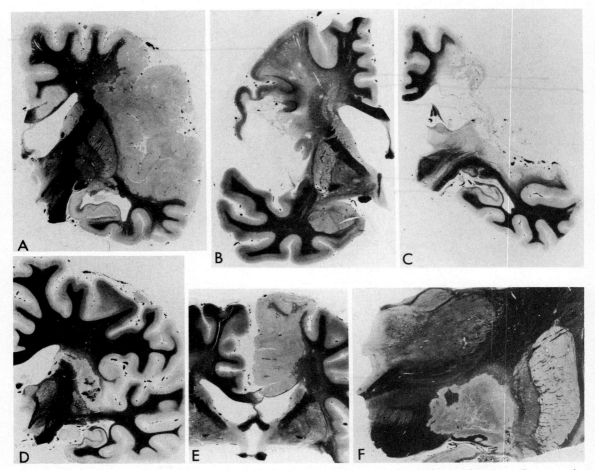

Figure 118. *Chief topographical areas of distribution of infarcts in the internal carotid territory* (Loyez stain for myelin).

A, Recent right-sided superficial middle cerebral infarct. Note the presence of a small associated infarct involving the corpus callosum and the cingulate gyrus (territory of the anterior cerebral artery).

B, Old left-sided superficial middle cerebral infarct, sparing the temporal lobe.

C, Old total right-sided middle cerebral infarct.

D, Recent deep right-sided middle cerebral infarct. Note its hemorrhagic character and its association with older, more superficial lesions (insula and claustrum).

E, Right-sided anterior cerebral infarct.

F, Right-sided anterior choroidal infarct.

atherosclerosis is responsible for isolated deep middle cerebral infarcts (Fig. 118D). Most often, infarction involves only part of the vascular territory (e.g., territory of the ascending branches). This may result from occlusion of the terminal branches, but more often results from proximal occlusion of the internal carotid artery coupled with ade-

quate reirrigation of the proximal territory through vascular anastomoses at the base of the brain.

c. Infarct of the anterior choroidal artery territory (Fig. 118F). The posterior part of the internal capsule, pallidum, and optic tract are located within this region.

Infarction of this deep area of supply, especially when recent, is often difficult to detect because of the limited extent of the territory.

Isolated infarction of this area is seldom seen. In most cases it accompanies total infarction of the middle cerebral territory and is therefore part of a massive infarct.

d. Massive hemispheric infarct. This infarct affects the entire relevant territory of vascular supply. It is produced as the result of sudden occlusion of the terminal portion of the internal carotid artery, either by an embolus or by an extension of an internal carotid thrombus beyond the terminal bifurcation of the artery, when all potential substitution byway of supply is denied. The large extent of the zone of ischemia accounts for the severity of the edematous reaction and for the risk of temporal herniation (Fig. 105).

e. Watershed or boundary zone infarcts (Fig. 119). These involve mostly the boundaries between the anterior and middle cerebral territories, especially posterior to the interparietal sulcus. Likewise, watershed

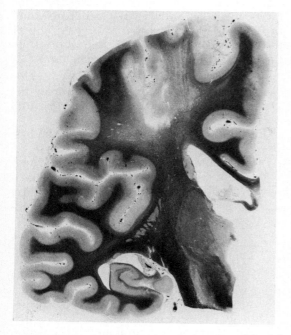

Figure 119. *Old infarct at the junction of the left anterior and middle cerebral territories.*

infarcts may occur in the center of the white matter, between the deep anterior and middle cerebral territories.

They may follow internal carotid thrombosis, particularly when thrombosis is bilateral.

2. Infarcts of the Vertebrobasilar Territory

The development of these infarcts depends on the same general pathophysiological mechanisms as those already described, to which should be added the special anatomical features of the posterior vascular arterial system and of its substitution byways of supply. Indeed the system consists of a median axis, the basilar artery, formed by the junction of two vertebral arteries originating low from the subclavian arteries and undergoing a tortuous course through the foramina transversaria, and of two terminal branches, the posterior cerebral arteries. It is important to stress the following:

The considerable anatomical variations of this vascular arrangement, especially in the size of the respective vertebral, posterior communicating, and posterior cerebral arteries, whose territories of supply may, as the result of narrowing or hypoplasia of their proximal segments, ultimately depend on one of the internal carotid arteries;

The variable extent of the numerous anastomotic communications that exist with the internal carotid arteries, through the posterior communicating arteries, with branches of the external carotid and subclavian arteries, and between the vertebral arteries themselves through the spinal perimedullary arterial network:

Finally, the lateral anastomotic rings formed by the cerebellar arteries, which complete the anatomical picture. The great variation of these arteries and their asymmetry, at least as far as the posterior cerebellar artery and its branches are concerned, should also be taken into consideration.

These special anatomical features therefore account for

The frequent bilaterality and asymmetry of the nervous tissue lesions observed;

The usually disseminated character of the lesions along the vertebrobasilar axis.

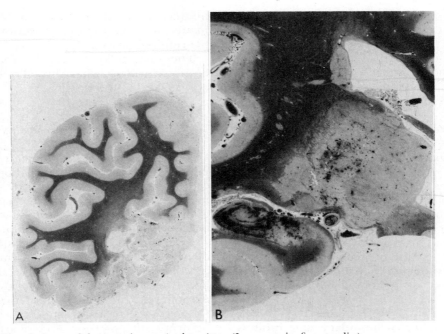

Figure 120. *Infarcts of the posterior cerebral territory* (Loyez stain for myelin).
A, Old temporo-occipital infarct. *B*, Recent infarct of the thalamogeniculate territory; note involvement of Ammon's horn.

a. Infarcts of the posterior cerebral artery territory. Infarcts of this hemispheric territory (Fig. 120) are often bilateral, producing necrosis of the inferomedial surface of the occipital lobe, of the cuneus, and especially of the calcarine cortex as well as part of Ammon's horn.

They follow occlusion of the posterior cerebral artery beyond its junction with the posterior communicating artery. Such an occlusion is generally embolic in origin; it is then most often secondary to underlying vertebrobasilar thrombosis (Fig. 115).

The most frequent infarcts of the deep territory of the posterior cerebral artery affect either the thalamogeniculate territory (Fig. 120*B*) (i.e., the ventrolateral formations of the thalamus and the pulvinar) or the thalamoperforating territory (i.e., the intralaminar formations), giving rise in the latter case to a bilateral butterfly-shaped lesion associated with a variable involvement of the mesencephalon (i.e., a tegmentothalamic infarct).

b. Infarcts of the brainstem (Fig.

121). In the vast majority of cases these infarcts are secondary to atherosclerotic thrombosis of the basilar artery. Although they often defy consistent classification, they fall roughly into the following scheme:

1. Localized lesions, corresponding to necrosis of a particular vascular territory served at each level:

Either by paramedian branches of the basilar artery, with the production of:

A midline infarct of the peduncular tegmentum with or without associated thalamic lesions (thalamoperforate infarct through involvement of the retromamillary peduncle);

A paramedian infarct of the pontine tegmentum and massive softening;

A paramedian infarct of the medulla;

Or by short circumferential branches of the basilar artery, with the production of:

An infarct of the middle cerebellar peduncle; or, especially,

An infarct of the lateral medullary region (Wallenberg syndrome).

2. Multiple and diffuse lesions. These may

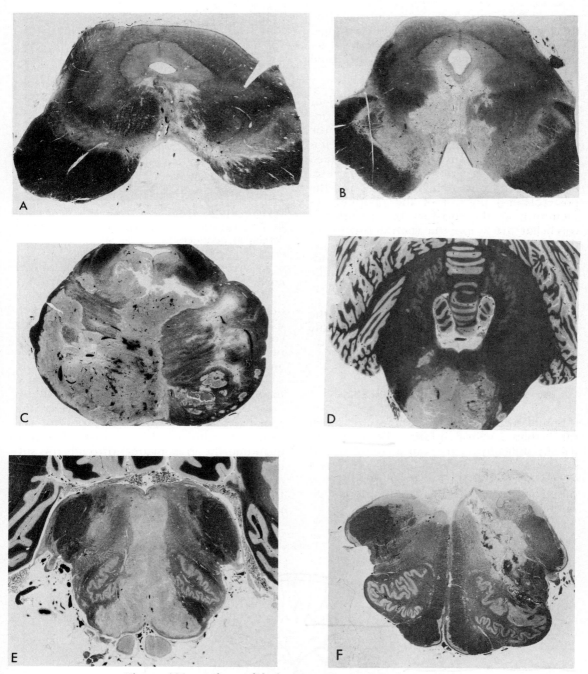

Figure 121.   *Infarcts of the brainstem* (Loyez stain for myelin).

A, Midpeduncular infarct.
B, Massive infarct of the peduncular tegmentum.
C, Massive upper pontine infarct with right-sided paramedian predominance.
D, Massive infarct of the basis pontis.
E, Central medullary infarct.
F, Lateral medullary infarct (Wallenberg syndrome).

involve all vascular territories and may furthermore consist of lesions of different age. They may also form relatively localized lesions which may extend beyond the usual topographical limits.

c. Cerebellar infarcts. In this type of circulation the lesions present as distal infarcts. These may involve the territory of the superior cerebellar artery (Fig. 122), which is usually the most constant anatomically (i.e., comprising the superior portion of the cerebellum down to the dentate nucleus and the posterolateral portion of the pontine tegmentum), or the territory of the inferior cerebellar artery on the ventral surface of the hemisphere.

Watershed infarcts situated at the boundary of these territories, i.e., in the middle zone of the cerebellum, are not uncommon. They are accounted for by the presence of cerebellar arterial rings derived from the vertebrobasilar axis and by the usually slender size of the cerebellar arteries that directly supply this area.

II. SPINAL INTRAMEDULLARY INFARCTS

Spinal intramedullary infarcts are much rarer than cerebral infarcts. Because it is usually difficult to carry out a complete and satisfactory anatomical study of the blood supply of the spinal cord, these infarcts may raise complex problems of pathophysiological interpretation.

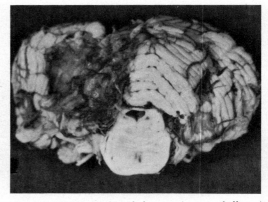

Figure 122. *Right-sided superior cerebellar infarct* (upper view). Note lesions in the superior cerebellar peduncle.

a. Arterial organization of the spinal cord. A number of distinguishing features in the arterial organization of the spinal cord determine the chief pathological varieties. The general pattern is that of a relatively constant and simple arterial intramedullary network associated with a highly variable and complex extramedullary network.

The *intramedullary network* depends on a major anterior spinal artery, which extends downward along the ventral aspect of the spinal cord and ensures the supply of the ventral two-thirds of the cord (therefore including the gray matter) through the sulcocommissural arteries; two posterior spinal arteries, which irrigate the dorsal three-fourths of the posterior columns; and a perimedullary anastomotic network, which

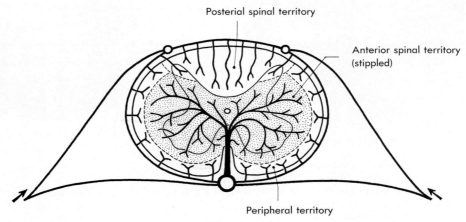

Figure 123. *Diagram of the three transverse arterial territories of the spinal cord.*

Posterial spinal territory

Anterior spinal territory (stippled)

Peripheral territory

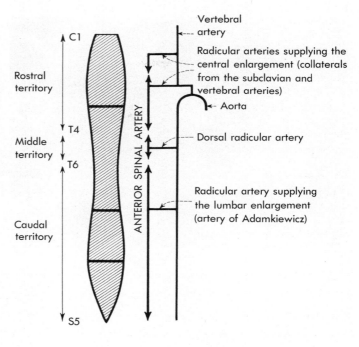

Figure 124. *Diagram of the three principal longitudinal arterial territories of the spinal cord.*

gives off a few branches to the periphery of the cord (Fig. 123).

The extramedullary network, which is highly complex and variable, depends on the presence of radicular arteries. Schematically, the following territories are recognized (Fig. 124):

A superior, or cervicothoracic, territory corresponding to the cervical and upper two or three thoracic segments and supplied by arterial twigs originating from the vertebral arteries or from branches of the subclavian arteries;

An intermediary, or middle thoracic, territory extending from T4 to T8, with a poor blood supply;

An inferior, or thoracolumbar, territory whose abundant vascularization is ensured by a single lumbar artery, i.e., the artery of the lumbar enlargement, or artery of Adamkiewicz. This artery is situated on the left and most frequently accompanies one of the lower thoracic or upper lumbar nerve roots, and is sometimes reinforced by an upper or a lower branch.

b. Topographical features. *1. Massive infarction* (Fig. 125A) usually occurs in the middle thoracic zone, which is normally poorly vascularized. It is presumably the result of sudden total ischemia, when reirrigation of the middle thoracic segments by the abundant cervical and lumbar networks is inadequate. The infarct extends over several metameric segments and is often lengthened into a distal and a caudal fusiform pencil of centromedullary softening (Fig. 125B and C) which is situated in the ventral part of the posterior columns, at the boundary between the anterior and posterior spinal territories.

2. Anterior spinal artery infarction (Fig. 126A) involves a greater or lesser portion of the anterior spinal territory and especially the ventral horns. It is the most frequent type of infarct in the spinal cord. It is found in the cervical region, and more often in the lumbar region because of the special vulnerability of this territory, which depends on a single artery without potential substitution byway of supply from an invariably slender middle thoracic arterial network.

3. Infarcts of the posterior spinal territory are considerably rarer (Fig. 126B).

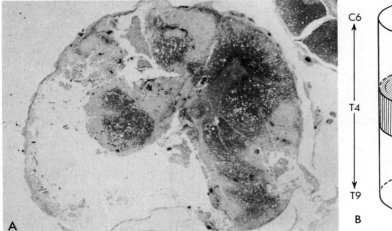

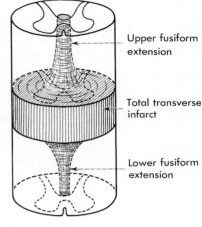

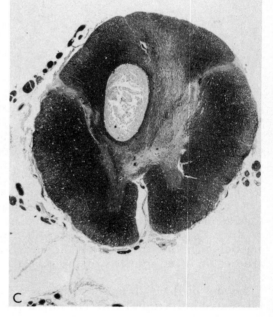

Figure 125. *Transverse infarct of the spinal cord.*

A, Maximal extent of the lesion (Loyez stain).
B, Diagram of fusiform extensions of the lesion.
C, Upper fusiform extension of the lesion (Loyez stain).

c. Microscopic features. The microscopic lesions are identical with those of cerebral infarcts; i.e., they consist of an initial edematous stage and of secondary processes of liquefaction and tissue resorption through the mobilization of compound granular corpuscles.

d. Chief etiological factors. *1.* Atherosclerosis and arterial thrombosis play an important role whether they involve the feeding vessels or the aorta itself. The pathological changes may operate either by obstructing the orifices of the intercostal and lumbar arteries or by causing an aortic aneurysm.

2. Arterial embolism can seldom be demonstrated to be an etiological factor.

3. Compression of bony and meningeal origin plays an important role, and in medullary compression of epidural origin, a

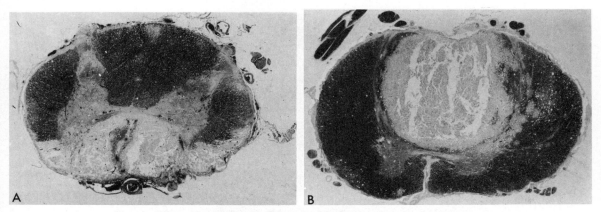

Figure 126.   *Focal infarcts of the spinal cord* (Loyez stain for myelin).

A, Anterior spinal artery infarct. *B*, Posterior spinal artery infarct.

vascular component is always associated to some degree with simple mechanical compression.

4. Thoracic surgery and aortography may be special etiological factors in vascular disorders of the spinal cord.

III. OTHER CEREBROVASCULAR LESIONS OF ISCHEMIC NATURE

Aside from cerebral and intraspinal medullary infarcts, which account for the most frequent manifestations of ischemic neurovascular pathology, other lesions may be observed which are determined by a different pathophysiological mechanism.

1. Lacunae (Fig. 127). These lesions consist of limited foci of cerebral necrosis with irregular borders and form cystic cavities which are surrounded by a zone of reactive gliosis. They are most often pale, but are sometimes orange-yellow because of the presence of old hemorrhages. Their size usually ranges from 2 to 10 mm, rarely exceeding 15 mm. The lenticular nuclei, pons, thalamus, internal capsule, and caudate nuclei are the sites of election in decreasing order of frequency. Lacunae are most frequently multiple.

Microscopically, discrete sequelae of acute

hemorrhagic lesions are frequently noted. These lesions contain hemosiderin pigment within scattered or grouped compound granular corpuscles, which tend to surround hyalinized blood vessels in the immediately adjacent areas.

In other words, lacunae are circumscribed cerebral infarcts that are characteristically found in older subjects suffering from long-standing hypertension. They are the result of thrombotic occlusion of small intraparenchymatous arterioles measuring less than 150 μm in diameter, in which the walls have been altered by the raised blood pressure and exhibit lesions of hyalinosis and sclerosis comparable to those that culminate in the formation of microaneurysms. It is therefore not surprising that these lacunae are often associated with intracerebral hemorrhagic lesions of various type and age.

They may also be found in association

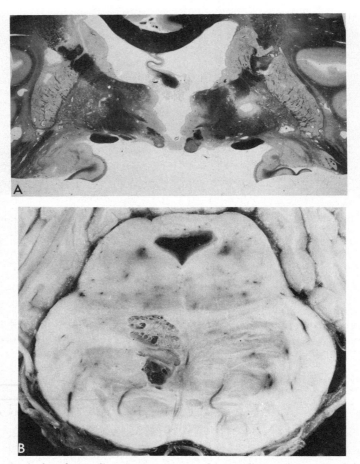

Figure 127.   *Lacunae* in basal ganglia (*A*) (Loyez stain for myelin) and in central fibers of pons (*B*).

with cerebral infarcts of atherosclerotic origin. These may be of variable size.

Status lacunatus ("état lacunaire") represents a pathological process characterized by multiple foci of lacunar disintegration. It may give rise to a variable clinical picture, in which a pseudobulbar syndrome is the most frequent presentation.

Status lacunatus must not be confused with *status cribratus* ("état criblé"), which is likewise found in the basal ganglia and sometimes in the white matter. The latter condition simply represents a dilatation of the perivascular spaces, which may contain a few macrophages. Like status lacunatus, it may be seen in the aged. The two processes may coexist.

2. *Granular atrophy of the cerebral cortex of arteriopathic origin* (Fig. 128). The pathological picture designated by this term is seen in certain forms of arteriopathic dementia. It is characterized by the presence of small punched-out foci of cavitated cicatricial softening, situated entirely in the cortex and accompanied by focal glial scars and zones of thinning of the cortical ribbon. The lesions, which are bilateral, are often remarkably distributed along the crests of the gyri, from the frontal to the occipital pole, along the superior frontal and interparietal sulci at the junction of the middle and anterior cerebral territories, and on the inferior surface of the temporal lobe at the junction of the middle and posterior cerebral territories.

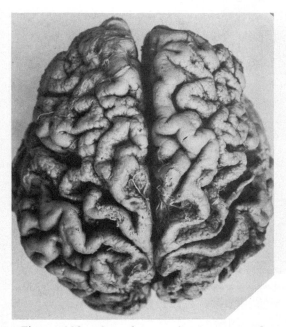

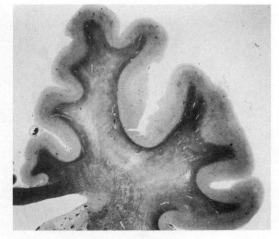

Figure 129. *Binswanger's subcortical encephalopathy* (Loyez stain for myelin).

Figure 128. *Granular atrophy* (upper surface of cerebral hemispheres).

The systematic distribution of this lesion is indicative of previous total circulatory ischemia related either to bilateral internal carotid thrombosis or to cardiac insufficiency.

The frequent presence of arteriolar changes over the cerebral convexity points to distal circulatory stasis as the etiological mechanism rather than to a cerebral form of Buerger's disease, which has been an alternative suggestion for this pathological process. However, a third possible hypothesis, namely the end stage of distal embolic migrations, cannot be absolutely excluded.

3. Binswanger's subcortical encephalopathy (Fig. 129). Binswanger's encephalopathy is characterized by diffuse lesions in the white matter and is seen in certain forms of arteriopathic dementia.

The changes consist in diffuse demyelination of the white matter which spares the U fibers and affects mainly the parieto-occipital regions. In addition to the demyelinating process, numerous juxtaposed microscopic foci of lacunar disintegration associated with astrocytic gliosis are seen.

This form of subacute leukoencephalopathy of atherosclerotic origin is apparently due to selective involvement of the deep arterial branches that supply the white matter; the shorter course of the cortical arteries would account for the relative sparing of the cortical territories.

IV. VASCULAR PATHOLOGY OF VENOUS ORIGIN

The study of cerebral venous lesions cannot be separated from that of the pathology of infectious diseases in the brain, as cerebral phlebitis is most often secondary to infectious lesions. It may also be seen in a number of generalized, often malignant, conditions, in which it may be associated with disturbances of coagulation.

Venous occlusion leads to circulatory stasis, diapedesis of red blood cells, and

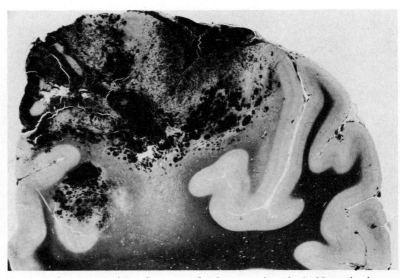

Figure 130. *Venous infarction resulting from superficial venous thrombosis.* Note the hemorrhagic involvement of the meninges, cortex and white matter (Loyez stain for myelin).

hemorrhages proximal to the site of vascular occlusion. A venous infarct is the final outcome of this process. It is characterized by the severity of the hemorrhagic features and especially by their localization. In contrast to arterial hemorrhagic infarcts, which predominate in the cortex, hemorrhages in venous infarction involve at one and the same time the leptomeningeal spaces, the cortex, and especially the white matter. In the latter, they show a picture of more or less confluent rosettes and tend to be distributed in a trian-

gular fashion, with the apex oriented toward the ventricular cavity (Fig. 130).

In superior sagittal sinus thrombosis, hemorrhagic lesions involve symmetrically the hemispheric white matter and predominate in the centrum ovale. In thrombosis of the vein of Galen, they involve the periventricular regions and the thalamic areas. In superficial phlebitis, they are localized in a hemispheric territory, where they involve in particular the underlying white matter.

PATHOLOGY OF INFECTIOUS DISEASES

A wide variety of pathogenic organisms—bacterial, fungal, parasitic, rickettsial, or viral—may affect the central nervous system; some are selective, but not all.

BACTERIAL INFECTIONS

I. PYOGENIC INFECTIONS

Some pyogenic infections may be localized to the epidural space (epidural abscess) or to the subdural space (subdural abscess or empyema); they are exceptional. Most often they involve the leptomeninges (purulent meningitis) or the cerebral parenchyma (cerebral abscess).

1. Purulent meningitis. This form of meningitis is due, in approximately 70 per cent of cases, to a *pneumococcus* or a *meningococcus;* less often, the causative agent is staphylococcus, *Listeria monocytogenes*, enterococcus, streptococcus, or various other bacteria.

The organism may reach the meninges:

Directly following open skull fracture or transgression of the dura and bone from a previous head injury with fracture of the base of the skull;

Through spread from an adjacent focus of suppuration (otitis, mastoiditis, sinusitis), either in direct continuity or through intermediary thrombophlebitis;

As a result of blood-borne dissemination from a distant infective focus (lung, skin, genitourinary tract).

Grossly (Fig. 131), a purulent exudate is seen in the leptomeninges.

Microscopically, large numbers of polymorphonuclear leukocytes are found to invade the leptomeninges and infiltrate the Virchow-Robin spaces (Fig. 132). Bacteria may be seen, lying either free or within polymorphonuclear leukocytes. Later, in the absence of early resolution, the polymorphonuclear leukocytes become altered and disappear, whereas a fibrinous exudate containing lymphocytes, plasma cells, histiocytes, and macrophages makes its appearance. After a few weeks, connective tissue proliferation begins.

All the central nervous tissue structures that are bathed by cerebrospinal fluid participate in the infectious process. Thus,

There is a polymorphic inflammatory cellular infiltrate in the walls of leptomeningeal arteries and veins, with the possible development of thromboses (which are likely to cause cerebral infarcts);

There is cellular infiltration of the cranial nerves and spinal roots, with the contingent development of demyelination;

There is invasion of the ependyma (Fig. 131*C*) and choroid plexuses;

There is possible infiltration of the subpial and subependymal neural parenchyma.

On the other hand, the production of a fibrinocellular exudate and the subsequent proliferation of connective tissue may obstruct the path of outflow of cerebrospinal fluid and result in the development of hydrocephalus, and even of pyocephalus.

Listeria infections deserve separate mention because of the frequency with which microabscesses ("listeria nodules"), distributed particularly in the brainstem, are associated with this type of purulent meningitis.

2. Brain abscess (Figs. 133 and 134). Brain abscesses fall within the definition of abscesses in general and are caused by pyogenic bacteria (most often streptococcus, staphylococcus, or pneumococcus) that have reached the cerebral tissue by

105

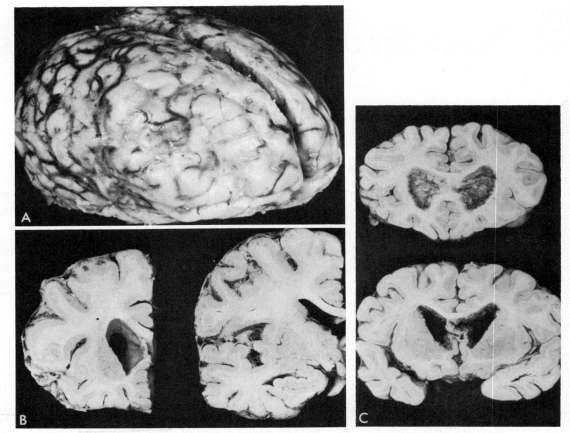

Figure 131.   *Gross features of purulent meningitis.*

A, External appearance of the brain.

B, Frontal coronal sections of the left hemisphere; note meningeal infiltration over the gyri and in the sulci of the cerebral convexity.

C, Involvement of the ependyma.

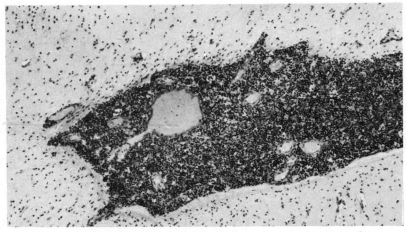

Figure 132.   *Microscopic features of purulent meningitis* (H. and E.).

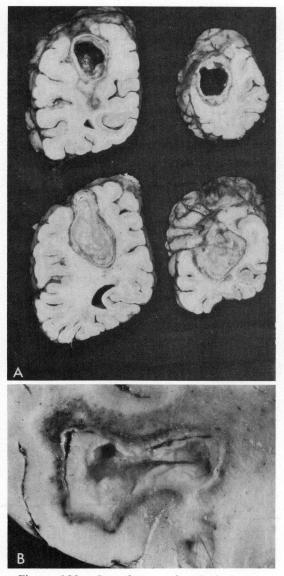

Figure 133. *Gross features of cerebral abscesses.*

A, Left parietal lobe abscess. *B,* Temporal lobe abscess; note the three distinct zones, consisting of purulent necrosis in the center, granulation tissue, and a peripheral capsule.

routes identical with those leading to meningitis.

a. Site. The localization of brain abscesses may suggest a particular mode of origin:

Post-traumatic abscesses occur *in situ* (craniocerebral wounds, neurosurgical operations);

Abscesses caused by direct spread from an adjacent suppurative focus are usually situated in the temporal lobe or in the cerebellum when they are secondary to otitis media or mastoiditis, or in the frontal lobe when they are secondary to sinusitis;

Hematogenous *metastatic abscesses* are usually multiple and deeply situated; they are most often secondary to bronchopulmonary suppuration or may be seen in congenital cyanotic heart disease, especially in Fallot's tetrad.

b. Microscopic features. In the initial stage (i.e., at the stage of presuppurative encephalitis, or cerebritis), the lesion is ill defined and characterized by early necrosis of cerebral tissue, with vascular congestion, petechial hemorrhages, microthromboses, perivascular fibrinous exudate, and infiltration by polymorphonuclear leukocytes. Surrounding cerebral edema may be associated with these lesions; it may spread for a considerable distance and may cause cerebral herniation.

Gradually within the next few weeks the abscess becomes circumscribed, and a shell becomes progressively organized around the central purulent necrotic focus. This shell is made up of granulation tissue including lymphocytes, plasma cells, monocytes and macrophages, numerous newly formed blood vessels, fibroblasts, and a considerable amount of collagen fibers. In its later stages the abscess, which is now truly encapsulated, is surrounded by a zone of perifocal astrocytic gliosis.

c. Complications. The two major, and most serious, complications of brain abscess are:

Raised intracranial pressure, with the risk of cerebral herniation;

Rupture of the abscess into a ventricle (ventricular empyema).

II. TUBERCULOSIS

Epidural tuberculous abscess is usually a complication of tuberculosis of the spine (Pott's

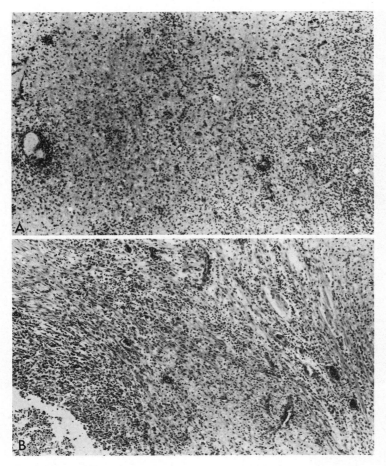

Figure 134. *Microscopic features of cerebral abscesses* (H. and E.).
A, The presuppurative encephalitic stage. *B*, Florid abscess: purulent necrosis in lower left; phagocytic reaction and granulation tissue in the center; reaction of the adjacent glia in upper right.

disease, involving either the vertebral bodies or the intervertebral discs).

Subdural tuberculous abscess is less frequent and is usually discovered incidentally either during surgery or at necropsy.

In fact, tuberculosis of the nervous system occurs most often in the form of a meningitis or, less often, a tuberculoma.

1. Tuberculous meningitis. The lesions in tuberculous meningitis differ from those in purulent meningitis in several respects:

The meninges over the base are predominantly involved (Fig. 135).

The meningeal exudate is essentially composed of lymphocytes, mononuclear cells, and small tubercles (Fig. 136). The latter consist of areas of central caseous necrosis surrounded by epithelioid cells and scattered

giant cells and by a peripheral ring of lymphocytes. They are situated in the leptomeninges and in the subpial layers[1] as well as in the ependyma and the subependymal parenchyma; acid-fast bacilli may be demonstrated in these tubercles.

Arterial lesions are constant and are fairly frequently responsible for the production of foci of ischemic necrosis in the neural parenchyma (Fig. 136).

These acute lesions are rarely seen now. Indeed, in most treated cases cicatricial fibrous lesions are found over the base and may result in blockage of the cerebrospinal fluid circulation (Fig. 135*C*).

---

[1]In these sites, larger tubercles are often also present. They are regarded as the source of origin of the meningitis.

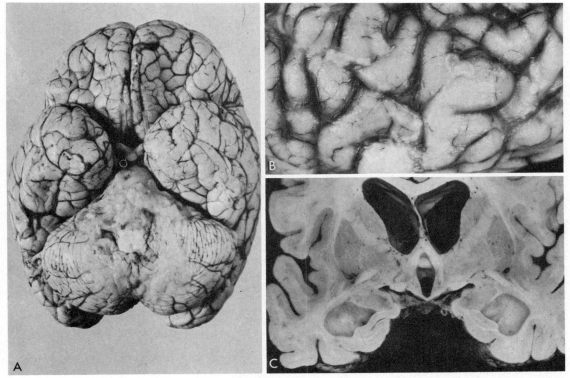

Figure 135.   *Gross features of tuberculous meningitis.*

A, Massive infiltration of the basal meninges; *B*, small tubercles on the cerebral convexity; *C*, basal obstruction, with ventricular dilatation.

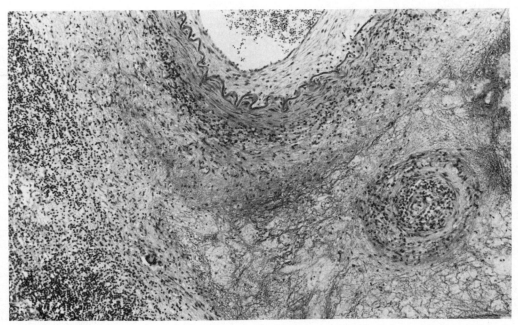

Figure 136.   *Microscopic features of tuberculous meningitis* (H. and E.). Note the marked vascular changes, characterized by occlusive endarteritis, and the exudative character of the lesions.

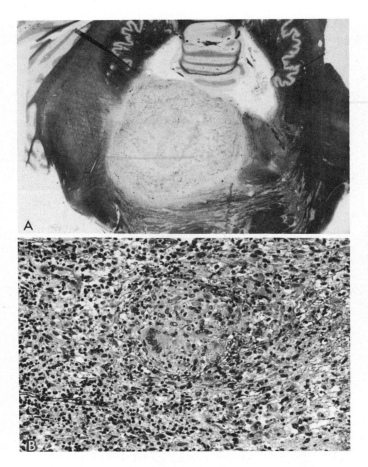

Figure 137. *Tuberculoma.*

A, Gross appearance of a tuberculoma of the pontine tegmentum (Loyez stain for myelin). *B,* Microscopic features at the periphery: note giant and epithelioid cells (H. and E.).

2. Cerebral tuberculoma (Fig. 137). This spherical or multiloculated lesion is composed of a caseous center surrounded by a ring of granulomatous tissue which includes epithelioid cells, giant cells, lymphocytes, and a collagen fibrosis of variable intensity.

Tuberculomas may be single or multiple. Their sites of predilection are the cerebellum, the pontine tegmentum, and the paracentral lobule.

They may spontaneously become cystic, fibrous, and calcified, but their chief risk lies in their liability to spill into the meninges.

III. SYPHILIS

Central nervous system involvement by syphilis is a sequel of primary luetic disease that either has escaped notice or has been inadequately treated.

1. Subacute secondary syphilitic meningitis. Leptomeningeal invasion by *Treponema pallidum* may result in a meningitis consisting of lymphocytes and plasma cells, with perivascular infiltrates.

2. Tertiary neurosyphilis. a. **Chronic meningitis** composed of lymphocytes and plasma cells, leading to fibrous organization and ultimate occlusion of the pathways of cerebrospinal fluid resorption, is virtually constant. Concomitant infiltration of the arterial vessel walls by lymphocytes and plasma cells (syphilitic arteritis) is frequent; it may result in ischemic parenchymatous lesions.

b. **Syphilitic gummas** are only exceptionally encountered today.

c. **In general paresis (general paralysis of the insane,** or GPI), inflammatory meningovascular lesions are associated with parenchymatous changes of encephalitic type. Involvement of the cerebral cortex is most striking. It is characterized by considerable cortical atrophy, neuronal depopulation, and a proliferation of rod-shaped microglia (see Fig. 20) which are distributed as scattered foci of different ages ("brush-fire appearance"). Pericapillary infiltration by lymphocytes and plasma cells may also be seen. Finally, *Treponema pallidum* may be demonstrated in these cerebral lesions with the help of special techniques.

d. Tabes dorsalis consists in degeneration of the posterior columns and spinal nerve roots, with involvement of the dorsal root ganglia. It is apparently the result of inflammatory meningovascular lesions localized to the subarachnoid portion of the dorsal nerve roots. Spinal cord involvement presents therefore as demyelination and gliosis of the posterior columns secondary to radiculoganglionic lesions. No inflammatory process is therefore demonstrable in the cord parenchyma, and *Treponema pallidum* is absent.

IV. BRUCELLOSIS

Leptomeningeal involvement is common in the septicemic phase of brucellosis (Malta fever). Either spontaneously or after inadequate treatment, the disease may give rise to subacute manifestations, either infectious or apparently hyperergic. The different forms of neurobrucellosis correspond to a variety of clinicopathological pictures, which include meningoencephalitis, meningomyelitis, and meningomyeloradiculitis, with fairly frequent involvement of the cranial nerves, particularly the acoustic nerve.

MYCOSES

Fungal infections of the central nervous system are seen mainly in special circumstances, such as following prolonged antibiotic treatment, in the course of hematological or lymphoreticular disease, or as a complication of immunosuppressive therapy.

The forms of fungal infection that are most frequently encountered in temperate climates are *candidiasis* and *torulosis* (or *cryptococcosis*). These infections may give rise to a granulomatous meningitis, with epithelioid and giant-cell formation, as well as to granulomas or to intraparenchymatous mycotic abscesses. Fungal organisms may be demonstrated microscopically in the lesions. Some have a characteristic appearance; others may be more difficult to identify (Fig. 138).

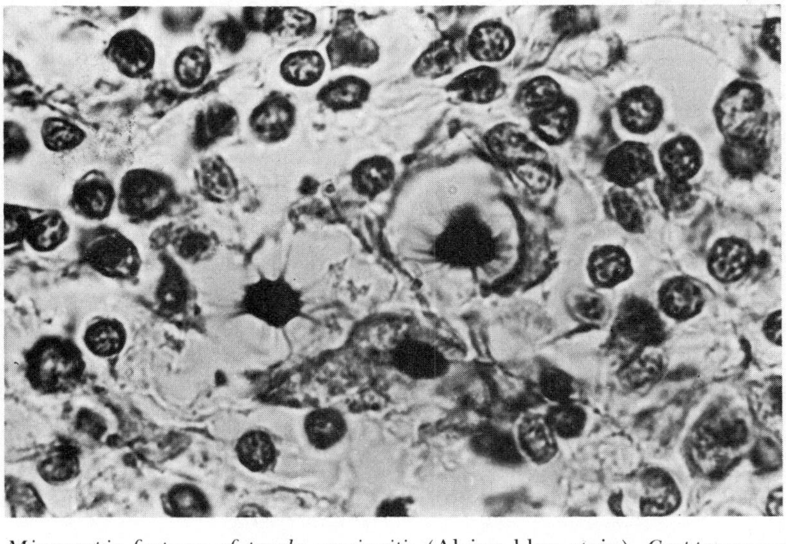

Figure 138. *Microscopic features of torula meningitis* (Alcian blue stain). *Cryptococcus neoformans* organisms are present.

Other, rarer, fungal infections that may involve the nervous system should also be mentioned:

Aspergillosis often presents as single or, more frequently, multiple cerebral abscesses in immunologically compromised hosts, especially after organ transplantation.

Mucormycosis (or *phycomycosis*) may complicate uncontrolled diabetes or acute leukemia. The organism may gain access to the brain by direct spread along the arterial vessel walls from a focus in the nose or the orbit. The lesion is characteristically a massive cerebral infarct due to thrombosis of the internal carotid or middle cerebral artery.

Coccidioidomycosis. This disease is endemic in California and the southwestern United States and causes a chronic granulomatous meningitis that resembles tuberculous or cryptococcal meningitis.

PARASITIC INFECTIONS
(Figs. 139 and 140)

The frequency of parasitic infections of the brain varies greatly in different geographical regions.

Such infections may involve the meninges and/or the brain (in the latter case forming cysts, granulomas, or abscesses), and the causative organism may be demonstrable in the lesions.

The chief causative parasites, protozoa and metazoa, are reviewed in the table reproduced in Figure 139.

	Parasitic diseases that may involve the nervous system	Pathogenic agent	Chief neuropathological lesions	Predominant geographical areas
Protozoa	Toxoplasmosis	*Toxoplasma gondii*	Diffuse or nodular granulomas	
	Amebiasis	*Entamoeba histolytica*	Amebic brain abscess, usually single	
		Naegleria (*N. fowleri*)	Primary amebic meningoencephalitis	
	Malaria	*Plasmodium falciparum*	Multiple necrotic and hemorrhagic foci	Tropical zones
	Trypanosomiasis	*Trypanosoma gambiense* and *T. rhodesiense*	Meningoencephalitis and Mott cells	West and East Africa
	Chagas' disease	*Trypanosoma cruzi*	Diffuse encephalitic lesions	Central and South America
Metazoa — **Platyhelminthes**	Cestodiasis (tapeworm infection)			
	Cysticercosis	*Taenia solium* (pig) *Cysticercus cellulosae* (larvae)	Multiple small meningeal and/or cerebral cysts	Latin America
	Echinococcosis (hydatid disease)	*Taenia echinococcus* (dog), or *Echinococcus granulosus*	Usually a single cerebral (hydatid) cyst (sometimes large)	Latin America Australia
	Coenurosis	*Multiceps multiceps* (tapeworm in dogs)	Single or multiple unilobular cerebral and/or meningeal cysts, containing larvae (*Coenurus cerebralis*)	South Africa
	Trematode (fluke) infection			
	Paragonimiasis	*Paragonimus westermani*	Single or multiple cerebral cysts	Far East
	Schistosomiasis (bilharziasis)	*Schistosoma japonicum*	Multiple small cerebral granulomas, containing *Bilharzia* ova	Far East
Metazoa — **Nemathelminthes**	Nematode (roundworm) infection			
	Filariasis (loaiasis)	*Loa loa*	Multiple small cerebral granulomas, containing microfilariae	Tropical regions
	Trichinosis	*Trichinella spiralis*	Multiple cerebral granulomas containing *Trichinella* larvae	
	Ascariasis	*Ascaris lumbricoides* (dog, cat)	Acute eosinophilic meningitis (granulomas containing *Ascaris* larvae in the brain)	

Figure 139. *Table of main parasitic diseases.*

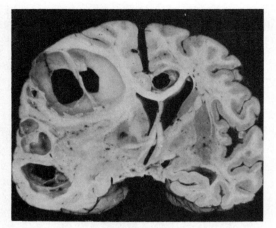

Figure 140. *Cerebral cysticercosis.* Gross appearance, showing numerous cystic cavities displacing brain tissue.

RICKETTSIAL INFECTIONS

Some forms of rickettsial infection (murine or endemic typhus, exanthematic or epidemic typhus, Rocky Mountain spotted fever) may cause nervous system lesions characterized by perivascular histiocytic and microglial nodules that preferentially involve the gray matter of the cerebral hemispheres and the brainstem.

VIRAL DISEASES

Nervous system lesions attributable to viral infection may show various forms.

1. Some lesions, which are nonspecific, are most often related to immunoallergic reactions that are secondary to viral infection. The lesions involve the meninges and especially the white matter (leukoencephalitis).

2. Other lesions are directly related to penetration of the central nervous system by the virus and involve chiefly the gray matter (polioencephalitis).

Some of the above forms have an acute course, as in the majority of "viral encephalitides." In others, special immunological phenomena play a role in the development of latent infection, as in herpes zoster, or persistent infection, as in the case of the measles virus presumed to be responsible for subacute sclerosing panencephalitis.

3. The last group is represented by disorders with very different histopathological features, but in which the demonstration of animal transmissibility and certain resemblances derived from comparative ·neuropathology suggest a special viral mechanism ("slow-virus diseases"). In such cases a slow-virus infection is considered to be responsible for neuronal and/or glial cell changes of degenerative character, without the usual inflammatory lesions that normally accompany acute and subacute viral encephalitis.

I. NONSPECIFIC NERVOUS SYSTEM MANIFESTATIONS OF VIRAL INFECTIONS

1. *Acute Viral Lymphocytic Meningitis*

This response is common to viral infections of highly multifarious origin:
Enteroviruses (poliovirus, Coxsackie B virus, echovirus)
Mumps virus
Herpesvirus
Varicella-zoster virus
Arboviruses
Lymphocytic choriomeningitis (LCM) virus
Encephalomyocarditis virus
Infectious mononucleosis virus
Hepatitis virus
Adenoviruses

2. *Postinfectious Perivenous Encephalitis*
(acute disseminated encephalomyelitis or acute disseminated leukoencephalitis)

Postinfectious encephalitis may complicate a variety of viral diseases, in particular exanthemas such as measles, chickenpox, rubella, and smallpox, or it may follow smallpox vaccination. It produces the clinical picture of an acute disseminated encephalomyelitis that may appear during the period of convalescence from the causative viral infection.

The histological features are characteristic and highly stereotyped, and consist of lymphocyte and plasma cell infiltrates around the venules of the neural parenchyma. These involve mainly the white matter, where they are associated with perivenous foci of demyelination, with relative sparing of the axons.

The close resemblance of the lesions to those of experimental allergic encephalomyelitis (EAE) and the infrequency with which a virus can be demonstrated in them have suggested that the basic mechanism of this postinfectious form of encephalitis must be immunoallergic. However, this hypothesis may have to be reconsidered in view of the recent detection of viral antigen in glial cells within the lesions.

The acute hemorrhagic leukoencephalitis of Weston Hurst[1] is characterized by the presence of hemorrhages in the white matter and by necrotizing changes in the blood vessel walls, consisting of fibrinous exudates and an infiltration by polymorphonuclear leukocytes. It is regarded as a hyperacute form of postinfectious encephalitis.

II. VIRAL ENCEPHALITIS

Viral encephalitis[2]—in the strict meaning of the term—is directly related to viral penetration of the central nervous system either as the result of direct spread along the peripheral nerves, and in particular along the olfactory nerves, or more often in the course of a viremia. This is followed by replication of the virus in the neurons and/or glia. Viral infection of the nervous system may be a sequel to infection elsewhere in the body at a site that has been directly exposed and therefore serves as a portal of entry. This

site may be the skin (exposed to infection by an animal or insect bite or through direct contact), the airway (after inhalation), or the alimentary tract (after ingestion).

Whatever the causative virus, the basic

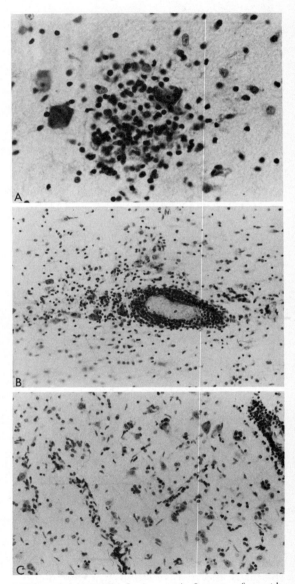

Figure 141. *Chief microscopic features of encephalitis.*

A, Picture of neuronophagia (Nissl stain). *B,* Lymphocytic perivascular cuffing (Nissl stain). *C,* Proliferation of rod-shaped microglia; note perivascular cuffing in upper right (Nissl stain).

---

[1]This form of hemorrhagic leukoencephalitis must not be confused with the type of "hemorrhagic encephalitis," more properly termed "hemorrhagic encephalopathy," that may accompany the neurological manifestations of malignant hypertension and is the result of circulatory, noninflammatory disturbances associated with cerebral edema, intense vasodilatation, and focal hemorrhages.

[2]Quite often the inflammatory process involves also the meninges (meningoencephalitis), the spinal cord (encephalomyelitis), or both (meningoencephalomyelitis), as well as the nerve roots (meningoencephalomyeloradiculitis).

neuropathological picture of viral encephalitis (Fig. 141) includes the following:

Involvement of the neuronal cell bodies, resulting in their destruction and engulfment by macrophages (neuronophagia);

Predominantly perivascular infiltrates composed of lymphocytes and plasma cells;

Microglial proliferation, with the formation of microglial nodules and the appearance of rod cells;

In some cases, intranuclear or intracytoplasmic inclusions, which are indicative of the presence of virus in the neurons and/or glia.

ant horn cell
frontal gyrus
hypothalamus
RF
post. horns

1. Encephalitides due to RNA Viruses

a. Encephalitides due to enteroviruses. Authentic meningoencephalomyelitides may be caused by the Coxsackie group of viruses or by echoviruses. They usually present as a lymphocytic meningitis. However, the central nervous system itself is more often involved by a *poliovirus.*

The most frequent form of the disease does not, admittedly, correspond to a typical encephalitis, but demonstrates the picture of *acute anterior poliomyelitis.*

The lesions selectively involve the *motor neurons of the anterior horns* and the cranial nerve nuclei, but may also involve other regions, such as the frontal gyri, the hypothalamus, the reticular formation, and the posterior horns.

The inflammatory infiltrates, vasodilatation, edema, and microglial and macrophage proliferation are often very severe. By electron microscopy, collections of viral particles may be found in the cytoplasm of the nerve cells.

Following resolution, the residual lesions consist of atrophy of the anterior horns, with neuronal cell loss and astrocytic gliosis.

An identical or fairly similar picture has also been reported with other enterovirus infections, in particular with *Coxsackie virus.* It is possible that the relative frequency of these cases may have been increased as the result of poliomyelitis vaccination.

b. Arbovirus encephalitides (arthropod-borne viruses). These encephalitides are transmitted by arthropods and have a distinct geographical distribution, often indicated by the name of the virus.

The best-known forms of *mosquito-borne* encephalitides include *St. Louis encephalitis* and the *eastern and western equine encephalitides* in North America; *Japanese B encephalitis* in the Far East; and *Murray Valley encephalitis* in Australia. The lesions in these various forms are widely distributed throughout the neuraxis.

Tick-borne encephalitis, which includes Russian spring-summer encephalitis and Central European encephalitis, is characterized by meningoencephalic lesions and by involvement of the lower cranial nerves and anterior horns, especially in the cervical levels.

c. Human rabies is due to a rhabdovirus and is transmitted to man by the bite of an infected animal, such as a dog, a cat, or a

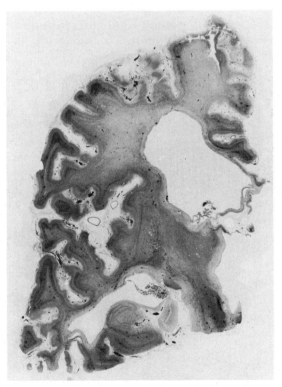

Figure 142. *Subacute sclerosing panencephalitis* (Loyez stain for myelin). Note massive demyelination of the white matter and severe cortical lesions.

wild animal. The disease is always fatal once it has declared itself. From the neuropathological point of view, it is identified by the presence of characteristic cytoplasmic inclusions in the neurons, or *Negri bodies,* accompanied by relatively discrete inflammatory cellular infiltrates.

The progressive extension of an epidemic of animal rabies transmitted by foxes has been reported in Western Europe. The animal reservoir includes foxes, skunks, coyotes and bats in North America, and jackals in India. However, the dog is the main source of human infection.

Polyneuritis and encephalomyelitis have been reported after rabies vaccination with either the attenuated or the inactivated virus which may or may not have been cultured on neural tissue. The pathophysiology of these complications is complex and may be related either to inadequate inactivation of the virus or to an immunopathological process.

d. Encephalitides due to paramyxoviruses. In addition to influenza and mumps, which may, exceptionally, be associated with different forms of encephalitis whose mechanism is debated, measles infection may cause two types of encephalitis that are quite different: acute postinfectious encephalitis (or perivenous leukoencephalitis; see p. 113), and subacute sclerosing panencephalitis.

Subacute sclerosing panencephalitis (SSPE)[1] occurs in children, several years after a known episode of measles.

The lesions involve the *gray matter* (cortex and basal ganglia), where inclusion bodies are found in neuronal and glial nuclei as well as in the cytoplasm of neurons; there is a considerable proliferation of microglial rod cells. Lesions also implicate the *white matter,* which is the site of a diffuse demyelination (Fig. 142) accompanied by marked astrocytic

---

[1]The term subacute sclerosing panencephalitis replaces today the name " subacute sclerosing leukoencephalitis" (SSLE) of van Bogaert, as well as the terms "Dawson's inclusion-body encephalitis" and "Pette-Döring's panencephalitis."

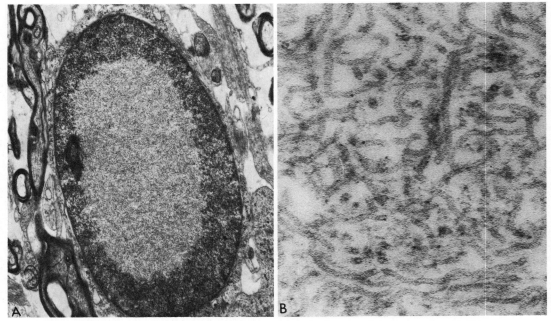

Figure 143.   *Electron microscopic features of subacute sclerosing panencephalitis.*

A, Oligodendroglial nucleus with inclusion (× 3000). *B,* High-power electron micrograph of intranuclear tubular formations, morphologically identical with measles myxovirus (× 90,000).

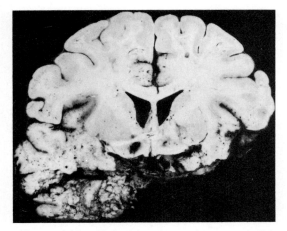

Figure 144. *Necrotizing herpesvirus encephalitis.* Necrosis of temporal lobe (the right temporal pole was surgically excised).

proliferation. Perivascular inflammatory infiltrates are present in both the gray and white matter.

Although the measles virus has been demonstrated to be the causal agent both by electron microscopy (Fig. 143) and by tissue culture, the precise mechanism of this type of prolonged viral infection is still poorly understood. Immunological factors, which are still undetermined, a defective virus, or possibly an associated virus may perhaps play a role.

2. *Encephalitides due to DNA Viruses*

a. Encephalitides due to the herpes virus group. 1. HERPES SIMPLEX ENCEPHALITIS is due to a subgroup A virus. It is remarkable by its *topography, involving predomi-*

Figure 145. *Herpesvirus encephalitis.* *A,* Light microscopic appearance; intranuclear inclusion bodies (H. and E.). *B,* Electron microscopy (× 3000); numerous intranuclear viral particles.

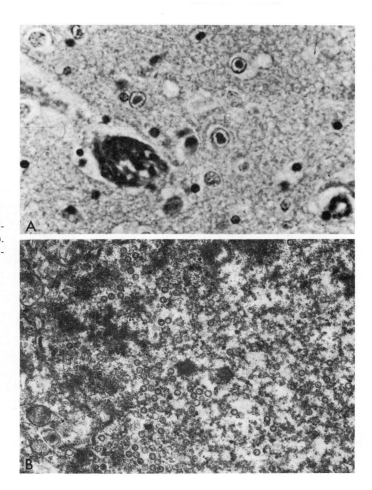

nantly the temporal lobes and the limbic regions (Fig. 144), and by the severity of the inflammatory infiltrates, which may culminate in actual hemorrhagic *necrosis* accompanied by marked cerebral edema (necrotizing encephalitis). *Intranuclear inclusions* may be found in the neurons and in some of the glial cells, and the virus can be identified in the electron microscope and by immunofluorescence (Fig. 145).

2. CYTOMEGALOVIRUS ENCEPHALITIS is due to a herpesvirus of subgroup B and may occur either as part of a multisystem viral infection or as an isolated central nervous system infection which is often associated with chorioretinitis.

The disease is usually due to early fetal infection and may result in microcephaly and, especially, hydrocephalus with intracranial calcifications that may be correlated with necrotic and inflammatory subependymal and subcortical lesions.[1]

3. HERPES ZOSTER-VARICELLA. The virus of shingles (zona), which is identical with that causing varicella, selectively involves the neurons of one or several *spinal root ganglia* and the *posterior horn* of the corresponding metameric segment. The inflammatory cellular infiltrates, which are composed of lymphocytes and plasma cells, tend to spill widely into the adjacent leptomeninges and spinal medullary levels.

---

[1]Discretely disseminated lesions due to cytomegalovirus, unaccompanied by necrosis, have also been reported in adults as examples of opportunistic infection in immunosuppressed hosts, in particular after organ transplantation (translator's note).

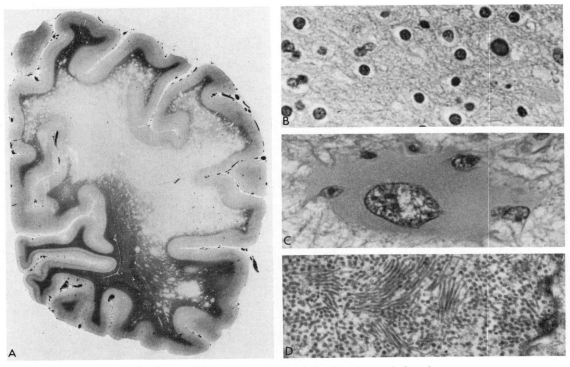

Figure 146. *Progressive multifocal leukoencephalopathy.*

A, Gross appearance. Note confluent demyelination (Loyez stain for myelin).
B, Abnormal enlarged oligodendroglial nuclei (H. and E.).
C, Giant astrocyte (H. and E.).
D, Intranuclear papovavirions (electron microscopy, × 20,000).

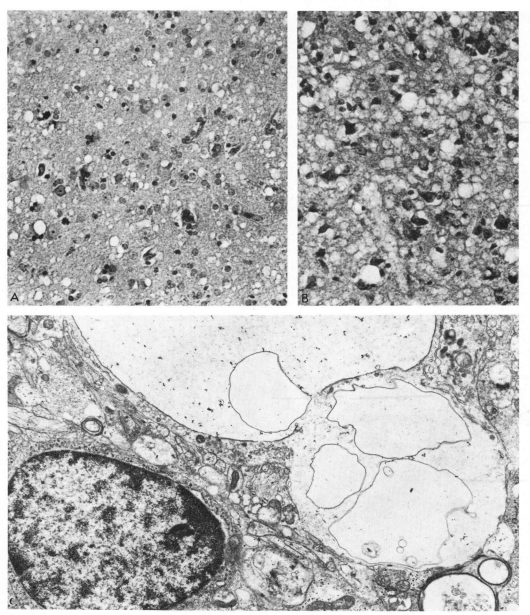

Figure 147. *Creutzfeldt-Jakob disease.*

A, Astrocytic gliosis (light microscopy). *B,* Spongiosis (light microscopy). *C,* Spongiosis (electron microscopy).

b. Encephalitis due to papovaviruses.

A papovavirus (JC virus and SV40-PML virus) is responsible for *progressive multifocal leukoencephalopathy* (PML). This disease occurs in special pathological circumstances.

It is indeed a complication of various diseases associated with immunodeficiency (e.g., chronic lymphatic leukemia, Hodgkin's disease). The hemispheric white matter, especially the occipital lobe, is the site of limited spotty foci of demyelination which may become confluent and amidst which giant atypical astrocytes and intranuclear glial inclusions, especially in the oligodendroglia, are characteristically found. The nuclei of the oligodendroglia at the periphery of the lesions are also markedly enlarged. Cellular inflammatory infiltrates may be present, and then only in moderate numbers (Fig. 146).

3. Encephalitides due to Nonidentified Viruses

a. Encephalitis lethargica (epidemic encephalitis of von Economo).

This disease, supposedly viral, was rampant from 1916 to 1930, but the viral agent was never demonstrated. It was characterized by preferential involvement of the midbrain and basal ganglia. Its main interest now lies in its sequel, a *postencephalitic parkinsonian syndrome.* The lesions in this late stage consist of loss of nerve cells in the substantia nigra, accompanied by neurofibrillary degeneration, but without Lewy bodies.

b. Uveomeningoencephalitides

present as inflammatory encephalitic, meningitic, and uveal lesions (choroid, ciliary body, and iris) of uncertain etiology.

Behçet's disease is characterized by recurrent uveitis, aphthous ulcers in the mouth and over the genitalia, and various visceral lesions that include a picture of encephalitis involving predominantly the thalamic, hypothalamic, and midbrain regions.

In this disease, as in other forms of uveomeningoencephalitis, a viral etiology has not been conclusively established.

III. TRANSMISSIBLE "SLOW-VIRUS" CEREBRAL INFECTIONS

This group of diseases, which is characterized by animal transmissibility (to chimpanzees and other primate species) after injection of cerebral biopsy fragments, includes two main disorders which were formerly classified as degenerative: Creutzfeldt-Jakob disease and kuru.

Creutzfeldt-Jakob disease is clinically characterized by a picture of dementia associated with various neurological manifestations and is fatal within a few months.

The neuropathological picture consists of neuronal cell depopulation, accompanied by spongiosis (Fig. 147) and by a dense astrocytic gliosis, involving mainly the cerebral cortex (especially the occipital cortex in some cases). However, the basal ganglia, thalamus, cerebellum, and anterior horns may also be affected.

Because of its resemblance to some animal virus diseases (such as scrapie in sheep and mink encephalopathy) and to kuru (a human disease observed in New Guinea) and because of its experimental transmissibility to primates, Creutzfeldt-Jakob disease is now regarded as a slow-virus infection. However, the pathogenic agent has not yet been isolated and the usual histopathological picture of encephalitis is entirely lacking.

MULTIPLE SCLEROSIS AND DISEASES OF THE WHITE MATTER

Diseases of the white matter result from pathological processes that are very dissimilar to each other. Some of these diseases, which by virtue of their genetic character belong to the group of leukodystrophies, display metabolic alterations in the myelin sheaths that are enzymatic in origin (described elsewhere on pp. 169 and 170). They include metachromatic leukodystrophy and globoid body leukodystrophy. Others, which like multiple sclerosis have inflammatory features, continue to be classified today within the traditional framework of "demyelinating diseases." The latter term corresponds to a major pathological characteristic that is common to various disorders of highly different nature; it retains its practical utility for the neuropathologist, despite the ambiguities and uncertainties with which it is beset from the etiological and pathogenetic points of view.

GENERAL CONSIDERATIONS

1. Demyelination

Demyelination is demonstrated histologically by a negative reaction of nervous tissue for stains that have a usual affinity for myelin. It is a frequently observed phenomenon in neuropathology.

a. Demyelination is found in various pathological conditions. *1.* It is one of the features of massive white matter lesions such as cerebral infarcts, hemorrhages, and cerebral tumors.
2. It may be secondary to processes, chiefly degenerative, involving neurons at the level of either the nerve cell bodies or the axons.
3. It constitutes the main feature of so-called demyelinating diseases, i.e., diseases in which the pathological process selectively involves myelin sheaths[1] and often spares, in a remarkable manner, the axis cylinders (myelin-axonal dissociation).

b. The demyelinating process. This has two aspects: biochemical and histochemical on the one hand, and histopathological on the other.

1. BIOCHEMICAL PHENOMENA AND THEIR HISTOCHEMICAL ASPECTS (Fig. 149). These consist in the liberation of the normal biochemical constituents of myelin (phospholipids, glycolipids, cholesterol, proteins) followed by the secondary formation of simple lipids (triglycerides, cholesterol esters) or neutral fats.

Normal myelin may—aside from its usual tinctorial affinities, which are rapidly lost as the result of pathological changes—show the

---

[1] It is important to recall that the myelin sheath (Fig. 148) results from the fusion of cell membranes of oligodendroglial origin that have become regularly wrapped around the axon. It is likely that enzyme systems responsible for myelin formation, maintenance, and turnover are present in the oligodendroglia, perhaps also in axons, and even in the myelin sheath itself. These systems appear to be selectively involved in demyelinating diseases. Their alteration by toxic, infectious, or allergic processes lies presumably at the basis of a number of myelinoclastic disorders. A deficit in these enzyme systems is the source of a number of leukodystrophic syndromes.

121

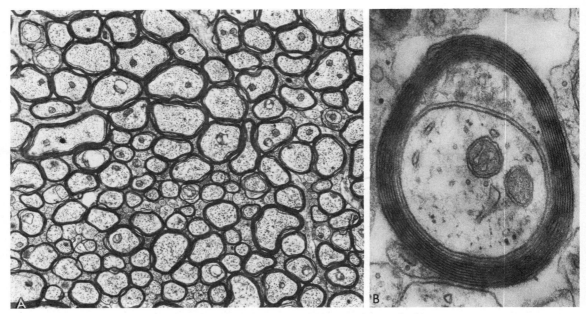

Figure 148.　*Electron microscopic appearance of normal white matter.*

A, Low magnification (× 10,500). *B*, Myelinated axon at high magnification (× 163,500). (Courtesy of Dr. B. Berger.)

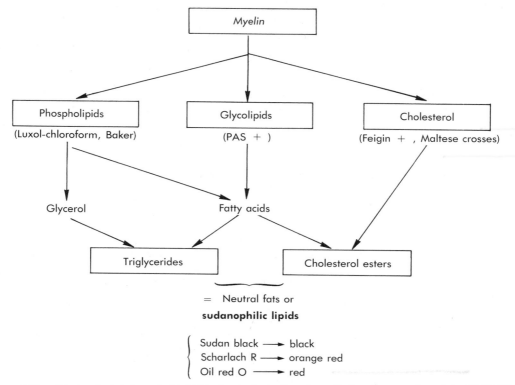

Figure 149.　*Biochemical data and chief histochemical reactions in wallerian degeneration of the myelin sheath.*

phenomenon of metachromasia, i.e., stain red with certain blue dyes such as toluidine blue and cresyl violet. Myelin breakdown products have this property at a very early stage only. Two final breakdown products, triglycerides and cholesterol esters, are easily identified by their black color when stained with sudan black and their red color when stained with scharlach R, sudan IV, or oil red O. These sudanophilic lipids, or neutral fats, make their appearance in foci of acute parenchymatous destruction after 48 hours, but the overall catabolic process may extend over several weeks.

This catabolic sequence, which culminates in the presence of sudanophilic lipids, is classically observed in the peripheral nervous system in wallerian degeneration (see below). Myelin disintegration of wallerian type is seen also in the central nervous system, in particular in some of the demyelinating diseases such as multiple sclerosis and Schilder's disease. In other pathological processes that may affect the white matter, especially in some of the leukodystrophies, myelin catabolism is altered, and a number of complex lipids, or prelipids, may be found which may give rise to the phenomenon of metachromasia.

2. HISTOPATHOLOGICAL ASPECTS. These include in succession:

Loss of normal myelin structures, with swelling, tumefaction, and breakdown of myelin sheaths;

Phagocytosis of breakdown products by compound granular corpuscles, which are first diffusely scattered and subsequently grouped in perivascular cuffs;

Inflammatory cellular lesions, which are reactive to the parenchymatous lesions and may be discrete or more intense, depending on the etiological factors;

Progressive disappearance of compound granular corpuscles *pari passu* with the catabolism of phagocytosed material;

Development of reactive gliosis of astrocytic type.

2. Classification of Demyelinating Diseases[1]

There are two main types of demyelinating disease that can be distinguished from both the etiological and the histopathological points of view.

a. From the etiological point of view. *1. Multiple sclerosis* and *Schilder's disease* are essentially the result of myelinoclastic processes. Their precise etiology is still un-

---

[1]Some of the general processes reviewed in other chapters may involve myelin sheaths in a fairly selective manner, but in view of the more diffuse character of the pathological process they cannot be regarded, strictly speaking, as "demyelinating diseases." This is so with the group of postinfectious encephalitides following acute exanthemata, with Grinker's myelopathy as a sequel of carbon monoxide poisoning, with central pontine myelinolysis and, to a lesser degree, with Marchiafava-Bignami's disease in chronic alcoholics, as well as with progressive multifocal leukoencephalopathy.

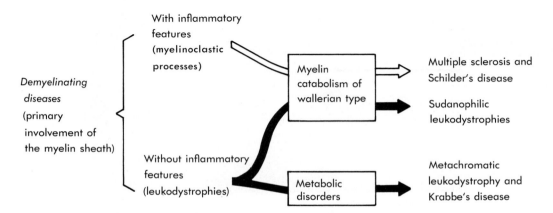

Figure 150. *Diagrammatic classification of demyelinating diseases.*

known, but an immunopathological process is generally suspected.

2. *Leukodystrophies* are familial conditions. Myelin sheath abnormalities appear to be caused by enzymatic disorders of genetic origin that are responsible for abnormal myelination. Consequently, the term "dysmyelinating disease" would appear to be more suitable, since they are characterized by an abnormal biochemical constitution of the myelin.

b. From the histopathological point of view. These diseases can also be distinguished according to whether they demonstrate *inflammatory cellular lesions* or not.

Myelinoclastic processes, such as in multiple sclerosis and Schilder's disease, frequently demonstrate these inflammatory cellular lesions, whereas they are absent in leukodystrophies.

While the concept of an inflammatory cellular reaction may provide an attractive distinction between these two groups, it cannot, however, be regarded as absolute. Indeed, inflammatory cellular lesions are usually present only in the early stages of some of the acute demyelinating processes, and tend to disappear in the course of the disease (i.e., in multiple sclerosis and Schilder's disease). The actual significance of these changes is also open to debate. Indeed, the inflammation may be primary, and therefore directly related to the etiological agent, such as infection or an immunological process, or it may be only symptomatic and secondary to the myelinoclastic process itself, and therefore compatible with some of the more rapid forms of demyelination of dystrophic origin. Consequently, this feature, which may be of considerable value in distinguishing the two groups when unequivocal, may be of uncertain significance when only discrete or altogether absent.

MULTIPLE SCLEROSIS AND SCHILDER'S DISEASE

I. MULTIPLE SCLEROSIS

Multiple sclerosis is the most common form of demyelinating disease. Its mechanism is probably immunological, but its etiology is unknown, possibly viral. The lesions are characterized by the formation of plaques of demyelination with gliosis (or sclerosis), as originally described by Charcot and Vulpian. The plaques are typical both in their structure and in their distribution, which is disseminated throughout the entire

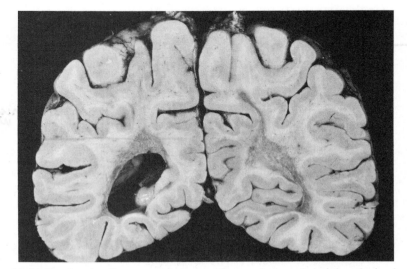

Figure 151. *Multiple sclerosis.* Gross appearance of a parieto-occipital hemispheric slice; note the periventricular distribution of the plaques.

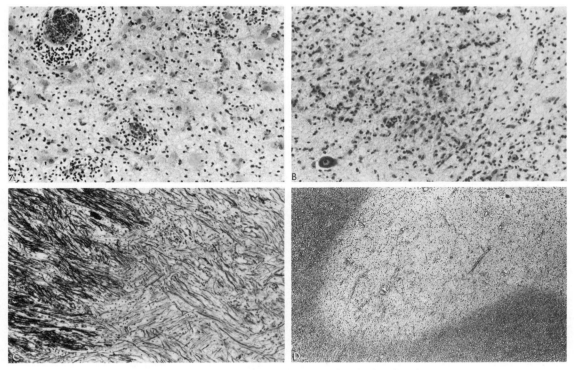

Figure 152. *Microscopic features of multiple sclerosis.*

A, Inflammatory features in a recent plaque; perivascular lymphocytic infiltrates; associated astrocytic gliosis (H. and E.).

B, Glial proliferation at the edge of a recent plaque ("glial wall").

C, Myelin-axonal dissociation, with preservation of axons (combined luxol fast blue and Bodian stain); note the normal staining of myelin on the left.

D, Old plaque (gliosis); absence of inflammatory features (P.T.A.H.).

neuraxis (disseminated, or multilocular, sclerosis).

1. Structure of the lesions. a. The plaques begin to be apparent from the moment of **gross examination** of the white matter and become more visible after a few minutes' exposure to air, when they present as rounded, well-limited areas, the older foci being grayish or translucent and the more recent being pink (Fig. 151).

b. On microscopic examination, three types of lesion are recognized in these plaques (Fig. 152).

1. Demyelination. Demyelination is characterized in myelin stains by a discoloration of the myelin with clear-cut and regular, practically punched-out borders. Sometimes, in so-called "*shadow plaques,*" where demyelination is less intense, myelin pallor is less obvious, although just as circumscribed (Fig. 152).

Myelin-axonal dissociation is a cardinal feature, and silver impregnations by the Bodian or Bielschowsky method demonstrate a tangled network of preserved axons in the plaque (Fig. 152). This accounts for the variable remissions that follow clinical episodes in the disease and for the absence of wallerian degeneration.

Myelin catabolism culminates in the formation of neutral fats, or *sudanophilic lipids.* These breakdown products are phagocytosed by numerous scattered compound granular corpuscles, which tend to group themselves around blood vessels.

2. Inflammatory cellular lesions. These lesions consist of perivenular lymphocytic cuffings, which are often conspicuous in recent plaques (Fig. 152).

3. Glial cell changes. Typically, the oligodendrocytes have disappeared. There is astrocytic proliferation, which is characteristic by its intensity. It is maximal at the periphery, where it forms the so-called "glial wall" and marks the limit of the centrifugal development of the plaque. Protoplasmic astrocytes, which are sometimes binucleated, and rod-shaped microglia are seen at that site, whereas gliosis becomes progressively more fibrillary toward the center.

c.   A number of special features must be stressed.   *1.*   Inflammatory cellular lesions, which are conspicuous in recent lesions, are absent in old plaques (Fig. 152D), where fibrillary gliosis predominates and where changes in the axis cylinders may occur.

The relapsing course characteristic of the disease is expressed morphologically by the coexistence of lesions of different ages at various levels of the neuraxis.

2. Some acute forms[1] have a necrotic character with a less obvious degree of myelin-axonal dissociation, but the outlines of the lesions are just as clear cut.

3. Subcortical *plaques* may encroach on the cortex (Fig. 153A). Neuronal cell bodies are then remarkably spared, as well as axis cylinders.

2.   *Distribution of the lesions.* While dissemination of the plaques throughout the entire neuraxis is an essential feature, there are, however, a number of preferential sites of involvement.

1. In the cerebral hemispheres (Fig. 153A) *the periventricular regions* (frontal and temporal horns) are the areas most frequently involved, especially posteriorly around the occipital horns, where some of the plaques may, not uncommonly, be unusually extensive (Fig. 153C).

2. The optic pathways: optic nerves, chiasm, optic tracts, tend to be selectively affected (Fig. 153B).

3. In the *brainstem* (Fig. 153D), the periventricular regions are the most frequently involved. The superior cerebellar peduncles and the posterior longitudinal bundles are frequently altered, accounting for the wealth of cerebellar signs, ataxic symptoms, oculomotor disturbances, and nystagmus.

4. The *central cerebellar white matter* and the middle cerebellar peduncles are often the site of numerous large plaques.

5. The *spinal cord* is involved in a random manner (Fig. 153E).[1]

3.   *Etiological factors.*   The *etiology* and the *pathogenetic mechanism* of multiple sclerosis are still unknown.

The disease, which is acquired by young adults, is seen with greater frequency in individuals with certain tissue-type antigens, in particular HLA-A3, HLA-B7, and HLA-Dw2. Because of its marked prevalence in cold wet temperate regions of the northern hemisphere and because of its higher frequency in persons who have recently immigrated in areas where its incidence is generally low, the role of a hypothetical *factor acquired* in early childhood has been proposed. So far, however, no data have confirmed the hypothesis of a slow or subacute virus infection, or helped to elucidate the possible role of an antecedent measles infection. The latter has been suspected because

---

[1]The lesions of *acute multiple sclerosis,* which has a more rapid clinical course, often with a single episode, are entirely comparable in their cardinal features to those in the more chronic forms of the disease. The severity of the inflammatory cellular reaction, the frequency of axonal changes, and the occasional presence of actual necrotic features emphasize the more destructive character of these lesions.

[1]The picture of *neuromyelitis optica acuta* has been variously interpreted. It is characterized by focal inflammatory demyelinating lesions that involve the optic pathways and the spinal cord. The extremely necrotic character of the spinal cord lesions, which cause actual myelomalacia over several segments, and the paucity of inflammatory cellular lesions are distinct features that are found also in some isolated forms of *acute necrotizing myelopathy.* The inclusion of the latter within the general framework of primary demyelinating diseases has been the subject of debate.

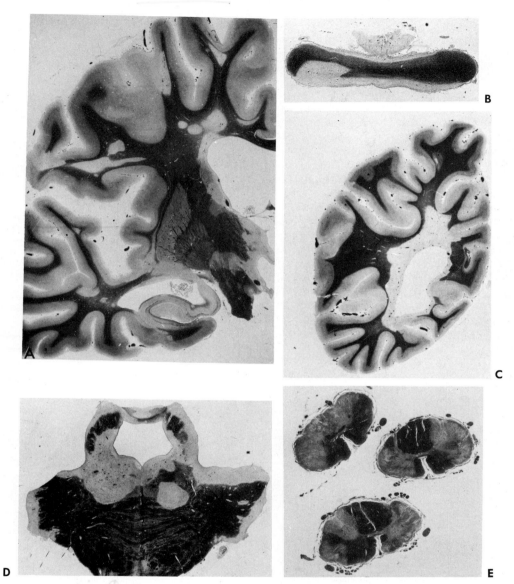

Figure 153. *Chief topographical features of multiple sclerosis* (Loyez stain for myelin).

A, Right cerebral hemisphere: disseminated plaques; note the periventricular distribution of the lesions.

B, Optic chiasm.

C, Parieto-occipital region.

D, Upper pons: plaque surrounding the rostral part of the fourth ventricle and involving the posterior longitudinal bundles and the superior cerebellar peduncles.

E, Plaques involving the spinal cord.

of the fairly significant rise of measles antibody titer in the cerebrospinal fluid of some cases.

Likewise the presence of structures resembling viral particles, noted by electron microscopy in a few cerebral biopsies and in tissue culture, has been reported in isolated cases, but their significance is debated.

On the other hand, the operation of an *immunological mechanism* appears highly probable in multiple sclerosis. The resemblance of the histopathological lesions to those of experimental allergic encephalomyelitis, in which certain myelin protein fractions are presumed to play the role of antigens, as well as to those that may follow rabies vaccination (after the injection of an attenuated virus cultured on cerebral tissues) has been stressed.

In addition, the raised γ-globulin titers in the cerebrospinal fluid and the effect of serum and/or lymphocytes from cases of multiple sclerosis on myelinating nervous system tissue cultures are further arguments in favor of an immunological hypothesis.

However, no clear explanation is so far available that can ascribe the various successive relapsing episodes of the disease to the triggering of an immunological disturbance, nor has the role of a viral infection been conclusively demonstrated.

II. SCHILDER'S DISEASE[1]

From the histopathological point of view, Schilder's disease consists of lesions whose structure is identical with that of lesions of multiple sclerosis (Fig. 155).

It is, however, distinct from multiple sclerosis:

---

[1] To contemporary workers this term must be restricted to those diseases of the white matter that are seen mainly in children and reproduce the description by Schilder in 1912 of encephalitis periaxialis diffusa. Two other cases were reported by the same author in 1913 and 1924 respectively and contributed to the establishment of cerebral sclerosis in children as a definite entity. Of the two, the first actually corresponds to an example of familial leukodystrophy, and the second to a case of subacute sclerosing panencephalitis.

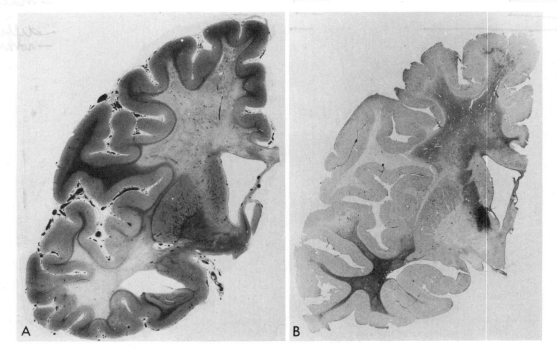

Figure 154. *Schilder's disease.*
A, Areas of massive hemispheric demyelination demonstrated with Loyez stain. *B*, Fibrillary astrocytic gliosis in affected areas (Holzer stain).

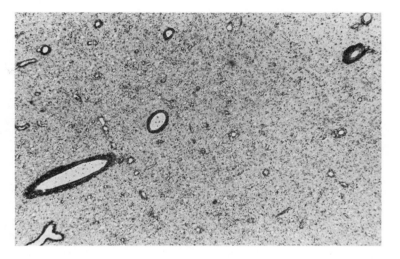

Figure 155. *Schilder's disease.* Microscopic appearance of recent lesions: inflammatory perivascular cuffings.

1. *By its more frequent occurrence in children and its continuous evolution.*

2. *By the characteristic distribution of the lesions.*[1] Indeed, the picture is usually that of a large area of bilateral and relatively symmetrical demyelination in the cerebral hemispheres (Fig. 154), which involves the corpus callosum — giving rise to the so-called "butterfly wing appearance" — and often the U fibers. The lesions predominate in the parieto-occipital regions. The gray matter is usually spared. The optic pathways are invariably involved. The brainstem and cerebellum are variously affected and often spared.

Fairly often these lesions are associated with isolated disseminated plaques that are remote from the main hemispheric focus ("transitional sclerosis").

In some cases, endocrine disturbances and especially *adrenal lesions* have been observed, and the frequency of cutaneous pigmentation or other clinical manifestations of adrenal insufficiency has been stressed. This association has been reported in examples of Schilder's disease that may or may not be familial, with or without inflammatory cellular infiltrates. The white matter lesions have been considered to be examples of either true Schilder's disease or sudanophilic leukodystrophy (adrenoleukodystrophy).[1]

THE LEUKODYSTROPHIES

Recognition of this group of diseases within the older framework encompassing the cerebral scleroses of childhood has gradually been achieved, with their separation from Schilder's disease by virtue of the lack of inflammatory cellular lesions and the frequency of genetic factors.

A number of characteristic features in the demyelinating process should be stressed: the frequently irregular character of the demyelination (Fig. 156); the sparing of U fibers; the frequent involvement of the cerebellum; the presence of a macrophagic reaction that is less intense than would be expected and whose distribution is diffuse

---

[1]*Balo's concentric sclerosis* is characterized by a heterogeneous appearance of the focus of demyelination which is produced by the alternation of concentrically arranged pale and darkly staining zones. Its histopathological structure is identical with that of Schilder's disease and multiple sclerosis.

[1]The view currently held by some authors is that the cases described in this section as showing the neuropathological picture of Schilder's disease are either examples of *transitional sclerosis* in which large multiloculated plaques of cerebral demyelination form a conspicuous element, or in reality examples of *adrenoleukodystrophy* occurring in males, either sporadically or more often as a familial disorder, and in whom the manifestations of addisonian insufficiency may either be evident, or minimal, or have escaped notice. According to this hypothesis therefore, Schilder's disease would no longer represent a distinct nosological entity and the eponym would lose all significance (translator's note).

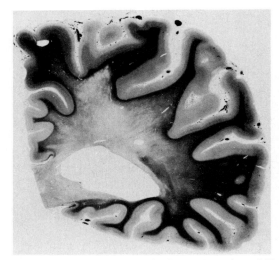

Figure 156. *Simple orthochromatic sudanophilic leukodystrophy.* Note the irregular distribution of the area of hemispheric demyelination.

rather than perivascular; and finally the distinct type of myelin catabolism in some forms, with the formation of nonsudanophilic and metachromatic prelipids.

In any event, this is a varied group of diseases in which very different conditions are included. Some of them are the result of a known disturbance of myelin metabolism. This has been demonstrated in *metachromatic leukodystrophy,* the most frequent in this group of disorders, consisting in a sulfatidosis due to absence of arylsulfatase A, and in *Krabbe's disease* or *globoid body leukodystrophy,* which is the result of a disturbance of cerebroside metabolism. These conditions are described in Chapter 9 in the section on nervous system diseases of metabolic and enzymatic origin (pp. 169–171).

Other leukodystrophies are still of uncertain pathophysiological origin, and it is therefore legitimate to retain them within the framework of diseases of the white matter. However, it should be stressed once again that most of them are, apparently, largely the result of a disturbance of myelin synthesis and that the term "dysmyelinating disease" is therefore preferable for these cases.

1. Sudanophilic leukodystrophies correspond to the group of diseases introduced in the preceding paragraph. They encompass a number of different disorders that have in

the past been grouped together solely because of the absence of inflammatory features and because of the sudanophilic character of the lipid material found in the white matter lesions.

a. The diffuse form, or **simple orthochromatic leukodystrophy** (Fig. 156), is the form that has generated the most extensive nosological debate about its separation from Schilder's disease. In sporadic cases, the distinction is particularly difficult. The absence of inflammatory cellular infiltrates and the frequent presence of axonal lesions are noteworthy features.

b. The tigroid forms are exemplified by *Pelizaeus-Merzbacher's disease,* which occurs at a very early age, i.e., from the first months of life, and has a very prolonged clinical course. Only male children are affected.

Essentially, the disease consists of a dysmyelinating process in which small islands of

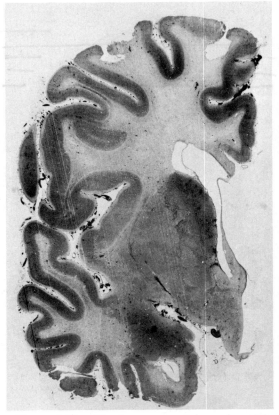

Figure 157. *Massive congenital sudanophilic leukodystrophy.* Complete absence of myelin (Loyez stain for myelin).

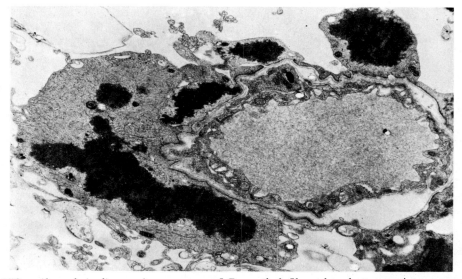

Figure 158. *Alexander's disease.* Appearance of Rosenthal fibers by electron microscopy. Electron-dense masses in pericapillary astrocytic cell processes. × 9300.

normal myelin, often perivascular in distribution, are found to persist along the main nerve fiber pathways. Axons are well preserved, and there is a striking contrast between the severity of the myelin changes and the paucity of the macrophagic reaction.

The cases of Lowenberg and Hill can be differentiated from the preceding form by their late onset in adult life and by the reverse distribution of the myelin changes, as a result of which demyelination presents a flecked appearance with irregular foci, often in a perivascular location.

c. The massive congenital forms (of Seitelberger type) give rise essentially to virtually total absence of central myelin (Fig. 157), with normal cranial and spinal nerves.

d. Sudanophilic leukodystrophies are *sometimes associated* with system degenerations, with phakomatoses such as meningeal angiomatosis, and with other metabolic changes (aminoacidurias, lipidoses, etc.).

2. Some authors also include two other diseases within the nosological context of the leukodystrophies. a. Alexander's disease is a rare condition characterized by mental retardation and, frequently, megalencephaly. The main pathological feature consists in the presence of elongated dense structures that are well demonstrated in

Mallory's phosphotungstic acid–hematoxylin (Rosenthal fibers or cytoid bodies). These structures as seen by electron microscopy are localized in the glial cell processes and consist of electron-dense osmiophilic masses closely related topographically to glial filaments. They often selectively involve the glial cells adjacent to the blood vessel walls (Fig. 158), to the ventricular cavities, and to the pial membrane. The precise relationship of these astrocytic lesions to the existence of myelin abnormalities, which are variable but often severe and associated with relative integrity of the axis cylinders, is now under discussion.

b. Spongy degeneration of the neuraxis (of van Bogaert and Bertrand; or Canavan's disease) is a familial condition occurring in the first years of life. Pathologically it consists in a spongy aspect of the subcortical layers of the cerebellar and cerebral white matter. By electron microscopy, the cavities seen in the areas of spongiosis appear to have been formed within the myelin sheaths following separation of the myelin lamellae: this appearance is similar to that seen in certain toxic forms of cerebral edema, especially following the use of tin salts.

On the other hand, spongiosis of the white matter may also be seen in various dysmetabolic processes of childhood.

Chapter 7

PATHOLOGY OF DEGENERATIVE DISEASES

Degenerative diseases of the central nervous system form a heterogeneous group of disorders in which the changes are chiefly neuronal and which occur sporadically, independently of any inflammatory, toxic, or metabolic factor known at this time. Genetic factors determine a large number of these conditions, which frequently have a familial character, but the pathogenetic mechanisms, which are probably enzymatic, are still unknown.

These diseases occur rather late in adult life, often in the presenile age group. To some extent the process tends to select certain neural structures: the cerebral cortex, when it gives rise to demential disorders; the basal ganglia, when it causes disturbances in which the symptomatology is extrapyramidal; or a number of spinocerebellar systems, as in the group of hereditary degenerative system diseases. However, many cases that show lesions predominating in certain selected anatomical areas may also demonstrate changes in other sites and thus present clinicopathological forms that are intermediary between the better defined nosological entities.

I. PATHOLOGY OF DEGENERATIVE CORTICAL DISEASES

Cortical degenerative processes constitute the most frequent neuropathological substratum of organic dementia.

Other disorders can, however, also cause symptoms of dementia. Some were in the past included within the framework of degenerative diseases, as for example *Creutzfeldt-Jakob disease*, which is today regarded as a slow-virus infection (see p. 120).

Inflammatory processes, as in general paralysis of the insane, and dysmetabolic disorders, like the lipidoses of late onset, may also give the picture of dementia associated with various neurological manifestations.

Vascular lesions, while liable to be responsible also for symptoms of dementia in the course of certain focal syndromes—as with some thalamic lesions, for example—are, however, more often found in association with the histological picture of senile dementia and may therefore be a constituent of mixed dementia.

Senile dementia and Alzheimer's disease account for approximately 80 per cent of cases in the group of degenerative cortical diseases.

1. Senile Dementia

Senile dementia causes only discrete cerebral atrophy, demonstrated by slight symmetrical thinning of the convolutions, predominant in the frontal lobes, and by a moderate degree of ventricular dilatation.

Microscopic lesions include senile plaques, neuronal cell changes, and vascular lesions of variable type and severity.

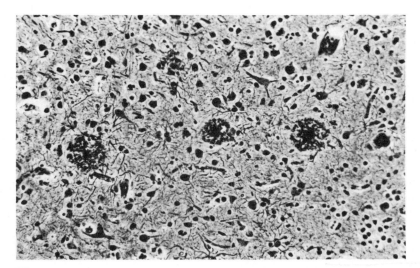

Figure 159. *Senile plaques in cerebral cortex of a case of senile dementia* (silver impregnation).

a. Senile plaques (Fig. 159) may occasionally be observed in physiological senescence. However, in senile dementia they are very abundant. They are best seen in silver impregnations, but are already visible in hematoxylin-eosin stains, where they form masses with a variable degree of eosinophilia surrounded by filamentous or microglial forms.

They present as rounded argyrophilic masses which may measure up to 50 μm.

They are arranged in a felt-like network of variable density, and suggest elements that are foreign to the central nervous system and displace preexisting structures. They are associated with only moderate glial reaction.

Plaques may have a target-like appearance, with a central amorphous part or nucleus, a peripheral felt-like filamentous rim, and a paler intermediary zone. However, the intermediary halo is often absent, and only the central nucleus and the peripheral rim may

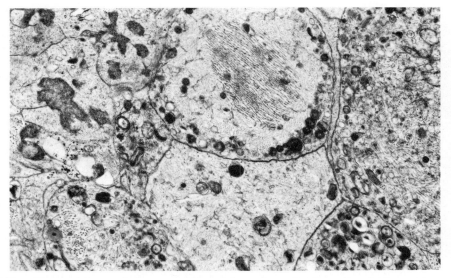

Figure 160. *Electron microscopic features at the periphery of a senile plaque.* Dendritic processes containing dense bodies, numerous mitochondria, and tubular profiles. ×12,000.

be demonstrated. In other places, plaques of smaller size (measuring 10 to 20 μm) simply form circular blobs with a fibrillary structure.

The central part demonstrates the features of amyloid, i.e., affinity for iodine, metachromasia with crystal violet, congophilia, birefringence, and PAS positivity. By electron microscopy filamentous structures identical with amyloid filaments have been seen. The peripheral portion of the plaque consists of a network of degenerated dendritic terminals and glial cell processes (Fig. 160).

Senile plaques are situated mainly in the superficial cortical layers. To a variable degree they are found in the entire cortical territories, with predominance in the frontal lobes and Ammon's horn. Preferential involvement of the latter site would seem to be more characteristic of certain forms of presbyophrenia or confabulating dementia of old age.

b. Among nerve cell changes, Alzheimer's neurofibrillary degeneration (see Fig. 9B) and granulovacuolar degeneration (see Fig. 9A), which were described in the chapter dealing with basic cellular lesions of the nervous system, are found with particular frequency, especially in Ammon's horns. The characteristic electron microscopic appearances of neurofibrillary tangles are shown in Figure 161. On the other hand, other nerve cell changes—especially excess of lipopigment and disappearance of Nissl bodies—are a commonplace finding with increasing age (see Fig. 7).

c. Vascular changes. *1.* A number of vascular alterations are part and parcel of the picture of senile degeneration and have the same significance as the changes previously described. This is the case with *dyshoric angiopathy,* a condition which is seen most frequently in the third layer of the calcarine gyrus and occasionally in Ammon's horn. This consists of an irregular moniliform thickening of the capillary and terminal arteriolar vessel walls, culminating in union of the vascular adventitia with the adjacent neural tissue. Dyshoric angiopathy is strongly argyrophilic and demonstrates the same tinctorial affinities as the centers of senile plaques, which explains why this condi-

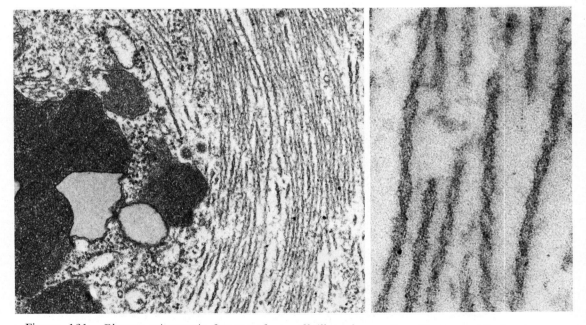

Figure 161. *Electron microscopic features of neurofibrillary degeneration.* Numerous "twisted neurotubules,"[1] near lipofuscin granules. *Left,* ×25,000. *Right,* ×120,000. (Courtesy of Dr. P. W. Lampert.)

[1] These structures are now believed to represent paired helical filaments. Their relationship to the normal neurofilaments is still uncertain (translator's note).

tion is regarded as a form of amyloid senile degeneration.

These features also align dyshoric angiopathy with *congophilic angiopathy,* a condition which is observed somewhat more frequently, especially in the superficial cortical layers, and involves arterioles of larger caliber.

2. Other vascular changes have no direct relationship to senility. These include *deep arteriolar hyalinosis* and *atherosclerosis* of the arteries over the convexity. Both vascular conditions may cause parenchymatous lesions, such as lacunae and cerebral infarcts.

The association of these vascular lesions and of senile degenerative lesions constitutes the pathological substratum of the group of *mixed dementias,* which occur just as frequently as pure senile dementia.

2. Alzheimer's Disease

Alzheimer's disease causes cerebral atrophy which is often very striking and affects diffusely the entirety of the cerebral convolutions (Fig. 162). Sometimes it may show a predilection for the parieto-occipital regions. It may also, though less often, give rise to circumscribed lobar atrophies which may present a clinical picture that is difficult to distinguish from Pick's disease when the frontal lobes are involved.

The microscopic lesions are those of senile dementia: they include senile plaques, and neurofibrillary and granulovacuolar degeneration, with absence of vascular changes.

They are, however, much more severe than in senile dementia.

In the eyes of most contemporary workers, the presence of features common to both conditions suggests an identical pathogenesis. The less severe changes of senile dementia are accordingly ascribed to a relatively late appearance of the process. In Alzheimer's disease, which occurs earlier and in which certain forms are known to occur in young adults — often on a familial basis — the lesions are of particular severity and culminate in a considerable degree of neuronal cell loss, accompanied by moderate astrocytic gliosis.

The lesions predominate in the parieto-occipital regions, where gross atrophy is most striking; this accounts for the wealth and early appearance of symptoms pointing to a combination of aphasia, apraxia, and agnosia associated with dementia. Less often, and to a lesser extent, the lesions may involve the basal ganglia and the reticular formation of the midbrain.

3. Pick's Disease

Pick's disease is frequently hereditary and presents a picture of circumscribed fronto-temporal cerebral atrophy which always spares the posterior third of the superior temporal gyrus (Fig. 163), thus accounting for the rarity of aphasic phenomena.

The parietal cortex is seldom involved and the occipital cortex is always spared. The an-

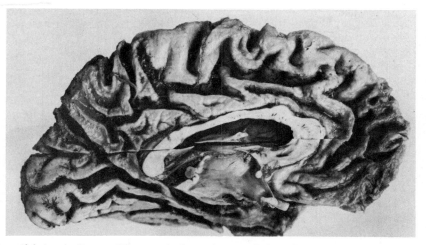

Figure 162.   *Alzheimer's disease, diffuse cortical atrophy.* (Medial surface of the left cerebral hemisphere.)

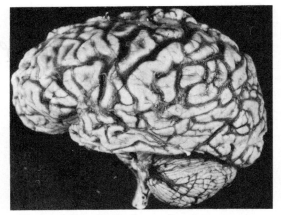

Figure 163. *Pick's disease.* Gross appearance.

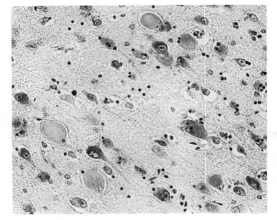

Figure 164. *Microscopic appearance of Pick's disease:* ballooned neurons in cerebral cortex (H. and E.).

terior frontotemporal ventricular dilatation, which is considerable, corresponds to the zones of cortical atrophy.

The microscopic lesions (Fig. 164), which occur at the above sites, include:

a. Cortical lesions, which are characterized by:

An extreme degree of neuronal cell loss associated with a frequently dense astrocytic gliosis and sometimes accompanied by a spongy state;

A picture of neuronal swelling (Fig. 164), which is seen in areas that are less severely affected (e.g., along the edges of the atrophied zones, in the deeper and secondarily altered layers of the cortex, and in Ammon's horn). This feature is regarded by some authors as corresponding to central chromatolysis resulting from retrograde degeneration. Such a view has been confirmed in the electron microscope, which in addition has sometimes demonstrated the presence of rounded granulovacuolar profiles containing filamentous structures measuring 20 nm (Pick's bodies) and other structures com-

posed of 10 nm filaments arranged in parallel and perpendicular arrays (Hirano bodies).

Intracytoplasmic argentophilic inclusions (see Fig. 10), which present as rounded bodies and are seen in only one-third of the cases, especially in neurons of Ammon's horn and of the amygdaloid nucleus.

b. White matter lesions, consisting in demyelination with gliosis of the centrum ovale and the temporal lobe, involving especially the frontopontine and temporopontine fascicles[1] and sometimes traceable down to the level of the brainstem.

c. Basal ganglia changes, which are frequent and involve the head of the caudate nuclei—often extremely atrophied—the rostral portion of the putamen, some of the thalamic structures and, less often, the pallidum.

---

[1]Some authors regard these white matter changes as the primary lesion and interpret the disorder as a systemic degenerative disease of these areas, with secondary involvement only of the cortex.

II. PATHOLOGY OF SUBCORTICAL DEGENERATIVE DISEASES

The subcortical degenerative diseases involve the basal ganglia to a variable degree and account for the majority of extrapyramidal syndromes.

1. Parkinson's Disease and Parkinsonian Syndromes

Besides Parkinson's disease proper, which is of degenerative origin, a number of processes of different etiology involve identical anatomical structures, thus resulting in a series of parkinsonian syndromes that are closely related clinically.

a. Parkinson's disease is the most frequent of the subcortical degenerative disorders. The lesions involve chiefly the pigmented nuclei of the brainstem, especially the substantia nigra, which is the origin of the dopaminergic nigrostriatal pathway.

Already on gross examination the substantia nigra appears pale (Fig. 165), especially in its lateral and medial ventral portions. Most of the neurons have disappeared, the scattered melanin pigment being frequently mobilized in a few macrophagic and glial cells, amidst which an astrocytic gliosis of variable severity may be found. In most cases, the residual neurons demonstrate rounded eosinophilic intracytoplasmic inclusion known as Lewy bodies (see Fig. 11). The *locus coeruleus*

and, to a lesser extent, the dorsal motor nucleus of X are the seat of comparable lesions. The neurons of the sympathetic ganglia are also often involved.

The globus pallidus demonstrates nonspecific changes only: these changes are pigmentary degeneration, with the presence of lipofuscin as commonly seen with increasing age, incrustation of the vessel walls by pseudocalcium, or enlargement of the perivascular spaces (status cribratus). Demyelination of the ansa lenticularis may also be present.

The putamen, which is the end-station of the nigrostriatal pathway and known to be the site of marked dopamine depletion in the disease, generally shows only discrete lesions that do not appear significant by light microscopy.

b. Nondegenerative **parkinsonian syndromes** to a variable extent show lesions in the same neural structures.

1. In postencephalitic parkinsonian syndromes involvement of the substantia nigra is the chief finding amidst more diffuse lesions. A few inflammatory cellular changes may be found. A fairly large number of cases show neurofibrillary degeneration in the residual neurons.

Lesions of the reticular formation in the midbrain and pons, with atrophy of the tegmentum, are frequently found.

2. Parkinsonian syndromes following carbon

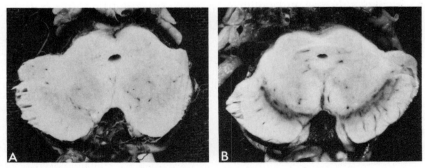

Figure 165. *Depigmentation of the substantia nigra in Parkinson's disease (A), compared with normal substantia nigra (B).*

monoxide poisoning are most frequently produced by necrotic pallidal lesions associated with cerebellar lesions. *Manganese* poisoning produces pallidal lesions in the same manner and frequently spares the substantia nigra, but the clinical picture is rather different from that of Parkinson's disease.

3. Parkinsonian syndromes of vascular origin are only exceptionally pure. In general, diffuse distribution of the lacunar lesions extends beyond the pigmented nuclei.

Parkinsonian syndromes of syphilitic origin have only seldom been systematically investigated from the pathological point of view.

2. Huntington's Chorea, or Chronic Chorea

Huntington's chorea is a familial disease of genetic origin which involves chiefly the corpus striatum and, to a variable degree, the cerebral cortex. The atrophy of the putamen and caudate nucleus selects preferentially the head of the caudate and is accompanied by ventricular dilatation of the frontal horns, which is often considerable (Fig. 166).

Microscopic lesions tend to predominate in the caudate nucleus and the anterosuperior portion of the putamen, and affect chiefly the small neurons. They are accompanied by dense fibrillary gliosis. Associated subcortical lesions which sometimes involve the subthalamic nuclei may be encountered.

The cerebral cortex, especially in the frontal and parietal regions, is most often the seat of neuronal cell loss, which predominates in the third and fourth layers and is accompanied by dense astrocytic gliosis. Transitional forms with Pick's disease and familial associations with the latter have been described.

3. Rarer Forms of Subcortical Degeneration

a. Striatonigral degeneration. This rare disease, in which the predominant clinical feature is extrapyramidal rigidity, is characterized by involvement of the substantia nigra and by considerable atrophy of the corpus striatum. The latter often presents

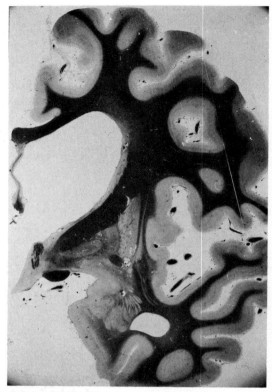

Figure 166. *Huntington's chorea. Gross appearance of the lesion in Loyez stain.* Atrophy of the caudate nucleus and putamen. Dilatation of frontal horn and cortical atrophy.

grossly with greenish discoloration due to the deposition of various pigments. In addition, it is the seat of neuronal cell loss which affects both large and small neurons, and of a marked gliosis. More discrete pallidal lesions are often associated.

b. Pure pallidal atrophy, which is often familial, is rare. It is associated most often with involvement of the subthalamic nuclei and sometimes with involvement of the striatum and substantia nigra.

c. Isolated atrophy of the subthalamic nuclei[1] is exceptional. It is most often associated with other pallidonigral degenerative lesions.

---

[1] In practice the symptomatology of hemiballismus is most frequently associated with a hemorrhagic lesion in the subthalamic nucleus.

d. Hallervorden-Spatz disease is characterized grossly by a rusty brown appearance of the pallidum and of the substantia nigra, and consists in the association of neuronal cell loss with the deposition of iron pigment. Axonal swellings in the shape of argyrophilic globular masses are sometimes visible.

The latter are especially characteristic of *neuroaxonal dystrophy,* a familial disease which, because of the similarity of this histological feature, is regarded by some authors as the infantile form of Hallervorden-Spatz disease.

e. Shy-Drager disease is a degenerative disorder in which an extrapyramidal syndrome is associated with orthostatic hypotension. It frequently involves the basal ganglia and particularly the striatonigral structures. However, the reported pathological picture is variable and may notably include ponto-cerebellar lesions.

The presence of lesions involving the vegetative nuclei in the floor of the fourth ventricle, the lateral horns of the spinal cord, and the peripheral sympathetic system accounts for the clinical picture of orthostatic

hypotension and indicates the diffuse nature of the degenerative process.[1]

f. Progressive supranuclear palsy, or **Steele-Richardson-Olszewski disease,** is responsible for a pathological picture that is characteristic for the type of lesions produced and for their topographical distribution.

These lesions consist of neuronal cell changes with neurofibrillary and granular degeneration, associated with astrocytic gliosis. They involve chiefly the nuclear structures of the reticular formation of the midbrain, the pretectal regions, the substantia nigra, the globus pallidus, the subthalamic nuclei, and the dentate nuclei. This topographical distribution accounts for the clinical picture of hypertonia, supranuclear ocular palsies, and disturbances of wakefulness.

---

[1]Some cases which show conspicuous lesions in the sympathetic ganglia and in the vegetative nuclei of the medulla and spinal cord, characterized by numerous Lewy bodies, apparently resemble Parkinson's disease.

III. PATHOLOGY OF CEREBELLAR DEGENERATIVE DISEASES

The complex group of cerebellar atrophies comprises all the degenerative disorders that involve the cerebellar cortex, its efferent pathways (cerebellofugal atrophies), and its afferent pathways (cerebellopetal atrophies). It includes a number of disorders that may vary according to whether the lesions show essentially a focal or a diffuse character, or according to which cerebellar system is affected.

A. CEREBELLAR ATROPHY WITH CHIEFLY CORTICAL INVOLVEMENT

1. Focal cerebellar atrophy. In the overwhelming majority of cases, this involves the

superior surface of the cerebellar hemispheres, especially the vermis, and produces *cerebello-olivary atrophy.*

The lesions include (Fig. 170*b*): *a. Cortical cerebellar lesions.* Already on *gross examination,* the atrophy demonstrates a characteristic systematic topographical distribution. It is localized to, or at least markedly predominates in, the upper surface of the cerebellum (Fig. 167*A*), where the cortical folia are shrunken and the sulci widened. Atrophy decreases in passing from the anterior to the posterior border and from the midline to the lateral borders, so that it is markedly preponderant in the superior vermis and adjacent portions of the lateral lobes, whereas appearances on the inferior surface are relatively normal.

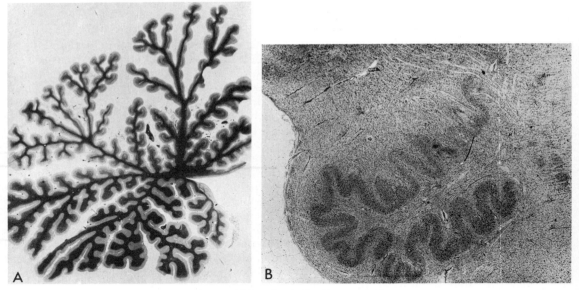

Figure 167.   *Cerebello-olivary atrophy.*

A, Atrophy of the vermis (Loyez stain for myelin). *B*, Cell loss in dorsal lamella of inferior olive (Nissl stain).

On microscopic examination, there is almost complete disappearance of Purkinje cells. Degeneration of their axons is indicated by demyelination in the fleece (amiculum) of the dentate nucleus. There is proliferation, of variable density, of Bergmann glia. A variable degree of neuronal cell loss in the granular and molecular layers is also seen.

b. *Lesions in the inferior olives* (Fig. 167*B*). These lesions consist of loss of neurons in the dorsal lamellae, accompanied by gliosis. This is generally regarded as the result of retrograde trans-synaptic degeneration, secondary to Purkinje cell loss.

c. Usually discrete *associated lesions* involving the spinal cord, the basal nuclei, or the substantia nigra are rather seldom observed.

The neuropathological picture described above is seen in: *a.* Holmes' *familial cerebello-olivary atrophy*, a rather infrequent disease.

b. *The late form of cortical cerebellar atrophy*, described by Marie, Foix and Alajouanine, in which cortical lesions would seem to be more concentrated and more marked in the vermis.

c. *Alcoholic cerebellar atrophy* (Fig. 189).

2. *Diffuse cerebellar atrophy.*[1] *1.* This is typically found in *paraneoplastic cerebellar atrophy*, the pathological picture of which has been dealt with elsewhere. Diffuse cerebellar atrophy seems to be more frequent when associated with neoplastic disease than as an isolated condition. In both instances there is characteristic cerebellofugal atrophy, with massive loss of Purkinje cells, sparing of basket cell fibers, and demyelination of the cerebellar white matter, which predominates in the region of the dentate nucleus. The dentate nucleus itself is spared (Fig. 170*c*).

2. *Congenital atrophy of the granular layer* is a familial disease found in children. It is

---

[1]The cerebellar cortex may be involved in a diffuse manner by various nondegenerative pathological processes. Thus, infantile lipidoses may cause atrophy of the granular layer with dendritic alterations of Purkinje cells that are comparable to those of congenital cerebellar atrophy. The presence of lipid neuronal storage products determines the differential diagnosis.

Anoxic processes and circulatory shock may produce changes in Purkinje cells and in the granular neurons. It will also be recalled that *postmortem* autolysis of the granular layer, which is a frequent finding and of artifactual origin, accounts in some cases for the picture of "état glacé" of the cerebellum.

characterized by massive loss of granular neurons (Fig. 170*d*). This causes global atrophy of the cerebellum, the abnormally slender folia of which are separated by widened sulci.

Loss of granular neurons and their axons (i.e., of parallel fibers) is virtually total. Purkinje cells are irregularly distributed, with ectopic displacements in the molecular layer. Their dendritic ramifications, which are often swollen, are deformed in the shapes of maces or cacti. Their axons are usually normal, but may sometimes show focal swellings in the form of torpedoes.

B. OTHER FORMS OF CEREBELLAR ATROPHY[1]

1. Olivopontocerebellar atrophy produces cerebellopetal atrophy which is remarkable by the involvement of fibers of pontine and olivary origin (Fig. 170*e*).

---

[1]"Crossed cerebellar atrophy" is not a degenerative disorder: it is secondary to massive involvement of the efferent corticopontine pathways at the level of the internal capsule and is characterized by general atrophy of the contralateral neocerebellar structures. It is rare and seen after a long period of survival, more often in children and young subjects than in adults, usually after certain forms of neonatal circulatory encephalopathy.

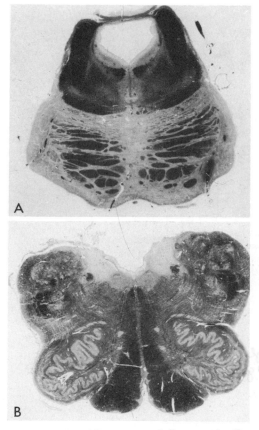

Figure 169. *Olivopontocerebellar atrophy* (Loyez stain for myelin).

A, Upper pons: massive demyelination of pontocerebellar fibers; sparing of the superior cerebellar peduncles, tegmentum, and pyramidal tracts.

B, Medulla: loss of olivocerebellar fibers; note the wedged appearance of the median raphe, due to loss of crossing fibers.

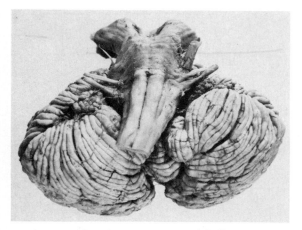

Figure 168. *Gross appearance of olivopontocerebellar atrophy.* Note severe atrophy of the basis pontis and of the middle cerebellar peduncles.

a. Olivopontocerebellar atrophy, which may occur in a sporadic form (Dejerine and André Thomas) or in a familial form (Menzel type), **is defined, as its name indicates, by lesions in the inferior olives, pons, and cerebellum:**

1. Atrophy of the inferior olives, with neuronal depopulation and degeneration of the olivocerebellar fibers (Fig. 169*B*).

2. Atrophy of the basis pontis (Figs. 168 and 169*A*), with loss of pontine nuclei and pontocerebellar fibers—which constitute the middle cerebellar peduncles.

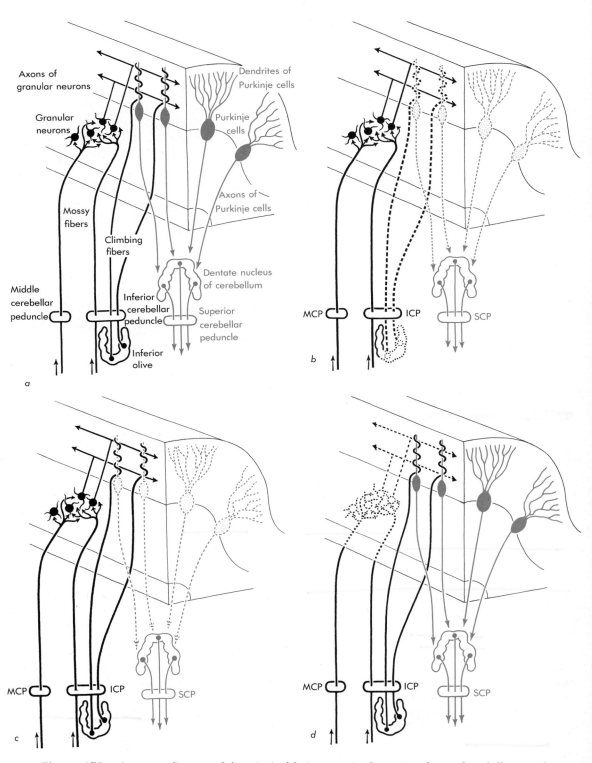

Figure 170. *Summary diagram of the principal lesions seen in the various forms of cerebellar atrophy.*

a, Normal cerebellum, *b,* cerebello-olivary atrophy; *c,* diffuse paraneoplastic cerebellar atrophy; *d,* congenital atrophy of the granular layer.

142

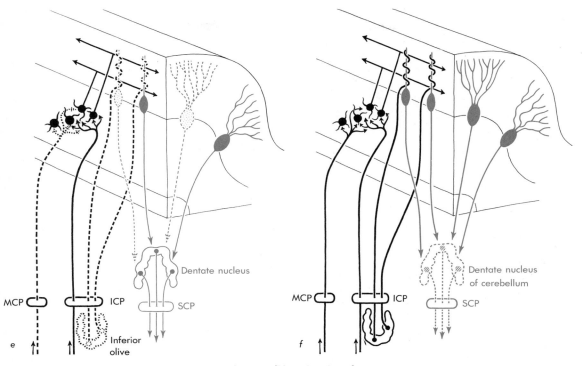

Figure 170. *Continued.*

e, Olivopontocerebellar atrophy; *f,* dentatorubral atrophy. *N.B.,* Main afferent pathways are shown *in black,* main efferent pathways *in red,* lost pathways are *stippled.*

3. Cerebellar atrophy, with a characteristic picture, consisting of:

Severe demyelination with gliosis of the central cerebellar white matter (to a large extent due to loss of olivocerebellar or pontocerebellar fibers);

Variable involvement of Purkinje cells, ranging from discrete rarefaction to complete cell loss:

Considerably less severe involvement or even sparing of granular neurons.

b. In actual fact, the triad of lesions described above are virtually never the only ones to be found in olivopontocerebellar atrophy, and other associated lesions, of variable severity, include:

1. Basal ganglia lesions, especially in the substantia nigra, which is affected practically constantly, less often in the corpus striatum, pallidum, or corpus Luysii.

2. Lesions in the dentate nuclei and their ef- *ferent fibers in the superior cerebellar peduncles,* of the kind seen in Ramsay Hunt syndrome.

3. Spinal cord lesions of the kind seen in Friedreich's ataxia, which are seen mostly in familial forms.

2. Dentatorubral atrophy (myoclonic cerebellar dyssynergia of Ramsay Hunt) is characterized by atrophy of the dentate nucleus and its efferent fibers in the superior cerebellar peduncles (Fig. 170*f*).

It is most often associated with lesions similar to those of Friedreich's ataxia and sometimes with lesions in the vestibular nuclei.

3. Opticocochleodentate degeneration is an exceptional condition. Primary degeneration of the optic pathways back to the superior corpora quadrigemina is associated with degeneration of the acoustic pathways, dentate nuclei, superior cerebellar peduncles, and frequently, spinocerebellar tracts.

IV. PATHOLOGY OF SPINAL MEDULLARY DEGENERATIVE DISEASES

Degenerative processes of the spinal cord affect, in various clinical conditions, a number of specific neuroanatomical fiber tract systems, but very often this systematic involvement of the spinal cord is accompanied by other lesions, especially in the cerebellum and basal ganglia. Similarly, it is frequently associated with lower motor neuron lesions involving the anterior horn cells and the ventral nerve roots, and with peripheral nervous system lesions involving the spinal root ganglia, dorsal nerve roots and peripheral nerve trunks. This accounts for the incidence of numerous transitional clinical and pathological forms, especially within the group of hereditary degenerative spinocerebellar diseases, and for the occurrence of different variants of system disorder within the same families.

1. Hereditary degenerative spinocerebellar diseases. Friedreich's ataxia is the most frequent and the best characterized of the group of spinocerebellar hereditary degenerative diseases (Fig. 174A).[1]

The most characteristic feature is involvement of the spinocerebellar tracts (Fig. 171). Chiefly affected are the dorsal spinocerebellar fascicle of Flechsig, which is demyelinated, and Clarke's columns, from which Flechsig's tract arises and from which the majority of nerve cells have disappeared. The ventral spinocerebellar tract of Gowers

is generally less severely involved, whereas neuronal cell loss in the posterior horns is more difficult to evaluate.

Involvement of the posterior columns is also constant and neuronal cell loss from the spinal root ganglia is frequently noted. The pyramidal tract is seldom intact and myelin pallor is frequently observed at that level.

Neuronal cell loss from some of the cranial nerve nuclei (XII, XI, VIII) is frequent.

In some cases, optic atrophy has been noted.

The cerebellum is fairly often altered, with irregular losses among the Purkinje cells. Involvement of the dentate nucleus is more frequent and is characterized by neuronal cell loss with demyelination of the superior cerebellar peduncles. These lesions, which are rather marked in some instances, constitute transitional forms with the Ramsay Hunt syndrome.

In a few examples there is atrophy of the anterior horn cells. This is accompanied by demyelination of the ventral nerve roots. This association with lower motor neuron and peripheral nervous system lesions suggests transitional forms to Charcot-Marie-Tooth disease.

2. Hereditary spasmodic paraplegia (Strumpell-Lorrain disease) (Fig. 174B). This is a rare condition, especially in its pure form. The lesions consist of bilateral atrophy of the pyramidal tracts throughout the entire length of the spinal cord. Involvement of the pyramidal pathways may be demonstrated higher up in the brainstem, and even degenerative cortical lesions restricted to the Betz cells have been described.

In actual fact, pyramidal tract disease, which is the dominant feature, is associated in most cases with involvement of the posterior columns and of the spinocerebellar tracts. Because of this association, this disorder appears related to the group of hereditary spinocerebellar degenerations.

---

[1]a. The nosological separation of the *hereditary cerebellar ataxia of Pierre Marie* is unclear from the pathological point of view. The few anatomically verified cases that seem to correspond to this clinical picture often show predominant involvement of the ventral spinocerebellar tracts. The cerebellum is often affected and the presence, in some instances, of associated olivopontocerebellar lesions has led some workers to include them within the group of olivopontocerebellar atrophy.

b. *Hereditary areflexic dystasia (Roussy-Levy syndrome)* is a purely clinical syndrome which, from the pathological point of view, appears to be an early form of either Friedreich's ataxia or Charcot-Marie-Tooth disease.

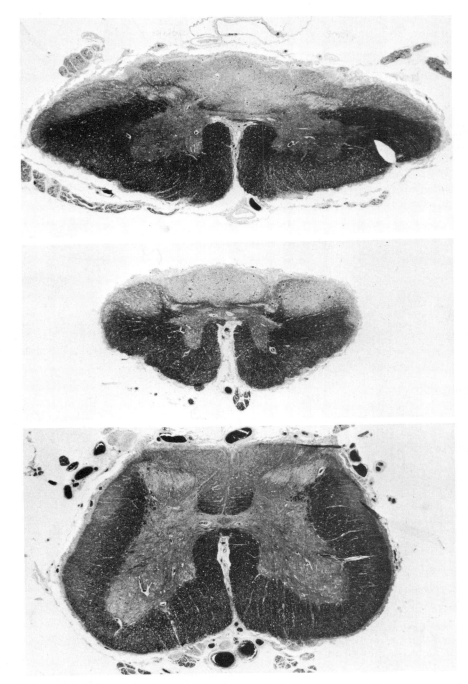

Figure 171. *Friedreich's ataxia* (Loyez stain for myelin). Involvement of the spinocerebellar tracts, mostly dorsal, and of the dorsal columns. Note discrete involvement of the pyramidal tracts in this case.

3. *Radiculospinal degenerative disorders.*
a. Charcot-Marie-Tooth disease. This condition, which is most often familial, involves both lower motor and peripheral sensory neurons (Fig. 174C).

Degenerative lesions affect chiefly the peripheral nerves, involving both axis cylinders and myelin sheaths, and are accompanied by interstitial fibrosis which is often of considerable severity. The spinal ganglia are often the seat of neuronal cell loss. Spinal cord lesions consist of nerve cell drop-out in the anterior horns, often accompanied by demyelination of the posterior columns.

Lesions in the more proximally situated neural structures are rare.

b. Hereditary sensory neuropathy of Denny-Brown. This disorder, which is associated with the picture of acropathia ulcero-mutilans (Thévenard), is often familial and involves peripheral sensory neurons. Degenerative lesions implicate the spinal ganglia, with massive neuronal cell loss, the dorsal nerve roots and the posterior columns (Fig. 174D).

The incidence of transitional forms to amyotrophic lateral sclerosis and to Friedreich's ataxia has been described, and cerebellar lesions have been noted in some cases.

c. Spinal hereditary amyotrophy, or Werdnig-Hoffmann disease (Fig. 174F). The

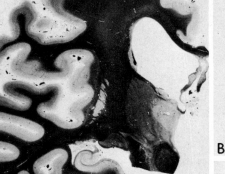

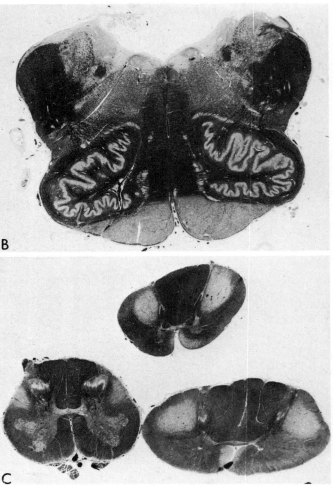

Figure 172. *Amyotrophic lateral sclerosis.* Pyramidal tract lesions are easily seen with the Loyez stain for myelin.

A, Cortical atrophy in frontal lobe; note also pallor in the centrum semiovale.

B, Demyelination of the medullary pyramids.

C, Demyelination of uncrossed and crossed spinal pyramidal tracts (cervical, thoracic, and lumbar).

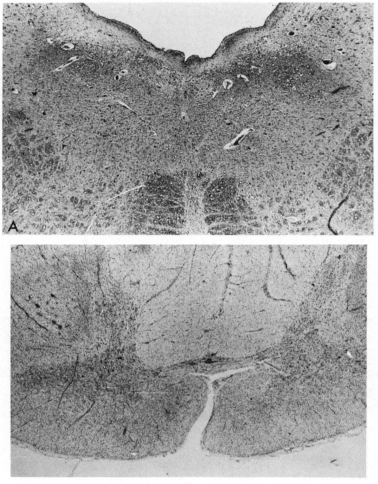

Figure 173. *Microscopic features of amyotrophic lateral sclerosis.*
A, Atrophy of twelfth cranial nerve nuclei (H. and E.). *B,* Atrophy of anterior horns of cervical cord; note also the gliosis in the lateral columns (Nissl stain).

lesions involve the anterior horns of the spinal cord and the nuclei of certain cranial nerves (VII, XII) and cause massive neuronal cell loss. A few residual neurons may show degenerative changes (cell retraction, neuronophagia) or the picture of chromatolysis. Fibrillary gliosis is present. The ventral nerve roots are atrophied and demyelinated. The posterior columns are not involved.

In some cases of arthrogryposis of nervous system origin, degenerative lesions are found in the anterior horns. However, this condition differs from Werdnig-Hoffmann disease by the presence of deformities in the extremities, which are noted from the time of birth, and by the absence of progression in the lesions.

d. Chronic anterior poliomyelitis (Fig. 174*F*). This disorder produces a degenerative lesion which evolves slowly in the adult. The changes caused are massive neuronal cell loss with gliosis in the anterior horns, and degeneration of the ventral nerve roots. Involvement of the medullary nuclei is a

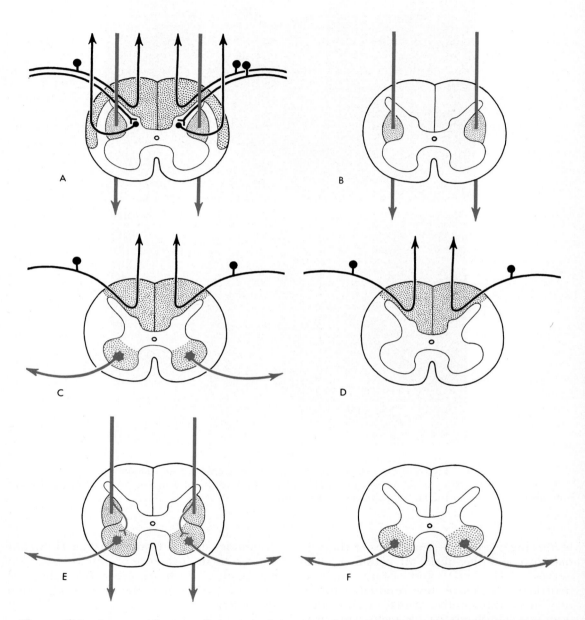

Figure 174. *Summary diagram of the main lesions seen in various forms of spinal and radiculospinal degenerative disorders.*

A, Friedreich's ataxia; *B*, hereditary spasmodic paraplegia; *C*, Charcot-Marie-Tooth disease; *D*, sensory neuropathy of Denny-Brown; *E*, amyotrophic lateral sclerosis; *F*, hereditary spinal amyotrophy and chronic anterior poliomyelitis.

late feature. Some of the more rapidly advancing forms are difficult to distinguish from amyotrophic lateral sclerosis.

4. Amyotrophic lateral sclerosis (Charcot's disease).[1]

This condition produces degenerative lesions of the pyramidal tracts associated with lesions of the lower motor neurons (Fig. 174E).

a. Pyramidal involvement (Fig. 172) is characterized by demyelination and gliosis of the lateral and anterior columns. In the lateral columns myelin pallor, which is often massive, spreads to a greater or lesser degree to involve the spinocerebellar tracts. Pyramidal tract involvement is often well seen in the

---

[1] Special variants of this condition have been recorded. Thus, familial forms have been described in Guam, which are characterized by the presence of neuronal cell changes with neurofibrillary degeneration and by the association of variable lesions in the basal ganglia and in a number of cortical and spinal cord structures. This familial form of amyotrophic lateral sclerosis appears to be restricted to a particular ethnic group in Guam, who may also develop a picture of dementia with extrapyramidal involvement (parkinsonian dementia syndrome of Guam).

medulla and, to a lesser degree, in the posterior limb of the internal capsule. Cortical lesions are usually found in the motor cortex and involve the Betz cells and the pyramidal neurons of the third and fifth layers, which either have disappeared or may present chromatolytic changes followed by cell retraction and atrophy. In some cases, the lesions spread over the remainder of the cerebral cortex, thus accounting for a form of dementia which, from the nosological point of view, is difficult to distinguish from Creutzfeldt-Jakob disease and Pick's disease.

b. Involvement of the anterior horns is typical. Grossly, they appear gray and retracted and are accompanied by atrophy of the ventral nerve roots. Microscopically, there is massive neuronal cell loss with gliosis, especially in the cervical and lumbar enlargements (Fig. 173B).

c. Involvement of cranial nerve nuclei of the medulla (XII, XI, and dorsal motor nuclei of X) is the predominant feature in bulbar forms, which are characterized clinically by labioglossopharyngeal paralysis (Fig. 173A).

Chapter 8

NEUROPATHOLOGY OF GENERAL PATHOLOGICAL PROCESSES

A number of major general pathological processes—namely, metabolic disturbances, certain intoxications, and various visceral lesions—can produce changes in the central and/or peripheral nervous system. These changes, which are usually nonspecific, depend on the interplay of various factors, which may be contributed by anoxia, deficiency disorders and, less often, toxicity.

CEREBRAL LESIONS OF ANOXIC NATURE

1. *Cerebral Anoxia*

In anoxia there is selective involvement of some of the cerebral territories. Two main theories have been proposed to account for this selectivity: the first postulates that there is predominant involvement of some of the cortical structures because they are better vascularized and metabolically more active; the second theory presupposes specific vulnerability, probably enzymatic, on the part of particular neuronal cell groups.

Cerebral anoxia, or decrease in the amount of oxygen available to nerve cells, may be the result of three principal mechanisms:

Anoxemic anoxia, following a drop in the partial pressure of oxygen (asphyxia, respiratory paralysis, anesthesia, etc.);

Anemic anoxia, following exsanguination or cardiac arrest;

Histotoxic anoxia, following inhibition of intracellular respiratory enzyme systems (e.g., in cyanide poisoning).

a. Anoxemic anoxia. Hyperacute forms, especially rapidly fatal asphyxia, produce a picture of meningeal and cortical congestion with venous and capillary dilatation which gives to the cortical ribbon and the basal ganglia a characteristic lilac appearance (Fig. 175). Hemorrhages with a perivascular distribution are frequent and predominate in the white matter and corpus callosum.

In less sudden forms of anoxia, when death is delayed, the lesions are remarkable by their systematic distribution. They consist of neuronal ischemic cell changes (see Fig. 1) which culminate in neuronal cell loss with gliosis. They often produce a spongy state with edema, capillary proliferation, and endothelial swelling (see Fig. 22). Less often,

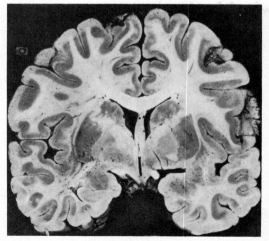

Figure 175. *Cerebral anoxia.* Lilac discoloration of cortex and basal ganglia.

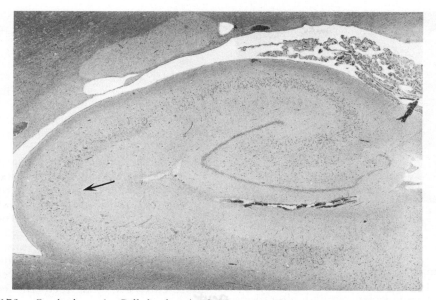

Figure 176. *Cerebral anoxia.* Cellular loss in the Sommer sector (see arrow) of Ammon's horn.

when the course is prolonged, actual necrotic foci may be found, which culminate in the formation of cavities in which areas of astrocytic glial proliferation may be present.

These lesions, which are chiefly cortical, predominate in the third layer. Occasionally in severe cases the whole of the cortical ribbon is involved. The superficial layers, which are spared, are often the seat of an intense astrocytic gliosis.

There is a special tendency for the Am-

mon's horn to be affected, especially the Sommer section (Fig. 176).

In the basal ganglia, the globus pallidus is the seat of the most severe changes, and cavitating necrotic lesions may be seen (Fig. 178).

The Purkinje cells of the cerebellum, the dentate nuclei, and the inferior olives are also highly vulnerable to anoxia.

The white matter is usually better preserved.

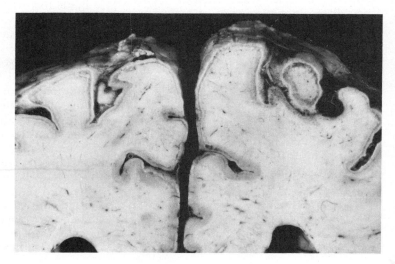

Figure 177. *Cortical laminar necrosis in cardiac arrest.* Gross appearance.

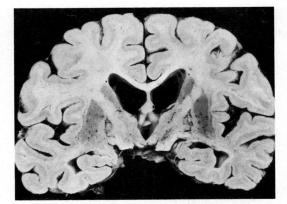

Figure 178. *Gross appearance of carbon monoxide poisoning:* bilateral necrosis of the pallidum.

b. Anemic anoxia. Anemic anoxia, which may result from circulatory arrest, as in cardiac arrest, causes similar alterations. The laminar cortical lesion may, however, be more severe and more diffuse (Fig. 177). These changes predominate mostly in the posterior parieto-occipital areas, whereas Ammon's horns are sometimes less severely affected. They often result in diffuse decortication.

Among the subcortical structures, the caudate nucleus and the putamen are more frequently involved than the globus pallidus.

c. Histotoxic anoxia. Histotoxic anoxia, of the kind produced by cyanide poisoning, frequently causes lesions that predominate in the white matter. This is especially so in some forms of experimental poisoning, which may result in demyelinating lesions in which the corpus callosum is chiefly involved.

In fact, this separation of cerebral anoxia into three types is rather arbitrary and, most often, the various lesions described above are found in association. However, the selective vulnerability of certain areas of the central nervous system remains a fairly constant feature. This is illustrated, for instance, in the case of carbon monoxide poisoning.

2. *Carbon Monoxide Poisoning*

Three main types of cerebral lesion are recognized.

1. Vascular congestion and hemorrhage may be the only lesions that are seen in rapidly fatal *hyperacute poisoning.*

2. Characteristic gray matter changes are visible when survival exceeds 48 hours. They consist of:
a. Laminar cortical lesions, which predominate in Ammon's horn (Fig. 176).
b. Pallidal lesions (Fig. 178). Necrosis of the globus pallidus, which is characteristic of anoxic damage, is seen here at its most typical and accounts for the extrapyramidal syndromes that follow carbon monoxide poisoning. The necrosis is localized to the superomedial portion of the external pallidum. It most often consists in an elongated slit which contains a few compound granular corpuscles, but occasionally presents as a more extensive cystic focus of necrosis. The vascular lesions, in which the vessel walls are encrusted with pseudocalcium and which are regarded as a classic feature, may be seen also in other pathological processes.

3. White matter changes are frequent. They may be caused by several mechanisms.

They may consist of acute initial lesions with a hemorrhagic character, of the kind seen in acute asphyxia.

In other instances, a circulatory factor may be invoked, as in the case of elongated necrotic lesions in the white matter of the inferior portion of the centrum ovale. These may culminate in the formation of actual cystic foci when survival has been sufficiently prolonged.

More characteristic are the features of diffuse demyelination known by the name of Grinker's myelopathy (Fig. 179). These are characterized by a spongy state with demyelination, often of spotty appearance, extending along white matter tracts and accompanied by sudanophilic myelin breakdown and an astrocytic gliosis that is often striking. Some degree of sparing of the perivascular myelin is frequently noted. This picture seems to be related, in most cases, to a late delayed stage of carbon monoxide poisoning following a variable "silent" time interval. The part played by anoxia has been the subject of debate, and it has been suggested that carbon monoxide may have a direct toxic effect on the interfascicular oligodendroglia. Contingent circulatory factors or changes resulting from the evolution of edematous lesions initiated by anoxia appear to be the more likely pathogenetic mechanism.

PATHOLOGY OF DEFICIENCY DISEASES

Deficiency disorders, especially avitaminoses, may cause lesions in the central nervous system that are frequently associated with changes in the peripheral nervous system.

1. Wernicke's Encephalopathy[1]

a. The pathological process (Fig. 180) is characterized by the association of the following lesions, which may vary in extent from case to case:

Microscopic or sometimes more extensive petechial hemorrhagic foci, which have an orange-yellow color in relatively late cases;

A spongy state with glial astrocytic and microglial proliferation; and, especially,

Capillary proliferation with hyperplasia of the blood vessel walls. This has often been noted to be a conspicuous feature, but its primary nature has been debated (Fig. 180A).

By contrast, and paradoxically, neurons are often spared and may demonstrate only the late lesions of central chromatolysis.

b. The topographical distribution of the lesions (Figs. 182 and 183) is the most characteristic feature of the disease. This ac-

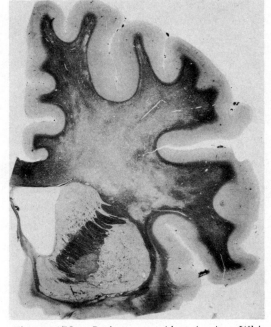

Figure 179. *Carbon monoxide poisoning.* White matter demyelination in a case of Grinker's myelopathy (Loyez stain).

counts for the symptoms, which include disturbances of wakefulness, hypertonic phenomena, and ocular palsies.

The periventricular regions, the medial formations of the thalamus and the massa intermedia, the floor of the third ventricle, and especially the mamillary bodies (Fig. 181)—which present a yellowish orange appearance—are the most frequently involved. Similarly, the periaqueductal region at the level of the third cranial nerve nuclei, the reticular formation of the midbrain, and the posterior corpora quadrigemina are typically affected. Involvement of the floor of the fourth ventricle at the level of the medulla (dorsal motor nuclei of the tenth cranial nerve) accounts for the terminal vegetative disturbances in some cases.

Peripheral nerve lesions often complete the pathological picture.

c. The principal causes of Wernicke's encephalopathy are
1. Vitamin B_1 deficiency in beriberi.
2. Starvation due to fasting or famine.

---

[1]Because of the resemblance of the lesions described by Wernicke in 1881 in "acute superior hemorrhagic polioencephalitis" to those of an earlier case reported by Gayet in 1875, this disease is sometimes referred to as Gayet-Wernicke's encephalopathy in the French literature. On the other hand, in order to underscore the etiological and histopathological relationship of these lesions to those of Korsakoff's alcoholic syndrome, which was described in 1884, other workers, particularly in English-speaking countries, prefer the term "Wernicke-Korsakoff encephalopathy."

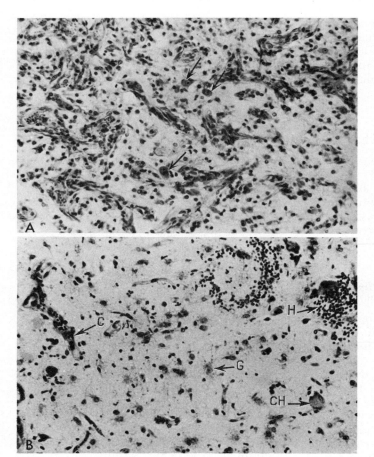

Figure 180. *Microscopic appearance of the lesions of Wernicke's encephalopathy.*

A, Capillary lesions, with swelling of endothelial capillary walls; note the normal appearance of a few neurons (see arrows) (Nissl stain).

B, Microhemorrhages (*H*), neuronal chromatolysis (*CH*), moderate astrocytic gliosis (*G*), and endothelial capillary swelling (*C*) in mesencephalic tegmentum.

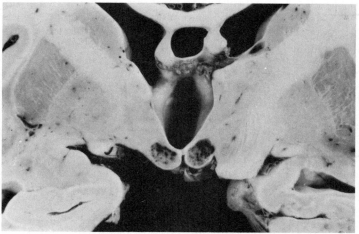

Figure 181. *Wernicke's encephalopathy.* Recent hemorrhagic lesions in the mamillary bodies.

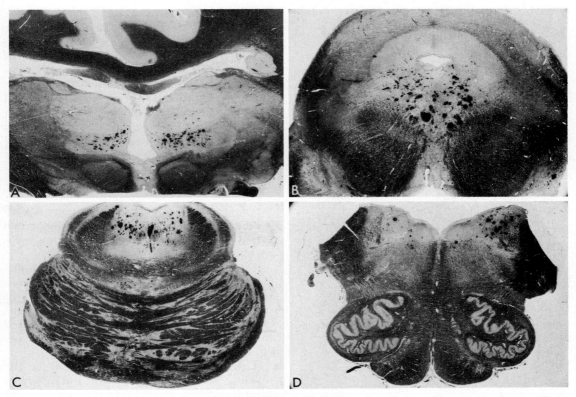

Figure 182. *Wernicke's encephalopathy; topographical distribution of the lesions* (Loyez stain for myelin).

A, Periventricular hemorrhagic thalamic lesions.
B, Lesions in the tegmentum of the midbrain at the level of the third cranial nerve nuclei.
C, Hemorrhages in tegmentum of upper pons.
D, Hemorrhagic lesions in the medullary floor of the fourth ventricle.

3. Inadequate intake resulting from esophageal stenosis or uncontrolled vomiting.

4. Secondary nutritional deficiencies resulting from alimentary tract lesions in the course of certain intoxications, as in chronic alcoholism.

2. Pellagra Encephalopathy

a. The lesions (Fig. 184) consist of isolated neuronal changes characterized by cellular chromatolysis, without associated glial or vascular alterations.

The lesions affect, in decreasing order of frequency, the Betz cells of the motor cortex, the pontine nuclei, the dorsal nuclei of the vagus, the nucleus ambiguus, the trigeminal

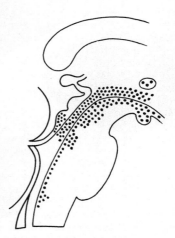

Figure 183. *Diagram showing topographical distribution of the lesions in Wernicke's encephalopathy.*

[handwritten notes:]
– motor cortex (Betz)
– pontine n
– dorsal n of X, n. ambig
– V, III VIII (vestib)
– ant horn cells

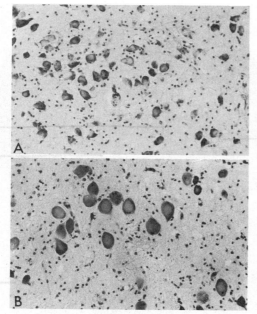

Figure 184. *Pellagra encephalopathy. Microscopic picture of cell chromatolysis* (Nissl stain). *A*, In nuclei pontis. *B*, In vestibular nucleus.

nerve nuclei, the oculomotor nuclei, the vestibular nuclei, the nuclei of the reticular formation, and the anterior horn cells of the spinal cord.

b. The chief causes are:

1. Pellagra produced by lack of PP factor;

2. A number of deficiency disorders observed in the course of complex states of malnutrition or in a number of chronic alcoholics (i.e., so-called "pseudopellagra encephalopathy," since lack of PP factor has not been conclusively established in these cases);

3. So-called "endogenous pellagra," due to a disturbance of tryptophan metabolism.

3. Avitaminosis B_{12}

Avitaminosis B_{12} elicits the picture of subacute combined degeneration of the spinal cord, which is seen in neuroanemic syndromes.

The lesions consist in a type of symmetrical bilateral demyelination which begins centrally to involve at first the posterior columns of the spinal cord and then spreads to the lateral columns, which are evenly affected throughout their entire length. A small peripheral zone is often spared (Fig. 185).

The primary lesion seems to involve the myelin, with swelling and degeneration of myelin sheaths, which present an edematous, spongy and areolar microscopic appearance. There is rapid secondary degeneration of

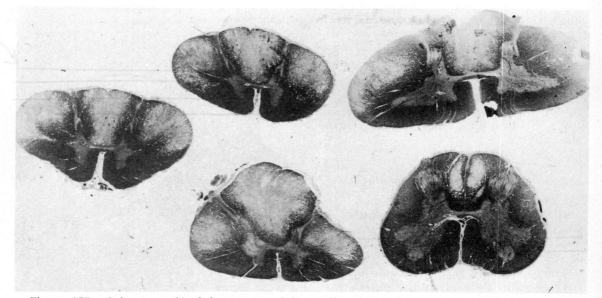

Figure 185. *Subacute combined degeneration of the spinal cord* (Loyez stain for myelin). Note demyelination and spongy appearance of the lateral and posterior columns.

the axis cylinders with contingent gliosis, which is often moderate and late.

ENCEPHALOPATHIES OF METABOLIC ORIGIN

The term "metabolic encephalopathy" is often used in a clinical setting to describe a number of cerebral disturbances secondary to general metabolic disorders. Because of its intense metabolic activity, the brain may be exquisitely sensitive to highly different biological conditions. Nevertheless, the lesions that may be seen are mostly nonspecific, and then usually related to various visceral lesions or to anoxic disturbances, which may be direct or indirect.

a. Respiratory encephalopathies are generally secondary to chronic bronchopulmonary disease and essentially attributable to hypoxia and hypercapnia. They are characterized by diffuse vasodilatation, microscopic hemorrhagic features, and anoxic neuronal lesions of variable intensity (see p. 150).

b. Hepatic insufficiency. *1. The lesions* consist of glial changes which involve astrocytic nuclei and present the picture of Alzheimer type II glia or "naked nuclei gliosis" (see the discussion on basic cellular lesions of the glia on p. 9) (see Fig. 16).

These lesions predominate in the globus pallidus, but may also be seen in the dentate nucleus and the cerebral cortex.

2. Principal causes include:

Severe hepatic insufficiency, as in terminal coma in cases of hepatic cirrhosis and in a number of cases with severe hepatitis.

Portocaval encephalopathy.

Wilson's disease (hepatolenticular degeneration).

c. On the other hand, **pancreatic encephalopathy** shows only nonspecific terminal changes. White matter lesions, especially in the cerebellum, have occasionally been described, but they are exceptional.

d. Hypoglycemic coma. Hypoglycemic coma, due to excessive insulin therapy or to insulin-secreting tumors, causes fairly specific cerebral lesions. The disturbance in glucose metabolism, which culminates in cessation of glucose consumption and in nonutilization of oxygen, produces changes that have been compared with those seen in cerebral anoxia.

Indeed, the cortical involvement is similar. It may result in necrosis of the entire cortical ribbon, but most often has a laminar distribution and implicates the third or the fifth cortical layer. Neurons are often pale, ballooned, and homogenized, rather than shrunken and hyperchromatic as in true ischemic and anoxic processes. Involvement of Ammon's horn is particularly conspicuous; the caudate nucleus and putamen are greatly altered—the small neurons being more vulnerable than the large—and the Purkinje cells of the cerebellum are less often involved than in anoxia.

e. Disorders of iron metabolism. In primary or secondary *hemochromatosis*, the blood-brain barrier provides an efficient protection against the diffusion of iron pigment into the central nervous system, and consequently cerebral lesions remain very restricted.

The sole regions affected are those in which there is no blood-brain barrier. Thus, the only areas impregnated by hemosiderin and therefore showing a reddish orange aspect to the naked eye and a marked microscopic Prussian blue reaction with ferrocyanide are the choroid plexuses, the area postrema in the medulla, the pineal gland, and a number of vestigial remnants such as the paraphysis and the subfornical organ.

f. Disorders of calcium metabolism. A number of instances of hypoparathyroidism may, exceptionally, be at the origin of the pathological picture of so-called *Fahr's disease*, which is characterized by massive perivascular deposits of pseudocalcium in the basal ganglia, especially in the caudate nuclei.

TOXIC ENCEPHALOPATHIES

The central nervous system displays a varying degree of sensitivity toward toxic substances which is attributable in part to the protective presence of the blood-brain barrier. Two general features should, moreover, be emphasized:

The selective vulnerability of some of the neural structures;

The diversity of lesions observed and of their different mechanisms.

The neuropathological picture is highly variable, and it is difficult to correlate a particular type of lesion with a specific etiology. Thus, in some of the hyperacute forms of poisoning the course may be so rapid that there is no time for histological changes to appear. In other instances, the changes that are seen often have no diagnostic significance by themselves, as for example, in the case of edematous or hemorrhagic lesions. Furthermore, in the majority of cases these lesions are actually to be ascribed to multiple visceral disturbances due to toxic damage. The latter may include cardiovascular disorders, which may present with sudden generalized circulatory collapse or with acute hypertension; cardiopulmonary difficulties, which may be responsible for cerebral anoxia; severe hepatic or renal damage; or secondary deficiency disturbances, such as those that follow damage to the digestive tract in chronic alcoholism. Finally, it is necessary to stress the frequent presence of associated peripheral nervous system lesions. These, as in lead poisoning, for instance, are apparently due to direct toxic damage.

Intoxications produced by heavy metals and by certain metalloids and organic compounds are essentially responsible for edematous and hemorrhagic lesions which are associated with acute neuronal changes. Direct toxic effects chiefly interfere with intracellular enzymatic processes, especially with those concerned with oxidation-reduction mechanisms. Visceral lesions are the rule.

a. Lead poisoning may cause acute encephalopathy, in which cerebromeningeal edematous lesions due to hypertensive episodes are associated with purpuric hemorrhagic extravasations and with lesions in the optic pathways.

In addition to changes in the peripheral nervous system, tetraethyl lead may produce cerebral lesions that are comparable to those of Wernicke's encephalopathy.

b. In acute arsenical poisoning the lesions, which are characterized by hemorrhagic diapedesis, predominate in the white matter and are associated with foci of necrosis and demyelination. It is likely that increased capillary permeability and allergic hypersensitivity play a part in the genesis of these lesions.

c. Bismuth salts may, after prolonged intake by mouth, be occasionally responsible for a picture of encephalopathy in which the lesions are most often nonspecific and of which the pathophysiology is still poorly understood.

d. Various organic compounds may similarly produce cerebral lesions in which edema is conspicuous (e.g., poisonous fungi, tin salts).

e. Various drugs [e.g., isoniazid (INAH) nitrofurantoin, vincristine, iodoquinoline] may, in certain conditions, cause peripheral nervous system lesions by affecting either the myelin sheaths or the neuronal cell body and the axon.

CHRONIC ALCOHOLISM

Chronic alcoholism illustrates perfectly the intricate role played by the various visceral lesions caused by alcohol in determining cerebral lesions. Whereas the general assumption that alcohol has a direct toxic effect on the nervous system has not been clearly established, the part played by hepatic changes and by deficiency disorders secondary to avitaminosis is, on the other hand, quite evident.

1. Cerebral Lesions Due to Hepatic Insufficiency
(see p. 157)

These lesions are essentially the result of a state of decompensated cirrhosis that has culminated in hepatic coma.

2. Cerebral Lesions of Deficiency Origin

a.   Wernicke's alcoholic encephalopathy. The lesions of Wernicke's encephalopathy are indeed most frequently observed in chronic alcoholism. They are secondary to deficiency of vitamin B_1 absorption, due to alcoholic gastritis (see above).

b.   Korsakoff's syndrome. Korsakoff's syndrome in alcoholics is regarded today as a late chronic stage of Wernicke's encephalopathy.

Predominant involvement of the mamillary bodies, which are orange-yellow and atrophied (Fig. 186), accounts for memory disturbances, with fixation amnesia, confabulation, and temporospatial disorientation. Other lesions, especially in the dorsomedial nucleus of the thalamus and in the midbrain, are often noted.[1]

The association of peripheral nervous system lesions (polyneuritis) with psychotic disturbances completes the final picture of nervous system involvement in this deficiency disorder.

c.   Pseudopellagra encephalopathy of chronic alcoholism. The predominance of chromatolytic neuronal lesions (Fig. 184) in a number of instances of deficiency encephalopathy associated with alcoholism has suggested, without definite proof, that lack of PP factor may play a part.

3. Alcoholic Encephalopathies of Undetermined Nature

a.   Marchiafava-Bignami disease. Marchiafava-Bignami disease is a rare disorder the pathophysiology of which is unknown and which is observed only in chronic alcoholism of long duration and great severity.

It produces, in various cases, either a *necrosis* (Fig. 187A and B), the appearance and course of which are comparable to necrosis of ischemic origin, or *demyelination with atrophy of the corpus callosum*, with relative sparing of axons (Fig. 187C).

Involvement of the corpus callosum, *other white matter lesions* which is constant, is often associated with white matter lesions in other areas, especially the anterior commissure, the hemispheric white matter, the middle cerebellar peduncles, and the optic nerves and tracts.

b.   Central pontine myelinolysis. This

---

[1]The analogy has been drawn between involvement of the mamillary bodies in the causation of memory disturbances in deficiency disorders and their implication in other pathological processes, either alone or concomitant with involvement of the hippocampal formations, the trigonal formations and the thalamic nuclei, to which the mamillary bodies are connected by Papez's circuit (Korsakoff's syndrome due to tumors, vascular diseases, degenerative processes, etc.).

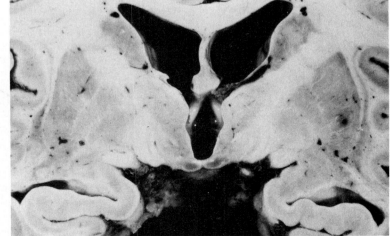

Figure 186. *Korsakoff's syndrome of alcoholic origin.* Note the atrophy and pigmentation of the mamillary bodies.

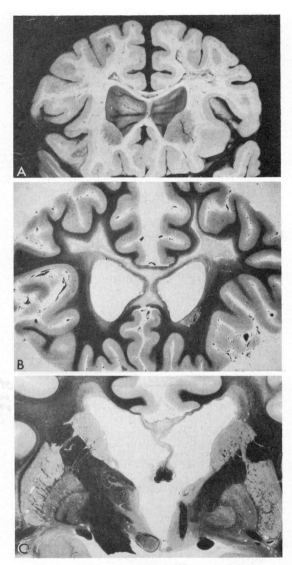

Figure 187. *Marchiafava-Bignami disease.*

A, Gross appearance showing necrosis of the corpus callosum.

B, Same picture with Loyez stain for myelin; note involvement of the adjacent white matter.

C, Atrophy of the corpus callosum.

is again a rare disease, whose pathophysiology is the subject of debate. It is seen mainly in chronic alcoholics, but may be met also in other conditions in which severe metabolic and electrolytic disturbances are present, as,

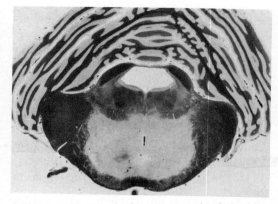

Figure 188. *Central pontine myelinolysis* (Loyez stain for myelin).

for example, in the course of treatment for severe renal or hepatic insufficiency.

The disease presents a histopathological picture with a type of demyelination which is similar to that seen in Marchiafava-Bignami disease, but with a characteristic site of predilection, namely the basis of the midpons (Fig. 188), and with the occasional association of lesions of the same type in the middle cerebellar peduncles and the anterior commissure.

c. Among cortical lesions, the picture of *Morel's laminar sclerosis* is the best known. This consists in a glial astrocytic band-like proliferation localized in the third cortical layer, especially in the lateral frontal cortex. The disease is frequently associated with the callosal lesions of Marchiafava-Bignami disease.

In addition, spongy lesions, cellular chromatolysis and neural cell losses are often seen in the cerebral cortex of chronic alcoholics. Their exact mechanism is probably variable.

d. Alcoholic cerebellar atrophy. Aside from Purkinje cell changes due to anoxic phenomena caused by episodes of coma, more specific cerebellar lesions have been described as characteristic.

They result in cortical cerebellar atrophy which predominates in the vermis (Fig. 189) and is associated with lesions of the dorsal laminae of the inferior olives. This is comparable to Holmes' cerebello-olivary atrophy.

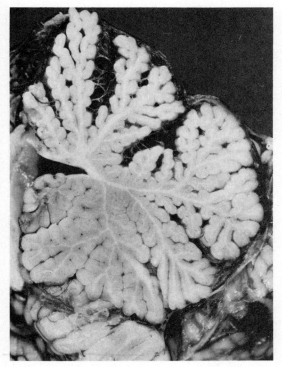

Figure 189. *Alcoholic cerebellar atrophy, with predominant involvement of the vermis.* Gross picture of a sagittal section through the vermis.

NERVOUS SYSTEM LESIONS DUE TO MALIGNANT VISCERAL DISEASE IN THE ABSENCE OF TUMOR DEPOSITS

Under the preceding heading, or more frequently under the term "paraneoplastic syndrome," various nervous system manifestations of a nonneoplastic nature have been described in which the development of pathological changes is attributable to distant visceral malignant disease. All types of cancer may account for these relatively infrequent lesions, but anaplastic bronchial carcinoma is most often the source.

Various skeletal muscle syndromes—e.g., polymyositis and dermatomyositis (which are discussed elsewhere) as well as so-called neuromyositis—are the most frequent in this group. Isolated nervous system lesions are less common, but may account for a clinicopathological picture that is highly characteristic. Their pathogenesis is still obscure: the mechanisms invoked include viral superinfection, carcinotoxic processes, deficiency disorders, competitive needs between the tumor and the rest of the body, and allergic responses.

a. Paraneoplastic sensory neuropathy, which is found in association with undifferentiated bronchial carcinoma, is characterized by spinal root ganglia lesions and demyelination of the nerve roots and posterior columns (Fig. 190).

Motor neuropathy has also been observed, but is exceptional. By contrast, *mixed sensorimotor neuropathy,* which is characterized by predominantly demyelinating lesions, is more frequent.

b. Necrotizing myelopathy, either resembling transverse myelitis and mimicking the picture of acute necrotizing myelopathy (see above, p. 126) or consisting of diffuse

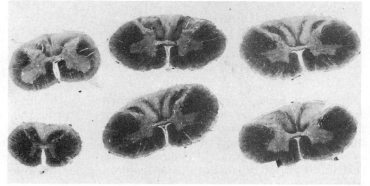

Figure 190. *Paraneoplastic sensory neuropathy in carcinoma of the bronchus.* Note demyelination of the posterior columns.

multiple lesions, has also been observed in the absence of spinal or epidural neoplastic deposits.

c. Paraneoplastic cerebellar atrophy is characterized by diffuse loss of Purkinje cells (see Fig. 191) without alterations in granular neurons. Inflammatory cellular lesions involving the meninges and the parenchyma, and consisting of perivascular lymphocytic cuffings and microglial nodules, are extremely frequent and may be noted at sites remote from the cerebellum.

d. Encephalopathic lesions have also been recorded. They appear to result from two main pathological processes, as follows.

1. A picture of *limbic encephalitis,* which is similar by its predominantly hippocampal distribution and its inflammatory features to that of necrotizing encephalitis (see p. 118). However, its course is slower and a viral etiology has never so far been conclusively established.

2. Vascular lesions, which are common, consist mostly of cerebral infarcts of embolic origin secondary to *nonbacterial thrombotic endocarditis,* a frequent occurrence in cancer patients. These infarcts are also often associated with visceral infarcts, especially in the spleen and kidneys, attributable to the same mechanism. *Cerebral phlebitis* is rarer. It, too, is presumably the sequel to a coagulative disorder which is a frequent feature of some visceral carcinomas, especially those originating from the pancreas.

HEMATOLOGICAL AND LYMPHORETICULAR DISEASES; DYSGLOBULINEMIAS

Malignant hematological and lymphoreticular diseases, in particular leukemias, may produce nervous system manifestations that are directly related to hemorrhagic phenomena, to venous thromboses, and to meningeal and cerebral infiltrative processes of a neoplastic nature.

The occurrence of lesions that have no direct causal relationship to the original disorder presents the same problem as the paraneoplastic syndromes already referred to.

The picture of progressive multifocal leukoencephalopathy, described elsewhere (p. 120), is seen mostly in chronic lymphatic leukemia and in Hodgkin's disease, when immunological disturbances favor the development of infection by a papovavirus.

Hodgkin's disease itself implicates the central nervous system only rarely. It may, however, give rise to a Hodgkin's leptomeningitis. Single cases of intracerebral granulomatous infiltration have also been recorded, but they are exceptional.

Sarcoidosis, which is more often responsible for lesions in the skeletal musculature or the peripheral nerves, may sometimes result in intracerebral infiltrates. The basal hypothalamic structures, and the optic and rhinencephalic pathways are most often involved.

Polycythemia vera and the various forms of *paroxysmal hemoglobinuria* may sometimes be the cause of cerebral infarcts and of venous thromboses by virtue of the coagulation disorders with which they are associated.

Thrombotic thrombocytopenic purpura, or *thrombotic microangiopathy* (Moschowitz' disease) may—as a result of the arteriolocapillary endothelial changes, thrombocytopenia, and hemolytic disturbances that characterize the condition—be the cause of small disseminated foci of hemorrhage and/or ischemia.

In *dysglobulinemias,* as in the case of hematological malignancies, infiltrates which are mostly epidural and of osseous origin may be found, especially in multiple myeloma (Kahler's disease). Central nervous system lesions of hemorrhagic nature, either cerebral or cerebromeningeal, may also be seen.

Some fairly rare types of infiltrative and proliferative lymphoreticular lesions are more characteristic of Waldenström's macroglobulinemia and of certain forms of agammaglobulinemia.

Peripheral nervous system lesions with demyelination and axonal lesions are most

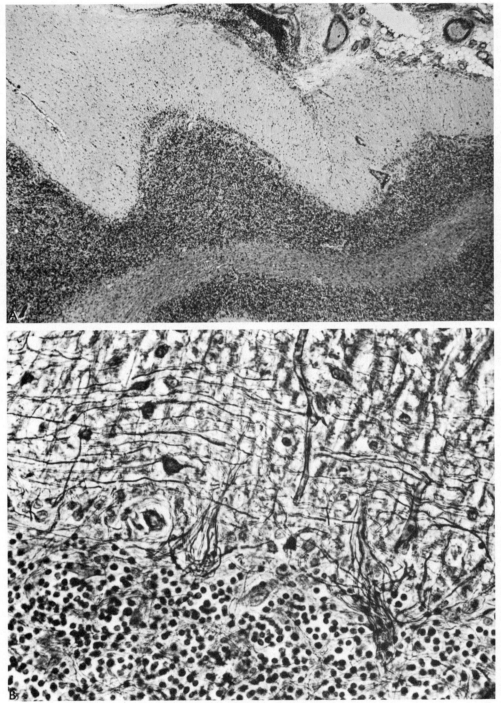

Figure 191. *Paraneoplastic cerebellar atrophy.*

A, Massive loss of Purkinje cells. Proliferation of Bergmann glia. Note the presence of a few inflammatory features (H. and E.).

B, Loss of Purkinje cells. Preservation of basket fibers and of granular neurons (Bielschowsky silver impregnation).

often related to an infiltrative process. Other lesions, seen mostly in Waldenström's macroglobulinemia, appear independent of such a process and raise the question of their dysmetabolic nature, to be ascribed either to a deficiency disorder such as avitaminosis B_1 or to amyloid infiltration.

AMYLOIDOSIS OF THE NERVOUS SYSTEM

When the nervous system is implicated, primary amyloidosis is mainly associated with peripheral nerve and skeletal muscle infiltration (see below) by amyloid material (see Fig. 237).

Involvement of the central nervous system is more exceptional, and the specific nature of the lesions has then been open to debate. Finally, the filamentous structures seen by electron microscopy in senile plaques as part of the picture of senile dementia are apparently of amyloid nature, but their presence appears to be secondary to the development of neuronal lesions.

DIABETES MELLITUS

The metabolic abnormalities resulting from diabetes may give rise to various types of nervous system lesion:

a. Terminal changes due to diabetic coma.

b. Vascular changes, especially arteriolar lesions, characterized by hyalinosis.

c. Peripheral nervous system lesions (see Fig. 238).

COLLAGEN DISEASES

Collagen diseases affect chiefly the skeletal musculature and the peripheral nerves (see below) through the mechanism of inflammatory vascular lesions, as in polyarteritis nodosa, chronic progressive polyarthritis, and systemic lupus erythematosus. They only exceptionally implicate the central nervous system.

Vascular lesions involving the small perimedullary or pericerebral arteries may be the source of disseminated infarcts, often of small size, in some cases of polyarteritis nodosa and systemic lupus erythematosus. Involvement of the intraparenchymatous arterioles themselves is exceptional. In addition, it may be difficult, in some cases, to distinguish the fibrinoid necrosis that may be present in the arteriolar vessel walls from the similar arteriolar lesions that are encountered in certain forms of malignant hypertension in young subjects.

Chapter 9

GENETIC METABOLIC DISEASES DUE TO AN ENZYME DEFECT

Various diseases that were previously classified as degenerative are recognized today to be due to a genetically based enzyme defect. The clinical picture is one of neuropsychiatric manifestations associated with a variety of systemic disturbances attributable to visceral lesions, which are often conspicuous.

In some of these diseases the enzyme defect results in an excessive accumulation (or thesaurismosis) that may implicate the neuronal cell bodies and their processes as well as the glia (as exemplified by the neurolipidoses) or the blood vessel walls and the

viscera. In other cases, the neuropathological lesions are the result of the metabolic disturbance itself, which may variously affect the white matter, the cerebral cortex, and the peripheral nervous system.

DISORDERS OF LIPID METABOLISM

These diseases are due to an abnormal accumulation, mostly within the neurons of the central nervous system, of a specific lipid

Lipids involved	Well-characterized neurolipidoses	Enzyme deficit
Sphingolipids		
Glycosphingolipids		
Gangliosides		
GM1	*GM1 gangliosidoses*	
	Variant O (Norman-Landing disease)	Galactosidase isoenzymes A, B, C
	Variant A (Derry's disease)	β-Galactosidase isoenzymes B and C
GM2	*GM2 gangliosidoses*	
	Variant B (type I) (classical Tay-Sachs disease)	Hexosaminidase A
	Variant O (type III) (Sandhoff disease)	Hexosaminidases A and B
Cerebrosides	*Glucosylceramide lipidosis* (Gaucher's disease)	Glucocerebroside β-glucosidase
	Galactosylceramide lipidosis (Krabbe's disease)	Galactocerebroside β-galactosidase
Sulfatides	*Sulfatidoses*	
	Metachromatic leukodystrophy	Arylsulfatase A
	Mucosulfatidosis (Austin's disease), variant O	Arylsulfatases A, B, and C
Trihexosylceramide	Fabry's disease	Ceramide trihexoside galactosidase
Ceramide	Farber's disease	Ceramidase
Sphingomyelin	Niemann-Pick disease	Sphingomyelinase
Less polarized lipids		
Phytanic acid	Refsum's disease	Phytanic oxidase
Cholesterol esters & triglycerides	Wolman's disease	
Lipoproteins		
α-Lipoprotein	Tangier's disease (α-lipoprotein deficiency)	
β-Lipoprotein	Acanthocytosis (β-lipoprotein deficiency) (Bassen-Kornzweig's disease)	

Figure 192. *Classification of the chief forms of neurolipidosis.*

metabolite. The abnormality may or may not be associated with peripheral nervous system lesions and visceral lesions. Current classifications (Fig. 192) specifically refer to the lipids involved and to the enzyme defect(s) responsible for their accumulation, rather than to the traditional clinical features (such as amaurotic idiocy, ocular lesions, "cherry-red macular spot," or gargoylism), to the tempo of their clinical course, or to their often contradictory and nonspecific associated etiological factors.

The chief lesions in the central nervous system consist of intense neuronal swelling (see Fig. 8), with distention of the cell bodies. Cerebellar lesions are common. They involve the Purkinje cells and the neurons of the granular layer, which is often markedly atrophied and gliosed. Involvement of the white matter and other associated lesions vary according to the different forms.

In some of these forms, the lesions are associated with changes in the peripheral nervous system, with implication of the Schwann cells and myelin sheaths. In some disorders, e.g., in Refsum's disease, the disturbance affects solely the peripheral nervous system.

Finally, visceral and ocular changes that are present may vary from case to case; they may involve the liver, lymph nodes, spleen, kidneys, etc. These changes result either from the same metabolic disturbance or from one that may be related to it.

The current study of these various disorders clearly extends beyond the context of classical neuropathology and cannot be undertaken without neurochemical and electron microscopic investigations, which must be performed on material freshly removed by cerebral or other visceral biopsy procedures.

I. THE SPHINGOLIPIDOSES

These disorders represent the most important group among the neurolipidoses and are characterized by an excess of sphingolipids. These lipids share as a common feature the presence of a ceramide moiety, which is derived from an unsaturated amino alcohol, sphingosine, in which one of the

hydrogens of the amino group is replaced by a long-chain fatty acid.

The Gangliosidoses

These diseases correspond roughly to the old entities forming the so-called "amaurotic idiocies." They are characterized by an accumulation of gangliosides, which are composed of one ceramide molecule; up to four hexoses (galactose and glucose); up to three molecules of sialic acid (N-acetylneuraminic acid, or NANA), thus resulting in the formation of mono-, di-, or trisialogangliosides*; and finally, one molecule of hexosamine (N-acetylgalactosamine).[1]

Aside from their recognizable histochemical features, gangliosides are characterized in the electron microscope by the presence, in the perikarya of neurons, of membranous cytoplasmic bodies, which are circular profiles measuring 1 μm and formed by alternating concentric electron-lucent and electron-dense bands 5 to 6 nm wide (Fig. 193).

1. The GM2 gangliosidoses are classified today according to their specific enzyme deficit.

a. Classical Tay-Sachs disease (also known as variant B, or type I GM2 gangliosidosis) occurs in Ashkenazi Jews. It is due to the accumulation of GM2 gangliosides and of an asialo derivative of GM2 ganglioside, namely ceramide trihexoside. It is caused by hexosaminidase A deficiency.

b. Sandhoff disease (also known as

---

*Monosialogangliosides are represented by the GM1, GM2, and GM3 gangliosidoses. The disialogangliosides are represented by the GD1, GD2, and GD3 gangliosidoses. Trisialogangliosides are represented by GT1 gangliosidosis.
[1]In the current nomenclature of the gangliosidoses, which was introduced by Svennerholm, the G stands for ganglioside; the letters M, D, and T indicate the numbers of sialic acid residues (mono, di, or tri); and the terminal arabic numeral indicates the order in which the compounds separate on thin-layer chromatography.

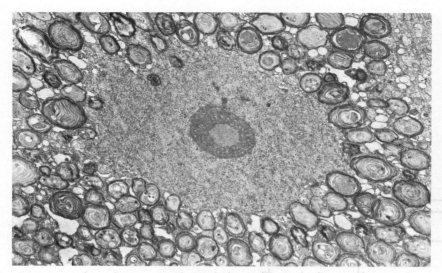

Figure 193. *Intraneuronal membranous cytoplasmic bodies in Tay-Sachs disease. Electron microscopy.* × 4000.

variant O, or type III GM2 gangliosidosis) does not show any particular ethnic predominance. It consists in the accumulation, within neurons, of GM2 ganglioside and, in the viscera, of both ceramide trihexoside and a globoside (a ceramide tetrahexoside: ceramide-glucose-galactose-galactose-*N*-acetylgalactosamine). It is caused by a deficit of both hexosaminidases A and B.

c. **Juvenile GM2 gangliosidosis** (also known as type II GM2 gangliosidosis) again does not show any specific ethnic prevalence. Essentially, it is due to an accumulation of the same GM2 ganglioside as in Tay-Sachs disease, but to a lesser degree, and the hexosaminidase deficit is only partial.

Likewise, **the AB variant,** which is rarer, is clinically identical with Tay-Sachs disease. However, there is normal hexosaminidase A and B activity *in vitro* as contrasted to their absence *in vivo*.

2. GD3 gangliosidosis (congenital amaurotic idiocy) and **GM3 gangliosidosis,** which involves the white matter in a manner similar to that of spongy degeneration of the neuraxis (Canavan's disease), are rarer, and their nosological position is debated.

3. GM1 gangliosidosis corresponds to some of the disorders that have previously been described as examples of late infantile amaurotic idiocy, Landing's generalized neurovisceral lipidosis, and pseudo-Hurler's syndrome.

The disease consists in the accumulation of two different compounds: a GM1 ganglioside within neurons of the central nervous system, demonstrated in electron microscopy by the presence of membranous cytoplasmic bodies and more heterogeneous bodies; and a mucopolysaccharide (glycosaminoglycan) in vacuoles of various reticulohistiocytic cells, especially pericytes.

Norman-Landing disease (also known as variant O, type I, or pseudo-Hurler syndrome) has an early clinical onset and a rapid course. It is due to a deficiency of the three A, B, and C isoenzymes of β-galactosidase. Visceral lesions involving the liver, spleen, cornea, bone, and lymphocytes (which contain vacuoles) are conspicuous.

Derry's disease (also known as variant A, or type II) is characterized by a later clinical onset and slower evolution. It is due to a deficiency of the B and C isoenzymes of β-galactosidase. Visceral lesions are discrete and usually clinically silent.

4. The traditional forms of late infantile,

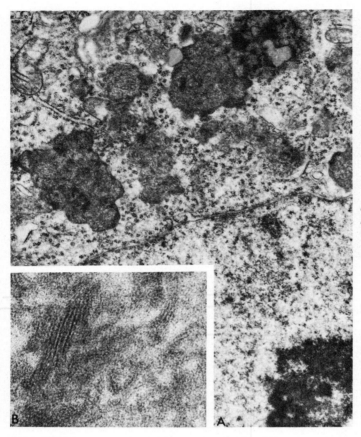

Figure 194. *Curvilinear bodies demonstrated by electron microscopy in ceroid-lipofuscinosis. A,* Low magnification. × 21,000. *B,* High magnification. × 110,000.

sphingolipidosis or peroxisomal ??

juvenile, and adult neurolipidosis (also referred to eponymically as the Jansky-Bielschowsky form, Batten-Mayou or Spielmeyer-Vogt disease, and Kufs disease, respectively) are currently regarded as a group of disorders for which the definition is debatable.

Some of these cases are authentic examples of neurolipidosis (GM1 gangliosidosis, juvenile GM2 gangliosidosis). Others, by virtue of their morphological features demonstrated by light and electron microscopy, seem to be examples of *atypical juvenile neurolipidosis,* but the actual neurochemical defect has not yet been established.

Finally, many cases in this group are in fact characterized by an abnormal accumulation of pigment. This pigment, which is autofluorescent by light microscopy, demonstrates by electron microscopy either a granulovacuolar appearance closely resembling typical lipofuscin pigment, or *curvilinear bodies* (Fig. 194), or a fingerprint pattern. The pigment accumulation is not limited to cells of the central nervous system, but also involves endothelial cells and the pericytes of the blood vessel walls and is found in most of the viscera. Its demonstration by electron microscopy in skin biopsies, appendectomy specimens, muscle biopsies, peripheral lymphocytes, and even urinary deposits, is at present of diagnostic value.

These disorders are currently grouped within the framework of the *ceroid-lipofuscinoses;* absence of peroxidase has been demonstrated in a few cases.

The Cerebrosidoses

1. Gaucher's disease, or glucosylceramide

lipidosis, is due to an accumulation of gluco-cerebroside (ceramide-glucose) resulting from a deficiency of glucocerebroside-β-glucosidase, which splits glucosylceramide into ceramide and glucose.

In the acute early infantile form and in some rarer forms of later onset and with a prolonged course characterized by dementia, the central nervous system is infiltrated by macrophages (Gaucher cells). These large (30 to 40 μm) cells are loaded with cerebrosides and are seen by electron microscopy to contain tubular, sickle-shaped profiles measuring 12.5 to 30 nm. The cells are found in large numbers outside the nervous system, e.g., in the liver, lymph nodes, bone, and especially the spleen. Within the central nervous system, they are distributed chiefly around blood vessels. Accumulation of glucocerebroside within the neurons themselves is variable and usually discrete.

In the more frequent chronic form, of later onset, the central nervous system is usually spared, and the lesions affect virtually only the viscera.

2. Krabbe's disease (or globoid body leukodystrophy, or galactosylceramide lipidosis) represents a more complex metabolic disorder. The disease chiefly implicates the galactocerebroside (ceramide-galactose) of myelin. The enzyme defect, which is still under discussion, seems to be a deficit of galactoside-β-galactosidase rather than one of cerebroside sulfotransferase (which mediates the synthesis of cerebroside sulfate).

The disease is characterized chiefly by conspicuous involvement of the myelin of the white matter, resulting in a picture of infantile *leukodystrophy* of usually rapid course and early onset. Demyelination, which is accompanied by astrocytic gliosis, is widespread throughout the cerebral and cerebellar hemispheric white matter, and is characterized by the presence of large multinucleated cells measuring 30 to 50 μm *(globoid cells)* (Fig. 195) and of numerous epithelioid-looking cells with a predominantly perivascular distribution; both these cell types are macrophages. Their phagocytic role in relation to the accumulated cerebroside is now well established.

Involvement of the peripheral nervous system, with segmental demyelination and the presence of lipid inclusions in the Schwann cells, may also be found.

The Sulfatidoses

These disorders are characterized from the biochemical point of view by an accumulation of sulfatide (ceramide-galactose-sulfate) due to a deficit of arylsulfatase.

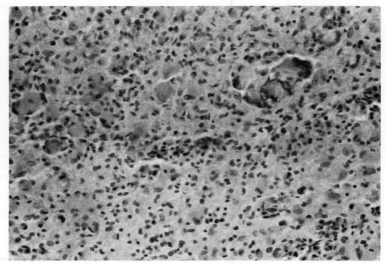

Figure 195. *Krabbe's disease.* Note the presence of numerous globoid cells and of smaller histiocytes (H. and E.).

*1. **Metachromatic leukodystrophy,*** which is due to absence of arylsulfatase A, is one of the most common neurolipidoses. It characteristically presents with myelin changes as a result of which the disease has become the best known and the most frequently identified of the leukodystrophies. Lesions of the central nervous system are associated with lesions in the peripheral nervous system and in visceral organs.

a. Lesions of the central nervous system. *1.* Hemispheric demyelination (Fig. 196*A*), which is irregular, often incomplete, and accompanied by fibrillary gliosis, is especially characterized by the presence of nonsudanophilic lipid breakdown products, which are metachromatic with cresyl violet (brown metachromasia) and with toluidine blue. These breakdown products consist of sulfatide material. They lie free in neuroglial

sparing U fibers

cells as well as in compound granular corpuscles and are found also in nondemyelinated areas. With the electron microscope they are seen to consist of complex lipid structures organized in parallel lamellae measuring approximately 6 nm in width, often piled up into prismatic formations mixed with mucopolysaccharides (Fig. 196*B* and *C*).

2. In addition, lipid neuronal storage of the same material is present in the basal ganglia, brainstem, and dentate nuclei.

b. Lesions of the peripheral nervous system. These lesions are typical of the disease, but are especially notable in affected children. They are characterized by the presence, demonstrated with cresyl violet, of metachromatic material in Schwann cells and macrophages, and by demyelination with relative sparing of the axis cylinders. The inclu-

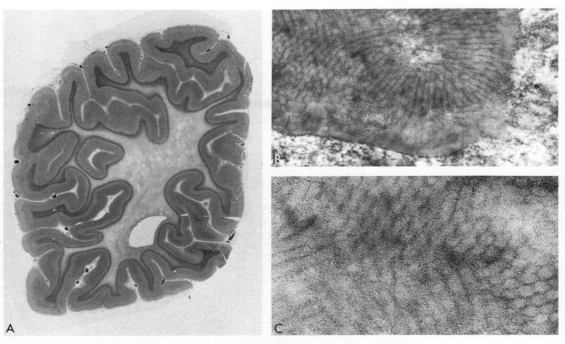

Figure 196.   *Metachromatic leukodystrophy* (sulfatidosis).

A, Massive demyelination sparing the U fibers in the left parieto-occipital region (Loyez stain for myelin).
B, Sulfatide inclusions (electron microscopy).
C, Hexagonal structure of sulfatide inclusions (electron microscopy at higher magnification). × 130,000.

sions with a prismatic structure, frequently seen in the central nervous system, are seen less often in the peripheral nerves, in which it is usually more common to demonstrate lamellar profiles of variable electron density within Schwann cells.

c.   The association of visceral lesions (atrophy of the gallbladder epithelium, renal tubular changes) with the presence of metachromatic material in these organs and the excretion of sulfatide in the urine complete the pathological picture and underscore the systemic character of this disorder of sulfatide metabolism.

In the *infantile* and *juvenile forms* the central and peripheral myelin are markedly involved.

In the *adult* and *late juvenile forms* dementia is often a conspicuous component of the clinical picture, and the white matter and peripheral nerves are affected less severely. On the other hand, the accumulation of sulfatides within neurons is much more marked.

2.   *Austin's disease* (or *mucosulfatidosis*, or variant O) is due to a total deficit of arylsulfatases A, B, and C. The sulfatide accumulation is accompanied by an accumulation of mucopolysaccharide.

The disease is characterized by the coexistence of the typical lesions of sulfatidosis with the neural and visceral lesions of mucopolysaccharidosis that somewhat recall those of Hurler's disease.

Niemann-Pick Disease

This condition displays several forms from the genetic and clinical standpoints. The nervous system is involved particularly in Crocker's acute infantile form (type A), which affects Jews. The juvenile form (type C), which is of slower evolution and less common, may also implicate the nervous system, but the neurological manifestations appear later in the course of the disease.

All these cases show a variable accumulation of sphingomyelin (ceramide-phosphoryl-choline), which is marked in types A and B. Cholesterol also accumulates. There is a deficit of sphingomyelinase.

Type D (the Nova Scotia variant), which may also implicate the central nervous system, is less clearly defined because there is no excessive sphingomyelin storage and sphingomyelinase activity is normal.

In those forms which affect the nervous system, neuronal involvement is accompanied by an infiltration of foamy cells (Fig. 197) and by variable changes in the endothelial and perithelial elements of the blood vessel walls. In a few cases the peripheral nervous system has also been involved.

Figure 197. *Foamy cells in Niemann-Pick disease.* Electron microscopic features. ×9900.

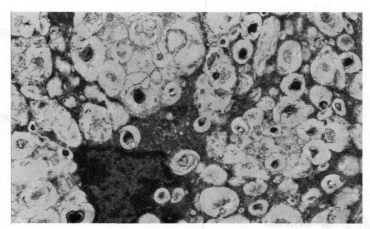

Fabry's Disease
(diffuse angiokeratosis, or juvenile xanthogranuloma)

X linked R.

This sex-linked recessive disorder is due to an accumulation of trihexosylceramide (ceramide-glucose-galactose-glucose) resulting from a deficiency of ceramide-trihexoside-α-galactosidase.

The disease consists in the development of cutaneous and mucous angiokeratomas and of corneal changes *(cornea verticillata)*. Foamy cells are found in the reticuloendothelial tissues of the liver, spleen, and lymph nodes as well as in the renal and cutaneous epithelia.

Nervous system involvement is apparently limited largely to some of the hypothalamic nuclei, the brainstem, and peripheral nerves.

Farber's Lipogranulomatosis

This rare disorder presents with multiple subcutaneous nodules resembling histiocytic granulomas and with hepatic, lymphatic, and renal lesions. In the nervous system, neuronal involvement occurs in the anterior horns, the brainstem, and the cerebellum. The disease is due to an abnormal accumulation of ceramide. Occasionally ceramidase deficiency has been demonstrated.

II. REFSUM'S DISEASE

This condition results from excessive storage of phytanic acid, which may be either free or associated with triglycerides and phospholipids. Phytanic acid accumulates in the tissues because of the absence of phytanic oxidase, which oxidizes phytanic acid to pristanic acid.

In this disease the peripheral nervous system is affected by a demyelinating neuropathy (see p. 210). In the later stages neuropathy is associated with onion-bulb Schwann cell hypertrophy. Osmiophilic lipid inclusions, which may be heterogeneous or crystalline, may be found within Schwann cells.

In the central nervous system cerebellar and posterior column lesions have been observed.

retinitis pigmentosa

The presence of raised levels of albumin in the cerebrospinal fluid and of retinitis pigmentosa completes the pathological picture.

III. OTHER NEUROLIPIDOSES

1. Among the **cholesterol** or cholesterol esters **neural storage diseases** (xanthomatoses), only *Wolman's disease* seems to correspond to the definition of a neurolipidosis as it is understood at this time. In the central nervous system there is accumulation of cholesterol associated with excessive storage of triglycerides. Calcification of the adrenals is accompanied by lesions in the intestinal mucosa and by pathological changes in the liver, spleen, and lymph nodes. In the central nervous system the choroid plexuses, the leptomeninges, and the Purkinje cells are often affected.

In *Hand-Schüller-Christian disease,* cholesterol storage appears simply to be secondary to reticulohistiocytic proliferation.

2. The group of **essential familial hyperlipidemias** are not apt to cause nervous system lesions except as the result of vascular changes. The same may be said of the group of **familial hypercholesterolemias,** although they may also give rise to a number of cerebellar and spinal cord changes whose nature is still obscure.

IV. THE LIPOPROTEINOSES

1. **Acanthocytosis,** due to a deficiency of β-lipoprotein, consists of abnormalities in the blood (acanthocytes) and retinitis pigmentosa (Bassen-Kornzweig's disease).

In addition the myelin of the peripheral nerves, the posterior columns and the spinocerebellar tracts may be involved, recalling the picture of Friedreich's ataxia.

2. **Tangier's disease,** which is due to a deficit of α-lipoprotein, is characterized by hypertrophy of the tonsils, hepatomegaly and splenomegaly, and hypocholesterolemia.

The peripheral nervous system may be affected in a manner that recalls Refsum's disease.

DISORDERS OF MUCOPOLYSACCHARIDE (GLYCOSAMINOGLYCAN) METABOLISM

The nervous system, and especially neurons, are involved only in certain forms of mucopolysaccharidosis.

In such cases a systemic disturbance of acid mucopolysaccharides, or glycosaminoglycans (which are excreted in the urine), is accompanied by a lipid neuronal storage disorder that essentially implicates gangliosides. Because of the secondary nature of the gangliosidosis, this group of diseases is usually excluded at this time from the neurolipidoses as a whole, but it should be stressed that in some forms the neuronal changes dominate the picture.

The histopathological findings consist of an association of nervous system changes with alterations in the blood vessel walls. In the cerebral cortex and cerebellum, the appearance of the swollen neurons is comparable to that seen in gangliosidoses, with the presence of zebra bodies (Fig. 198*A*) and other structures that are intermediary to the membranous cytoplasmic bodies of Tay-Sachs disease. Capillary pericytes may show marked vacuolation (Fig. 198*B*), which corresponds to the excessive accumulation of glycosaminoglycans. Vacuolization is found in the central nervous system, in various visceral organs (including the liver, myocardium, and bone marrow), and in lymphocytes. The vacuoles appear to be of lysosomal origin, as suggested by the demonstration of acid phosphatase.

In *Hurler's disease,* or type I mucopolysaccharidosis (mucopolysaccharidosis with excessive chondroitin sulfate B and heparan sulfate), the systemic picture of facial and skeletal deformities (gargoylism) is more conspicuous than the nervous system lesions, which are usually discrete. Hydrocephalus may be present.

Hunter's disease, or type II mucopolysaccharidosis, is biochemically identical with Hurler's disease, but differs by its sex-linked recessive character and the absence of corneal opacities. The nervous system is only discretely involved.

In *Sanfilippo's disease,* or type III mucopolysaccharidosis (in which only heparan sulfate accumulates in excessive amounts), the nervous system lesions are conspicuous, whereas the facial and skeletal deformities are discrete.

According to some workers, the excessive accumulation of both gangliosides and glycosaminoglycans could be accounted for by a deficiency of β-galactosidase, the same enzyme being capable of degrading both products. According to others, the enzyme deficit is one of L-iduronidase in Hurler's disease, *N*-sulfatase in Sanfilippo's disease type I (or

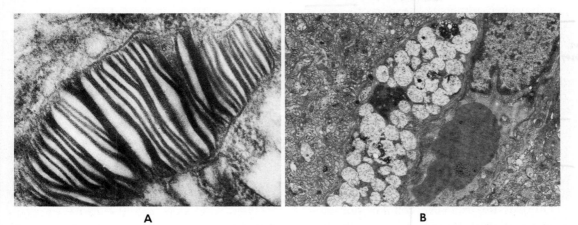

A   **B**

Figure 198.   *Electron microscopic appearances in mucopolysaccharidosis. A,* Zebra body in Hurler's disease. × 65,000. *B,* Vacuoles in a pericyte in mucopolysaccharidosis. × 6000.

A), and *N*-acetylglucosaminidase in Sanfilippo's disease type II (or B), both types being distinguished on the basis of fibroblast tissue culture.

Under the term **mucolipidoses** a number of diseases have been described in which there is a disorder of lipid and glycosaminoglycan metabolism without urinary excretion of the latter. The central nervous system is often involved. This group of diseases, which is still controversial, includes:

Type I mucolipidosis, or lipomucopolysaccharidosis, as described by Spranger;

Type II mucolipidosis, or I-cell disease, which has been said to resemble mannosidosis and fucosidosis;

Type III mucolipidosis, or pseudopolydystrophy.

In mucosulfatidosis (see p. 171) and in GM1 gangliosidosis (see p. 167) a similar double metabolic abnormality is also present.

DISORDERS OF CARBOHYDRATE METABOLISM

1.   The glycogenoses.   Some forms of glycogen storage disease, such as Pompe's disease, MacArdle's disease, and Forbes' disease (p. 202), involve chiefly the skeletal musculature. The central nervous system is affected only exceptionally.

Pompe's disease (or type II glycogenosis), which is caused by acid maltase deficiency, can, however, implicate the nervous system. The neurons of the anterior horns, of some of the brainstem nuclei, of the cerebellum and, to a lesser extent, of the cortex, are vacuolated and swollen, and may, like the glia, show an excessive storage of type α glycogen when examined by electron microscopy.

2.   Galactosemia.   A deficit of galactose-1-phosphate-*N*-uridyltransferase, which results in an accumulation of galactose-1-phosphate, may, especially in slowly progressive cases, produce nervous system lesions.

There is no excessive cellular storage of galactose phosphate, but secondary neuronal cell loss accompanied by gliosis may occur, involving the cerebral cortex and the cerebellum, associated in some instances with pallidonigral degeneration.

3.   Lafora's disease.   This condition is characterized by the presence of rounded structures, measuring 0.5 to 30 μm, which are PAS-positive and found in the perikarya and processes of neurons. These structures are known as *Lafora bodies* (see Fig. 12). They are scattered very widely throughout the cerebral cortex and gray matter in general, but chiefly involving the basal ganglia and dentate nuclei. They apparently consist of acidic glycoproteins, acid mucopolysaccharides, or α-polyglucosan. The exact metabolic disturbance, which might be due to excessive storage of amylopectin, is still debated.

The neuropathological lesions account for the clinical picture of progressive familial myoclonic epilepsy of the Unverricht-Lundborg type.

4.   Subacute necrotizing encephalopathy. Subacute necrotizing encephalopathy, or Leigh-Feigin disease, is seen most often in early childhood, but variants with late onset have been described. The condition is characterized by the presence of symmetrical spongy necrotizing lesions that affect the cortex and sometimes the hemispheric white matter. Involvement of the basal ganglia (putamen, thalamus), the tegmentum of the brainstem, the corpora quadrigemina, and the inferior olives is characteristic.

The relative sparing of the neurons, the presence of gliosis, and especially the endothelial proliferation closely resemble the lesions of Wernicke's encephalopathy and beriberi.

The precise metabolic disorder responsible for the lesions is still poorly understood. It is likely that a disturbance of the Krebs cycle may be at fault.

Congenital lactic acidosis may likewise cause necrotizing lesions in the hemispheric white matter.

DISORDERS OF AMINO ACID METABOLISM

These disorders are the cause of many syndromes of mental retardation in childhood which may be associated with various neurological manifestations.

1. Phenylketonuria is due to absence of phenylalanine hydroxylase, which hydrolyzes phenylalanine to tyrosine. The neuropathological findings are variable and rather poorly defined: they include microcephaly, status spongiosus, and alterations in the myelin of the hemispheric white matter resembling leukodystrophy.

2. Tyrosinosis is related to a deficiency in the oxidation of parahydroxyphenylpyruvic acid.

3. Leucinosis, or maple syrup urine disease, is identified by the presence of α-hydroxybutyric acid in the urine, which has a characteristic odor. It is due to a decrease of decarboxylase activity.

It may cause spongy lesions in the white matter resembling those of Canavan's disease.

4. Homocystinuria is due to a deficit of cystathionine synthetase, which normally couples homocysteine to serine so as to form cystathionine.

The disease may apparently cause alterations in the blood vessel walls, with fibrosis of the intima and degeneration of the elastic fibers. Foci of cerebral necrosis, suspected to be of vascular origin, are often found.

5. Hartnup's disease, which is due to a disorder of tryptophan absorption, produces a picture that resembles pellagra.

DISORDERS OF METAL METABOLISM

1. Wilson's disease. Hepatolenticular degeneration, or Wilson's disease, is related to a deficiency of ceruloplasmin, and causes characteristic lesions in the basal ganglia. These culminate, in advanced stages, in actual necrosis of the putamen with cavitation, whereas the globus pallidus, the thalamus, and the cerebral cortex are involved to a lesser extent.

Less severe lesions consist in spongy state, with glial changes that involve the astrocytic nuclei. These are voluminous, pale, and multilobulated, and present the picture of Alzheimer type II glia (see Fig. 16). More voluminous cells with eccentric nuclei, or Opalski cells, are also found in the basal ganglia in places.

Microscopic copper deposits are found to incrustate the astrocytes.

2. Kinky hair disease. Kinky hair disease (Menkes' disease or trichopoliodystrophy) is due to a defect of intestinal copper absorption and presents with low levels of copper in the blood and low levels of blood ceruloplasmin.

The disease causes abnormality in the hair and neuropsychiatric manifestations. Pathologically, there are changes in the hemispheric myelin and lesions in the cerebellar cortex and in the blood vessel walls.

DISORDERS OF PIGMENT METABOLISM

1. Porphyria. Acute intermittent porphyria, which is due to a deficiency of porphobilinogen deaminase (uroporphyrinogen I synthetase) and secondary accumulation of both δ-aminolevulinic acid and porphobilinogen, chiefly causes peripheral nervous system lesions (see Fig. 238).

In the central nervous system, neuronal chromatolysis in the anterior horn cells and in the motor nucleus of the vagus may be associated with cerebellar lesions that are not very specific.

2. Nuclear jaundice (kernicterus). *Nuclear jaundice* in its acute form mainly shows characteristic lesions in the basal ganglia; these lesions consist of a yellowish infiltration of the globus pallidus, corpus Luysii, dentate nuclei, and Ammon's horns by bilirubin pigment.

In the late subacute form of the disease, the sequelae are characterized by gliosis and demyelination of these structures.

Nuclear jaundice, which is most often secondary to a hemolytic process, either fetal-maternal Rh incompatibility or hereditary hemolytic anemia, may sometimes be related to an enzyme deficiency; this consists in absence of glucuronyltransferase in the case of a recessive familial form of congenital hyperbilirubinemia (Criggler-Najjar syndrome).

Chapter 10

CONGENITAL MALFORMATIONS OF THE NERVOUS SYSTEM AND PERINATAL PATHOLOGY

ETIOLOGY OF CONGENITAL MALFORMATIONS

Malformations of the nervous system may, like those of the rest of the body, be due to three groups of factors:

Exogenous factors:

Infections, especially rubella, toxoplasmosis;

Radiation (x-rays, atomic exposure);

Chemical agents (especially various drugs).

Genetic and chromosomal factors, in particular trisomy 21 or mongolism (Down's syndrome), trisomy 13–15.

An interaction of the two main factors above.

The relatively late completion of brain development in fetal life accounts for the protracted effects of some of these teratogenic factors.

DISTURBANCES DUE TO DEFECTIVE CLOSURE OF THE NEURAL GROOVE (OR DYSRAPHIC STATES)
(Fig. 199)

These defects constitute the most frequent malformations of the nervous system. If in the course of neural tube formation there is defective closure of the neural groove, various nervous system malformations will appear, depending on the localization and the extent of the closure defect. These malformations will to some extent be accompanied by developmental defects affecting the subjacent tissue planes (meninges, posterior arch of the vertebrae, dermis), whose

development is normally subject to inductive influences from the neural tube.

1. *Spinal Cord*

These malformations are most often localized to the lumbar and lumbosacral regions, and are subsumed under the generic term of spina bifida.

a. Spina bifida aperta (or myeloaraphia). This is the major form of dysraphism. The open neural groove is immediately exposed to the surface, with its borders in continuity with the adjacent epiblast. Because of nonclosure of the neural groove, no leptomeninges are formed, the vertebral arch does not close, and the topographically related skin fails to develop.

b. Myelomeningocele. In this lesser form of dysraphia the neural tube has undergone closure, whereas the posterior arch of the vertebrae has not, with the result that the meninges protrude directly under the skin, where there is, in addition, faulty development of the dermis. Various nervous tissue elements, i.e., spinal cord parenchyma and nerve roots, are present in the sac thus formed, which is filled with cerebrospinal fluid. These neural tissues may also be attached to the wall of the sac. Fairly often, such a myelomeningocele is associated with hydrocephalus due to a malformation involving the medulla and the cerebellar tonsils that impedes the passage of cerebrospinal fluid at the level of the fourth ventricle (Arnold-Chiari malformation) (see p. 184).

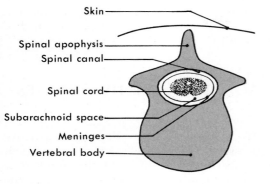

Skin

Spinal apophysis

Spinal canal

Spinal cord

Subarachnoid space

Meninges

Vertebral body

Normal

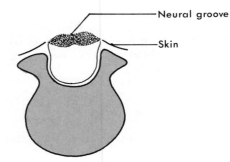

Neural groove

Skin

Spina bifida aperta

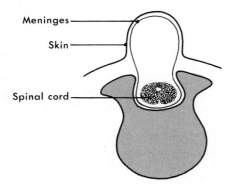

Meninges

Skin

Spinal cord

Meningocele

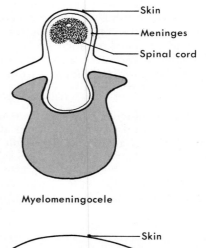

Skin

Meninges

Spinal cord

Myelomeningocele

Dermal sinus

Skin

Meninges

Spinal cord

Congenital dermal sinus

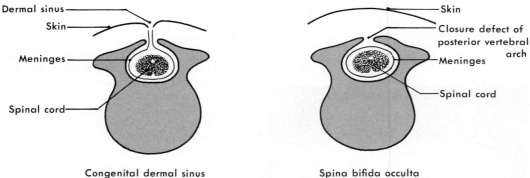

Skin

Closure defect of posterior vertebral arch

Meninges

Spinal cord

Spina bifida occulta

Figure 199. *The various closure defects of the neural groove.*

c. Meningocele. This malformation is essentially similar to the preceding defect, but the sac does not contain any nervous tissue.

d. Congenital dermal sinus. In this case the meninges are linked to the epidermal tissues by a narrow aperture across the incompletely closed posterior vertebral arch.

e. Spina bifida occulta. This highly frequent malformation does not give rise to any clinical manifestations and is usually discovered incidentally on radiological examination of the spine. It consists essentially in a closure defect of the posterior arch of the vertebrae, sometimes accompanied by discrete abnormalities in the overlying skin (e.g., tufts of hair).

2. Brain

Similar malformations may be found in the brain.

a. Anencephaly (or encephalo-araphia) (Fig. 200).[1] This condition is due to failure on the part of the neural tube to close at the level of the encephalon. There is lack of development of the meninges, of the cranial vault, and of the skin; such an "open" nervous system is therefore exposed to the air. This malformation is fatal within a few hours after birth.

b. Encephalocele. In this condition, part of the brain protrudes under the skin through a bony defect in the vault of the skull.

c. Meningocele. This malformation consists of a meningeal sac filled with cere-

---

[1]Exceptionally, spina bifida aperta involving the entire spinal cord may be associated with anencephaly, thus resulting in total encephalo-myelo-araphia (or craniorachischisis).

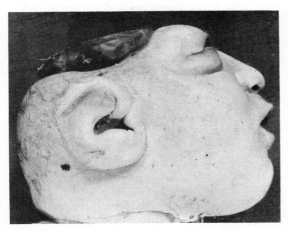

Figure 200.   *Anencephaly.*

brospinal fluid and protruding under the skin through a bony defect in the vault of the skull.

AGENESES AND DYSGENESES

1. Microencephaly.   Various destructive processes occurring before birth may result in a decrease in volume of the brain associated with other anomalies. However, the term "true microencephaly" (or small brain, which may coexist with microcephaly— characterized by decrease in size of the cranial perimeter) may be used only when referring to a brain of small size, weighing less than 900 gm in the adult, and without degenerative lesions. This picture, which is of obscure etiology, may be associated with the clinical picture of oligophrenia and idiocy, which is sometimes familial.

2. Megalencephaly.   This may be seen in normal subjects just as frequently as in mentally deficient subjects. The increase in volume (defined as that of a brain weighing more than 1800 gm) may be diffuse or localized.

The brain may sometimes be structurally normal, but most often there is either a diffuse glial proliferation or a variable pathological process; this may include tuberose sclerosis, various malformations, cerebral lipidoses, spongy degeneration of the white matter, and Alexander's disease.

3. Cyclocephaly.   This is a rare malformation which affects the tissues derived from the prosencephalon. In the major form, the telencephalon is not divided, and there is a single central ventricle which communicates with the third ventricle. The presence of a single median eye (cyclopia) or of a considerable degree of hypotelorism, absence of the pituitary, and aplasia of the nasal structures complete the picture. Minor forms are sometimes observed.

It is generally believed that the condition is due to an induction defect of the prochordal plate resulting from a chromosomal abnormality.

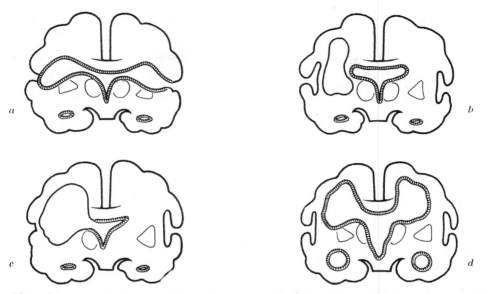

Figure 201. *Diagrammatic features of the main intracranial cystic malformations* (the ependymal lining is represented by hatched lines).

a, Porencephaly; *b*, false porencephaly; *c*, hydranencephaly; *d*, hydrocephalus.

4. *Porencephaly.* This consists in cerebral cavitation due to localized agenesis of the cortical mantle, leading to the formation of a cavity or a lateral slit through which the lateral ventricle communicates with the convexity. This term has often been erroneously used to designate all types of intracerebral cavities secondary to various destructive processes (Figs. 201 and 202).

In schizencephaly, the malformation is bilateral. Two cavities extend from the ventricle, which is often single, to the operculoinsular convexity. They are lined by ependyma or even by malformed gray matter and are covered along the convexity by a thin pia-ependymal layer which often ruptures into the subarachnoid space. Various malformations are frequently associated, especially heterotopias and foci of microgyria along the borders of the cavity.

In less severe forms the cavitation may be reduced to a lateral slit lined by ependyma.

5. *Hydranencephaly.* In contrast to the preceding malformations this condition is generally the result of destructive processes. Similar to porencephaly, it presents as a large intracerebral cavitation which may at

first mimic ventricular dilatation. However, in contrast to hydrocephalus, the cavity is not lined by ependyma but by a glial border, and the thin external wall is formed by leptomeninges and by a thin layer of superficial cortex which is the seat of glial proliferation. Hydranencephaly also differs from those porencephalic cavities that are lined by ventricular ependyma (Fig. 201).

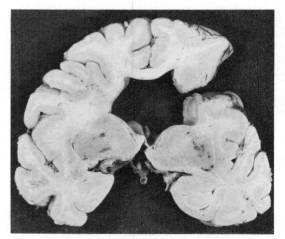

Figure 202. *Porencephaly with agenesis of the septum lucidum.*

The usual topographical distribution of this lesion, which generally involves the anterior part of the cerebral hemispheres, suggests a circulatory pathogenesis implicating the carotid artery system.

6. Ageneses and commissural malformations. a. Septal malformations. *1. Septal agenesis* (Fig. 202).   This malformation is not uncommon and gives rise to the picture of a single ventricle. It must be distinguished from septal ruptures that are secondary to severe forms of hydrocephalus.

2. Cyst of the septum (or double septum or fifth ventricle) (Fig. 203). This is a frequent finding, which corresponds to an abnormal persistence of the fetal cavum septi pellucidi.

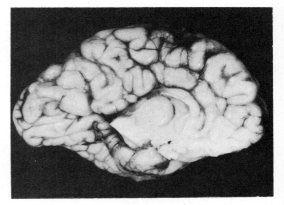

Figure 204.   *Partial agenesis of the corpus callosum.*

The presence of a "sixth ventricle" (cavum vergae) between the posterior half of the corpus callosum and the columns of the trigone is rarer. It may communicate with the third ventricle.

b.   Agenesis of the corpus callosum (Fig. 204). This may be partial or, less often, total. The corpus callosum may be reduced to a thin lamella or may be completely absent. The defect may be an isolated finding, but is often associated with other malformations.

Not infrequently, neoplastic lipomatous tissue, calcifications, or vascular abnormalities are observed at the site of an absent corpus callosum.

7. Arhinencephaly. This may involve only the olfactory bulbs (Fig. 205). The anomaly, which is associated with other malformations, especially of the cerebellum, is typical of trisomy 13–15. It may also involve the hippocampal formations and accompany other complex malformations such as holoprosencephaly (Fig. 206), which is characterized by a more or less complete fusion of the cerebral hemispheres, thus indicating a severe disturbance in the development of the fore-end of the telencephalic vesicle.

8.   Cerebral and cerebellar ageneses. *Hemispheric cerebral ageneses* are rare and seem related more frequently to early vascular disturbances than to a malformative process.

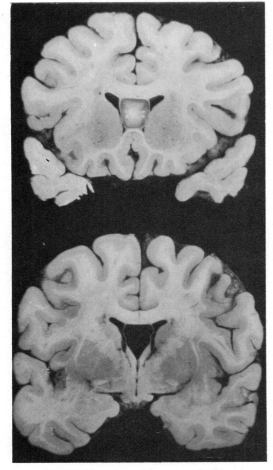

Figure 203.   *Cyst of the septum lucidum.*

Hemispheric cerebellar agenesis is associated with alterations in the contralateral inferior olive. It is to be distinguished from crossed cerebellar cortical atrophy secondary to a contralateral cerebral hemispheric lesion.

Paleocerebellar aplasia indicates a disturbance in posterior fusion of the rhombencephalon and may give rise to complete separation of both cerebellar hemispheres.

Pontoneocerebellar hypoplasia is rare. It consists in the association of hypoplasia of the pontine nuclei with that of the cerebellar hemispheres.

CORTICAL ANOMALIES

These anomalies are related to a disturbance in maturation of the germinative layer around the end of the second month of fetal life.

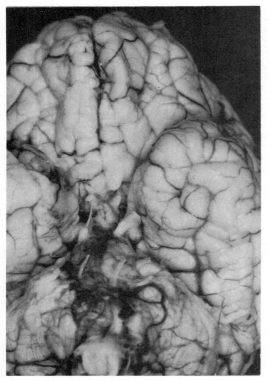

Figure 205. *Agenesis of olfactory bulbs in a case of trisomy 13–15.*

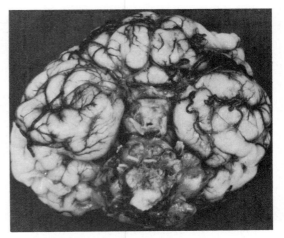

Figure 206.   *Holoprosencephaly.* Fusion of frontal lobes and agenesis of olfactory bulbs.

a.   Lissencephaly or agyria.   This is the normal state up to the seventh month of fetal life and is characterized by absence of fissures and convolutions. It may either be total or involve only part of the hemispheres. It is often associated with some degree of pachygyria.

b.   Pachygyria (Figs. 207 and 208).   In this condition, the convolutions are abnormally wide and thick, and the cortex demonstrates a four-layer type of lamination. The association of this condition with heterotopic nodules in the white matter indicates a disturbance in the migration of neuroblasts to the periphery of the brain.

c.   Heterotopias.   These are frequently observed as an isolated phenomenon in the shape of masses of gray matter in the centrum ovale near the caudate nucleus (Fig. 209), in the cerebellar white matter, in the brainstem, and in the inferior olives. They are very frequently associated with other malformations.

d.   Microgyria and polymicrogyria (Fig. 210). Both conditons are often associated with the malformations described above and are fairly commonly observed. They tend to involve certain cortical cerebral and cerebellar areas, with a distribution that is frequently bilateral and symmetrical.

They are characterized by the grouping of small convolutions that are reduced in size,

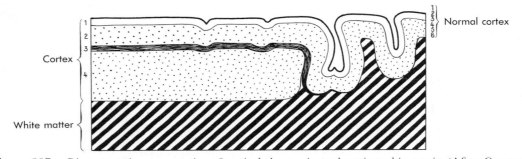

Figure 207.   *Diagrammatic representation of cortical changes in pachygyria and in agyria.* (After Crome and Stern, 1967.)

irregular, malformed, and with a verrucous appearance. They show large numbers of sulci and must be distinguished from the type of convolutional atrophy found in ulegyria (p. 188).

The cortex shows a four-layer structure, in which the second lamina has a festooned appearance.

e.   Other cortical anomalies.   These may be observed in a number of chromosomal aberrations, especially in *mongolism,* or Down's syndrome (trisomy 21). In the latter, there are posterior temporal abnormalities involving the superior temporal gyrus, which is reduced in size. An irregular decrease in the number of nerve cells in the third layer is often found, as well as cerebellar anomalies accompanied by a reduction in size of the cerebellum. The presence of neurofibrillary degeneration and of senile plaques has also been noted.

ARACHNOIDAL CYSTS

The above term refers to the formation of intracranial extraparenchymatous cysts *that*

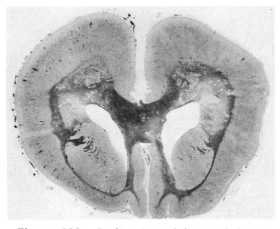

Figure 208.   *Pachygyria and lissencephaly.* Numerous gray matter heterotopias (Loyez stain for myelin).

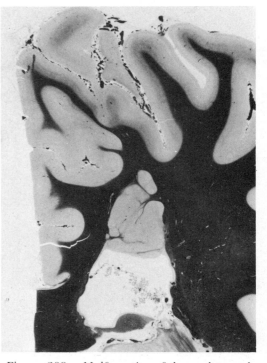

Figure 209.   *Malformation of the caudate nucleus with heterotopias of gray matter* (Loyez stain for myelin).

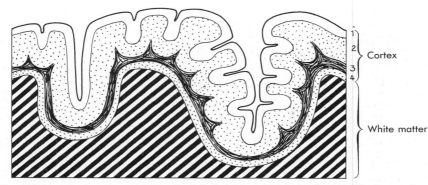

Figure 210.   *Diagrammatic representation of cortical changes in micropolygyria.* (Redrawn from Crome and Stern, 1967.)

are lined along their entire inner surface by arachnoidal tissue and which contain clear fluid (Fig. 211). The definition, however, excludes a number of cystic meningeal lesions with which arachnoidal cysts are often confused. The former include post-traumatic lesions, such as subdural hygromas, and postinfectious cysts resulting secondarily from the formation of loculations within the subarachnoid space (circumscribed arachnoiditis, serous meningitis). The inner lining of these cystic cicatricial lesions is quite different from that of genuine arachnoidal cysts.

Arachnoidal cysts are most frequently seen in children and are sometimes associated with underlying cerebral abnormalities, such as hypoplasia of the temporal pole. These abnormalities are attributed by some workers to a coexistent cortical malformation and by others to secondary changes resulting from the meningeal lesion.

HYDROCEPHALUS

Strictly speaking, hydrocephalus corresponds to an increase in cerebral mass caused by excessive quantities of cerebrospinal fluid. In practice, it corresponds to a variable degree of dilatation of the ventricular system. In children, where the cranial bones have not yet been united, excessive pressure of cerebrospinal fluid and ventricular dilatation result in a variable increase in skull circumference. In the long run the neural parenchyma undergoes thinning, and secondary cortical atrophy occurs if shunting procedures are not performed.

Noncommunicating hydrocephalus is secondary to narrowing of the aqueduct of Sylvius, which causes obstruction to the flow of cerebrospinal fluid. Aqueduct stenosis may be due to a tumor, most often glial, to ependymal changes secondary to an inflammatory process, or to a malformation with duplication of the ependyma, which is found particularly in von Recklinghausen's neurofibromatosis.

Communicating hydrocephalus corresponds to massive dilatation of the entire ventricular system. It may be secondary to:

Hypersecretion of cerebrospinal fluid from a choroid plexus papilloma (see Fig. 42);

Impairment of cerebrospinal fluid resorption in secondary meningeal scarring processes, such as may occur in the late stages of meningitis with basal obstruction, or as a sequel of subarachnoid hemorrhage or subdural hematoma.

However, the cause of hydrocephalus often remains obscure. A number of sex-linked familial forms are known.

Often the picture of hydrocephalus is associated with other cerebral malformations. This is particularly so in the following two conditions:

Dandy-Walker syndrome, in which there is occlusion of the foramina of Magendie and Luschka, and in which enormous dilatation

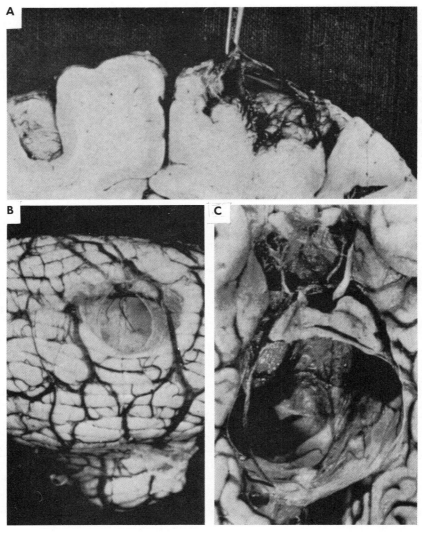

Figure 211.   *Arachnoidal cysts.*

A, Right parietal cyst. The stretched outer arachnoidal cyst wall, opened at operation, is held by a pair of forceps.

B, Left cerebellar cyst. The continuity of the outer cyst wall with the cerebellar arachnoidal membrane is well seen.

C, Cyst of the pineal region. Marked flattening of the cerebral peduncles and displacement of the pineal to the right by a voluminous cyst causing invagination of the medial temporal structures.

of the fourth ventricle (Fig. 212) associated with an occipital meningocele and agenesis of the cerebellar vermis—and sometimes of the splenium of the corpus callosum—appears to indicate a disorder of posterior fusion.

Arnold-Chiari malformation, in which hydrocephalus is often the result of malformations at the base of the skull, where the following lesions are associated:

Platybasia, with malformation of the occipitovertebral joint;

SYRINGOMYELIA

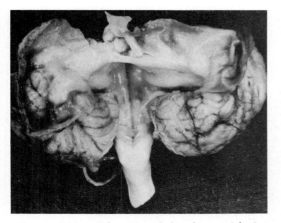

Figure 212. *Dilatation of fourth ventricle in a case of Dandy-Walker syndrome.* Note also the striking agenesis of the cerebellar vermis.

A cerebellar malformation frequently affecting the vermis and especially the tonsils, which are elongated and herniate in the foramen magnum;

Elongation of the brainstem at the level of the pons and medulla, which also herniates into the foramen magnum;

Lumbar spina bifida with myelomeningocele, which results in fixation of the spinal cord at its caudal end and is, according to some authors, responsible for secondary traction on the more rostral neuraxis concurrent with increase in length of the spinal canal. However, the presence of malformations involving the cerebellum and the base of the skull rather suggests dysplasia of the latter, and this seems confirmed by absence of the normal curvature of the pons.

Syringomyelia is the result of a cavitation of the spinal cord, or syrinx, which extends over several metameric segments (Fig. 213), most often involving the cervicothoracic segments. The spinal cord, which in the living is widened and swollen at that level, presents on the contrary a flattened appearance at postmortem examination. The syringomyelic slit or cavity, which is most often single but sometimes multiple, occupies the center of the spinal cord and is usually situated behind the ependyma, involving, in the midline, the crossing fibers of the ascending pain and temperature nerve fiber tracts. It may implicate the gray matter and fuse laterally with the entering sensory nerve roots or affect to a variable extent the anterior horns, resulting in lower motor neuron paralysis with amyotrophy. It may also extend transversely into the white matter of the lateral and posterior columns, as well as more caudally, but seldom involves the lumbar segments. It is limited by highly fibrillary glial tissue which often includes blood vessels with hyalinized walls. It may incorporate ependyma and, in these areas, the ependymal lining is then continuous with the lining of the syringomyelic cavity.

In the majority of cases the syrinx extends into the inferior portion of the brainstem, but seldom involves the pons. In the medulla *(syringomyelobulbia)* (Fig. 214), three types of syrinx may be found: a lateral slit, which is oblique and situated anteriorly and laterally to the floor of the fourth ventricle; an axial

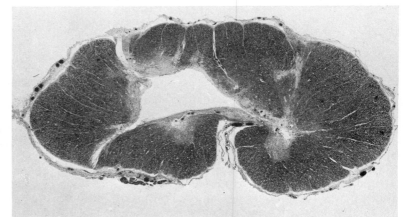

Figure 213. *Syringomyelia.* Centromedullary cavitating lesion encroaching upon the posterior horn and column (Loyez stain for myelin).

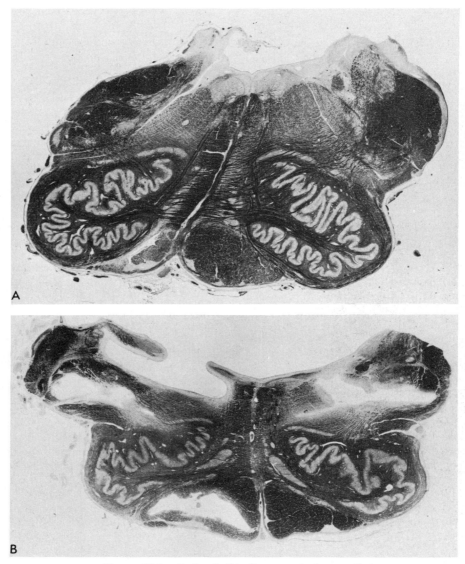

Figure 214.   *Syringobulbia* (Loyez stain for myelin).

A, Lateral right-sided slit extending from fourth ventricle and ventral slit in ipsilateral medullary pyramid. *B*, Several cavities. One of these communicates with the fourth ventricle.

and midline slit along the median raphe; or an anterior slit between the inferior olives and the medullary pyramid.

Syringomyelic slits must be distinguished from pseudosyringomyelia, which is the result of cavitation secondary to old hemorrhagic or necrotic foci or to cystic tumors of the spinal cord, such as hemangioblastomas or gliomas.

A number of pathogenetic theories have been proposed to explain the development of syringomyelia.

The *dysraphic theory*. According to this theory, there is a closure defect of the neural tube at the level of the posterior raphe.

The *hydrodynamic theory*. This hypothesis has more recently been suggested in an effort to account for the frequent coexistence of syringomyelia and Arnold-Chiari malformation. According to this theory, syringomyelia would be due to a disturbance in the outflow of cerebrospinal fluid from the fourth ventricle. The basic abnormality is postulated to consist in a failure on the part of the foramina of Lushka and of Magendie to open. Hydrocephalus would then occur, accompanied by herniation of the medulla oblongata and of the cerebellar tonsils (Chiari malformation), later followed, as the result of increased cerebrospinal fluid pressure, by dilatation of the ependymal canal (hydromyelia). A syringomyelic cavity might then subsequently develop as the result of a rupture in the wall of the dilated ependymal canal.

BLASTOMATOUS DYSPLASIAS AND PHAKOMATOSES

Within the context of malformative and neuroectodermal dysplastic processes, there is a group of diseases that have in common an association of distinctive malformations of the neuraxis with small tumors (phakomas, or lentil-like neoplasias) which involve the skin, the nervous system, or the eyes. Included within this definition are von Recklinghausen's neurofibromatosis and tuberose sclerosis (or Bourneville's disease). To these pathological disorders of dysplastic nature it is customary to add von Hippel–Lindau's disease, in which multiple tumors are the characteristic feature. Because of the presence of diffuse vascular malformations of angiomatous nature, Sturge-Weber's disease is also included in the group by analogy with von Hippel–Lindau's disease, although it does not, in actual fact, demonstrate the peripheral neoplastic manifestations which, by definition, justify the term "phakomatosis."

1. Von Recklinghausen's neurofibromatosis. This common familial disorder shows the following associations:

a. Cutaneous lesions. "Café-au-lait" spots and pigmentary nevi;
Pedunculated tumors of the "molluscum pendulum" or "fibrosum" type;

Nodular subcutaneous neurofibromas and so-called "royal tumors," which may sometimes be extremely voluminous.

b. Neural tumors. These tumors most frequently involve nerve roots. They may present either as neurofibromas or as schwannomas (or neurilemmomas) (see pp. 33–35; Fig. 48). They may involve the cranial nerves and in particular give rise to bilateral acoustic schwannomas.

Multiple meningiomas and a form of meningiomatosis are also characteristic.

Central nervous system tumors are less often encountered; they include especially optic nerve gliomas, gliomas of the chiasm or of the brainstem, and sometimes even glioblastomas.

c. Nervous system malformations. These malformations consist of heterotopias, cortical dysplasias, stenosis of the aqueduct of Sylvius, or syringomyelia. In association with bony malformations of the spine, they indicate the dysplastic nature of this process.

2. Tuberose sclerosis (Bourneville's disease). This condition is less common and shows an association of the following lesions:
Skin lesions, which include adenoma sebaceum involving the skin in the nasolabial fold, angiofibromas, and cutaneous and periungual fibromas.
Cortical cerebral malformations, consisting of circumscribed nodules containing voluminous cells which are often multinucleated and irregularly distributed, corresponding either to monstrous neurons or to giant glial cells. Heterotopic nodules of identical structure are also frequent in the white matter.
Cerebral tumors, of variable size and of glial nature, localized mainly to the striatothalamic fold.
Visceral tumors, including skeletal muscle neoplasms, cardiac muscle tumors, endocrine tumors, and pulmonary nodules.

3. Von Hippel–Lindau's disease (retinocerebellar angiomatosis). This disease, which is likewise familial, is characterized by the presence of multiple hemangioblastomas (see pp. 49–51) localized most frequently to the retina and cerebellum (Fig. 64), and less often to the spinal cord or the cerebrum.

In some cases the large size of draining vessels may lead to the erroneous interpretation of a vascular malformation.

Visceral tumors and cysts, involving especially the kidney and pancreas, may be associated with the disease.

4. Encephalotrigeminal angiomatosis or Sturge-Weber's disease. This condition shows the following association:

A flat extensive unilateral cutaneous angioma of the face.

A leptomeningeal encephalic angiomatosis, often predominating in the parieto-occipital region, of venous type, and accompanied by alterations in the underlying cortex. The alterations consist of gliosis of the superficial layers and especially in the presence of calcium concretions which extend throughout the thickness of the second and third cortical layers and account for the radiological picture of parallel linear calcifications.

PERINATAL PATHOLOGY

At the time of birth and during the first months of life, various etiological factors may result in definite cerebral lesions. These account for a number of various neurological syndromes, of which the most common are:

Infantile cerebral hemiplegia;

Infantile cerebral diplegia, or Little's disease;

Some forms of congenital epilepsy.

The determining lesions, which are most often traumatic, circulatory, or anoxic, are identical with those described in the relevant chapters dealing with these various pathogenetic mechanisms. However, their supervention on the immature brain gives rise to a highly distinct pathological picture. These lesions are obviously more frequent and more severe in premature infants.

It is customary to separate the cerebral damage related to the birth process itself (neonatal pathology) from that secondary to disturbances in the first months of life (post-

natal pathology), but the sequelae are often identical and the lesions are frequently of the same nature.

1. Neonatal pathology. a. The pathogenetic mechanisms that may alter the brain at the time of birth may be summarized into three main types:

Traumatic mechanisms, in which obstetric injury results in cerebral lesions that are direct or more often indirect, the effects being usually hemorrhagic as the consequence of blood vessel rupture, especially venous (often the result of difficult birth presentation).

Circulatory mechanisms, either venous and related to increase of intracerebral venous pressure at the time of birth, or arterial and secondary to a fall of blood flow resulting from circulatory arrest.

And finally, *anoxic* and *asphyxial mechanisms.*

b.   The lesions may be acute, leading to death, or cicatricial, resulting in the picture of secondary encephalopathy of neonatal origin.

ACUTE LESIONS are essentially of hemorrhagic nature:

Subdural hematomas, which frequently become organized.

Subarachnoid hemorrhage, which may ultimately lead to hydrocephalus as the result of secondary cicatricial arachnoidal lesions.

Intracerebral hemorrhage localized to the white matter, due to venous damage, or to the basal ganglia and, more precisely, to the germinative periventricular matrix layer, whose involvement is characteristic.

SECONDARY LESIONS responsible for the group of infantile encephalopathies are the sequel of hemorrhagic or necrotic lesions.

They may consist of

Extensive lobar or hemispheric atrophies that may suggest vascular occlusion, which is, however, difficult to prove;

Cortical changes, in which *ulegyria* (Fig. 215) has the most characteristic appearance. This consists in cortical atrophy involving the deeper part of the cortex of a cerebral gyrus,

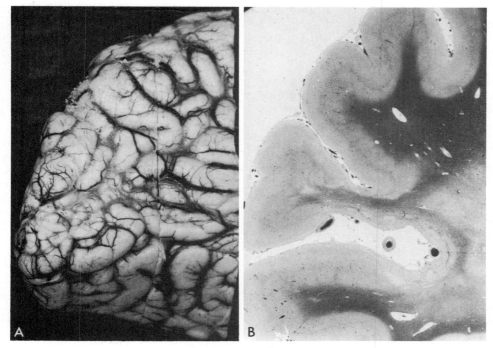

Figure 215. *Ulegyria.*

A, Gross appearance on the medial aspect of the occipital lobe. *B,* Microscopic appearance (Loyez stain for myelin); note atrophy of the base of the gyrus.

with relative sparing of its convexity. As a result there is a retractile, mushroom-shaped sclerosis of the altered gyrus. A picture of secondary hypermyelination may occur in the less severely affected part of the cortex. These atrophied convolutions are often grouped together. They may present a granular appearance. Their distribution in a vascular territory or in a boundary zone of arterial supply, particularly in the parieto-occipital convexity, suggests an ischemic circulatory mechanism.

The white matter may be the seat of extensive bilateral retractile glial scars, corresponding to the pathological picture of the *centrilobar sclerosis* of Charles Foix and Pierre Marie, a condition which is of venous circulatory origin and in the past has been confused with some of the demyelinating conditions of childhood.

Large cystic pseudoporencephalic cavitations (Fig. 216) may also be observed.

The basal ganglia may be the seat of various

lesions, of which *status marmoratus (état marbré),* due to a secondary phenomenon of hypermyelination along cicatricial glial le-

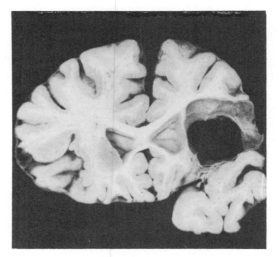

Figure 216. *Pseudoporencephalic cystic cavity of circulatory origin.*

sions of the corpus striatum, is the most characteristic. This pathological change is often associated with the neurological picture of double athetosis.

2. Postnatal pathology. The observed cerebral lesions may be secondary to numerous etiological and pathogenetic mechanisms.

1. EARLY VASCULAR ENCEPHALOPATHIES. Some of these are related to venous lesions, such as thrombosis of the vein of Galen or of the superior longitudinal sinus, and are often secondary to early meningeal infections.

Others are related to arterial occlusions whose embolic or thrombotic origin is difficult to prove. They may produce the picture of lobar or hemispheric atrophy.

2. POSTEPILEPTIC ENCEPHALOPATHY. This is characterized by gliosis with atrophy of Ammon's horn, secondary to episodes of anoxia due to repeated epileptic fits or to status epilepticus.[1]

Cerebellar changes involving the Purkinje cells, granular neurons, and the dentate nuclei may also be seen.

3. NUCLEAR JAUNDICE is the result of hemolytic neonatal anemia due to Rh incompatibility.

The lesions are characterized by their topographical distribution — involving the globus pallidus, the subthalamic nuclei and, to a lesser extent, Ammon's horns, the dentate nuclei, and the inferior olives — and by their yellow appearance due to the presence of bilirubin (see also above, p. 175).

---

[1]These lesions are regarded by some authors as being of circulatory origin, namely due to ischemia of the territory of the posterior cerebral artery at the time of birth, and as being the cause of the epileptic seizures.

NEUROMUSCULAR PATHOLOGY Chapter 11

For practical reasons neuromuscular pathology will be reviewed only within the context of information provided by muscle and peripheral nerve biopsy. Indeed, these procedures constitute one of the current methods of laboratory investigation in diseases of the peripheral nerves and of the skeletal musculature, and represent one of the most important aspects of daily neuropathological practice. Traumatic and neoplastic disorders of muscles and peripheral nerves are not dealt with in this manual, since they more properly belong to the field of general pathology.

HISTOLOGICAL EXAMINATION OF MUSCLE BIOPSIES

Muscle biopsy has now become common practice. It essentially permits the neurogenic or, alternatively, the primary myopathic nature of muscular atrophy to be determined and sometimes provides the clue to its etiology. In addition, the findings may be related to those obtained by a peripheral nerve biopsy, which can be performed at the same time.

The traditional histopathological techniques are usually adequate for most muscle biopsies carried out for the purpose of eliciting or confirming a diagnosis of some general pathological disturbances such as an inflammatory process, a collagen disease, amyloidosis. Enzyme histochemistry and more specialized techniques, such as those permitting the study of the motor nerve endings, as well as electron microscopy play a major complementary role when microscopic lesions no longer fall within well-established diagnostic frames of reference. These methods have now become essential for the investigation of those pathological processes involving the skeletal musculature, such as the "congenital myopathies," that are still incompletely understood today.

A. PRINCIPAL LESIONS

Complete histological examination of a muscle biopsy must successively take account of changes in the vascular and connective tissue components of the muscle, the extrafusal muscle fibers, the terminal motor innervation, the motor end-plates, and the neuromuscular spindles. Here we shall deal only with alterations in the extrafusal muscle fibers and in the vascular and connective tissue elements of the muscle, since the study of changes in the other elements listed above necessitates techniques and expertise that extend beyond the usual domain of current neuropathological practice.

1. Changes in Muscle Fibers

Examination of muscle fibers must be systematically carried out on sections that are

191

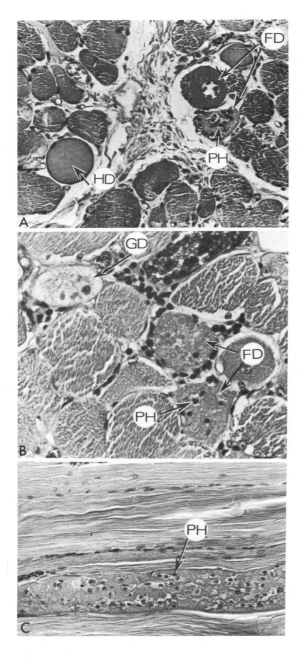

Figure 217. *Various types of necrotizing change in muscle fibers* (H. and E.).

A, Hyaline degeneration *(HD);* note the homogenized appearance of the involved fiber compared with normal fibers, in which myofibrils show a normal degree of dissociation. Note also phagocytosis and flocculent degeneration *(FD)* of other muscle fibers.

B, Granular degeneration *(GD).* Note also flocculent degeneration *(FD)* of two muscle fibers; a few macrophage nuclei are seen in one of them *(PH).*

C, Phagocytosis of a muscle fiber seen in longitudinal section *(PH);* note the isolated character of the lesion and the normal striation in the adjacent fibers.

Dissociation of fibers resulting from undesirable injection of anesthetic into the muscle;

Fractures and lacerations of muscle fibers resulting from ill-considered traction on the biopsy fragment;

Contraction artifacts resulting from poor fixation in overconcentrated formalin solution (Nageotte's bands);

Swelling, cloudy appearance and vacuolization due to immersion in fixing solution of insufficient concentration;

Retraction of fibers due to inadequate heating of the paraffin-embedding medium;

Laceration of fibers due to a blunt microtome;

Apparent inequality in size of muscle fibers due to poor orientation of the block or to selection of a biopsy sample too near the musculotendinous insertion.

Each type of pathological alteration must be listed for further analysis after all the sections have been examined, *as each of the observed changes may in itself be of no specific diagnostic value and may be seen in any form of neuromuscular disorder. Only the regrouping of these changes will have a diagnostic value.*

a. **Morphology of the lesions.** *1. Changes in muscle fiber size.*[1] The fibers may be atrophic

strictly transverse and longitudinal. Pathological changes must be carefully differentiated from the numerous artifacts due to various causes and resulting from the fragility of muscle tissue. These artifacts include:

Traumatic lesions due to previous electromyographic exploration;

[1]The size of muscle fibers varies according to the age of the subject and the muscle examined. In the adult, it ranges from 20 to 100 μm. It is therefore difficult to evaluate the degree of hypertrophy of a muscle fiber if its diameter is less than 100 μm or its degree of atrophy if its diameter is more than 20 μm.

or hypertrophic. This aspect can be gauged with precision only in perfectly transverse cross sections of the muscle biopsy, which must be selected well within the muscle mass, remote from the tendinous insertions. Other features to be noted are the variations in outline of the muscle fibers as seen in transverse sections, particularly the loss of their usual polyhedral shape, e.g., rounding of the muscle fibers or reduction of their caliber.

2. *Appearance and distribution of the nuclei* (Fig. 218).

Increase, apparent or real, in their number, i.e., more than four to eight nuclei for each muscle fiber seen in cross section;

Central displacement (i.e., involving more than 3 to 5 per cent of the nuclei as an average) or, inversely, marginal displacement along the sarcolemma;

"Chain-like" (or "tramcar") arrangement;

Hyperchromasia and small size of the nuclei or, inversely, vesicular nuclei.

3. *Changes in muscle fiber structure* (Fig. 217).

Necrotic changes essentially consist of loss of the normal cross-striated structure of the muscle fiber and are accompanied by variable phagocytic manifestations. The changes correspond to the classical picture of granular, hyaline, and floccular degeneration, and often have a segmental appearance.

Hyaline degeneration is characterized by swelling of the muscle fiber, which is filled by homogeneous eosinophilic material. In *floccular degeneration* the fiber has disintegrated into small eosinophilic masses, which are associated with discrete evidence of phagocytosis. In its extreme form, degeneration culminates in total necrosis.

Basophilic fibers. The fibers have a basophilic, either weakly striated or nonstriated, cytoplasm as seen in hematoxylin-eosin preparations, and vesicular nuclei with conspicuous nucleoli, often arranged in chains. They are thought probably to represent regenerating muscle fibers (Fig. 227*A*).

Target fibers (Fig. 219). The fibers have a heterogeneous central zone surrounded by a clear halo and are thought to be the result of secondary reinnervation in neurogenic muscular atrophy.

Vacuolated fibers. The presence, visible by both light and electron microscopy, of vacuoles in muscle fibers must be interpreted with caution in view of their often artifactual nature, contingent on the fixation procedure.

Striated annulets (Ringbinden) are formed by myofibrils which are normal in structure, but abnormally arranged so as to be perpendicular to the muscle fiber axis as seen on cross section (Fig. 220).

Lateral sarcoplasmic masses (Fig. 221) present as nonstriated clear areas situated between the sarcolemma and a central myofibrillary zone, which appears normal. The masses are often associated with striated annulets.

b. Distribution of the lesions. *1. A definitely fascicular distribution* is indicative of involvement of the lower motor neuron (Fig. 222).

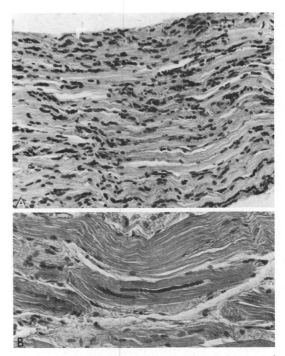

Figure 218. *Nuclear abnormalities in muscle fibers* (H. and E.).

A, Apparent increase in the number of sarcolemmal nuclei in neurogenic atrophy. *B*, Central displacement and *"tramcar"* appearance of sarcolemmal nuclei in myotonic dystrophy.

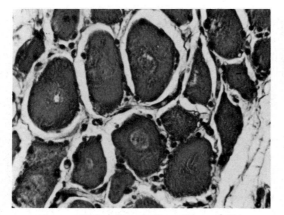

Figure 219. *Target fibers* (H. and E.).

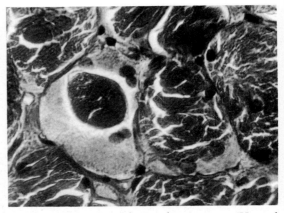

Figure 221. *Lateral sarcoplasmic masses* (H. and E.). Note the presence of lateral crescents due to myofibrillary disorganization.

2. A diffuse distribution, i.e., one in which all the fascicles are involved to the same degree, is seen in a number of dysmetabolic processes.

3. An uneven distribution, disorderly and nonsystematic (i.e., one in which all the fascicles are involved, but in which the fibers are unevenly and randomly affected within the same fascicle), is essentially observed in primary muscle disorders (myopathies).

4. A focal distribution, i.e., one in which the lesions are restricted but not systematic, suggests a vascular process.

5. A perifascicular distribution, i.e., one in which the most peripheral fibers of the muscle bundles are the most severely affected, suggests polymyositis.

c. Changes in the distribution of the various muscle fiber types as demonstrated with histoenzymological techniques. Generally speaking, enzyme histochemical studies have revealed:

In *neurogenic atrophy,* changes in the usual mosaic distribution of the motor units, with a tendency on the part of the muscle fibers of the same type to group themselves together. This rearrangement is apparently the result of reinnervation of denervated muscle fibers by collateral sprouts from neighboring axons that originally innervated muscle fibers of different histochemical types (*"type grouping"*) (Fig. 224);

In *atrophy from primary myopathic disease,* the two main histochemical muscle fiber types are affected unevenly (Fig. 226).

2. Interstitial Changes

Certain alterations seen in the interstitial tissue may sometimes have diagnostic importance and establish the etiology of the process with assurance; others have, on the contrary, no such diagnostic value.

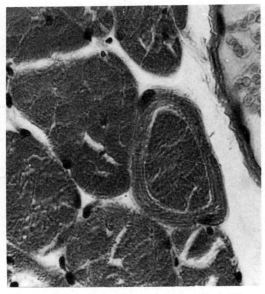

Figure 220. *Striated annulet (ring fiber)* (H. and E.).

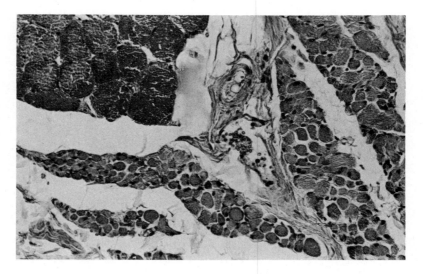

Figure 222. *Fascicular muscle fiber atrophy in peripheral neuropathy* (H. and E.).

a. Diagnostic changes. Chiefly notable are the granulomatous lesions of *sarcoidosis* (Fig. 229); the arteriolar lesions of *polyarteritis nodosa* (Fig. 228), which have characteristic necrotic and inflammatory features and a segmental distribution; and the deposits of *amyloidosis*, which are metachromatic when stained with crystal violet.

b. Nondiagnostic changes. These changes include infiltration by connective or adipose tissue, which is seen in the late stages of muscular atrophy regardless of its etiology.

Nondiagnostic changes also include inflammatory lesions composed of different cell types (lymphocytes, histiocytes, polymorphonuclear leukocytes), especially when they are discrete.

B. CHIEF ETIOLOGICAL PROCESSES

1. Muscle lesions secondary to lower motor system involvement (amyotrophy of neurogenic type or denervation atrophy).

a. General features include: *1.* Systematic fascicular distribution of the lesions (Fig. 222).

2. Simple atrophy of the muscle fibers, which maintain their angular polyhedral shape on cross section and in which cross striations remain identifiable for a considerable time in longitudinal sections. On the other hand, the nuclei, which preserve their normal lateral distribution, often appear more numerous than normal (Fig. 223). In very severe atrophy, this may culminate in the fragmentation of muscle fibers into multinucleated segments from which cross striations have disappeared.

3. Loss of the mosaic distribution of the muscle fibers demonstrated in enzyme histochemistry, and presence of large groups of fibers of the same histochemical type, resulting from reinnervation by collateral sprouting from intact axons ("type grouping"). This may lead to a preponderance of type I fibers[1] (Fig. 224) with atrophy of type II fibers.

4. Presence (especially in neuropathic disorders of recent onset) of target fibers, which are believed to result from attempts at collateral reinnervation (Fig. 219).

[1] Subsequent secondary degeneration of the originally spared motor units produces the picture of fascicular atrophy seen by conventional light microscopy; such an appearance therefore indicates a fairly advanced stage of neurogenic atrophy.

[handwritten] LMN – 1. Fascicular dist
2. Atrophy
3. Type grouping
4. Target fibers

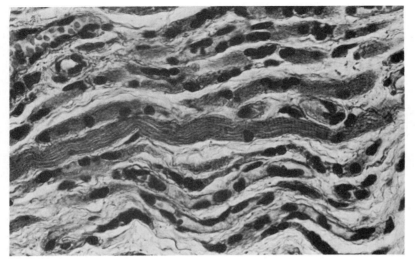

Figure 223. *Neurogenic atrophy* (H. and E.). Note the persistence of cross striations in the atrophied fiber in the center of the field, and apparent multiplication of the sarcolemmal nuclei.

5. Absence or paucity of interstitial changes.[1]

b. Special features. *1. According to the level of neurogenic involvement.* Involvement of

---

[1]Note also the presence of changes in the terminal motor nerve fibers and in the motor end-plates, as well as the classic sparing of neuromuscular spindles. By electron microscopy, an evolutionary sequence in the morphological changes of muscle fibers has been recognized, characterized by progressive decrease of myofilamentous material occurring *pari passu* with a reduction in muscle fiber size.

the anterior horn of the spinal cord is characterized by:

A clear-cut appearance in the fascicular distribution of the atrophy;

The paucity of degenerative changes.

By contrast, involvement of the spinal nerve roots or peripheral nerve trunks is characterized by:

A less clear-cut appearance in the fascicular distribution of the atrophy;

The possible presence of degenerative changes, especially necroses.

2. According to the rapidity of the neurogenic

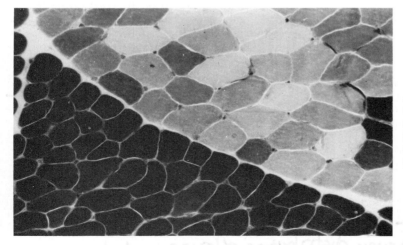

Figure 224. *Neurogenic muscular atrophy.* Grouping of type I muscle fibers demonstrated by enzyme histochemistry (ATPase at pH 4.65). (Courtesy of Drs. M. Fardeau and F. Tomé.)

involvement. In muscular atrophy resulting from protracted denervation, e.g., in Charcot-Marie-Tooth disease, the typical picture of fascicular atrophy often coexists with "pseudomyopathic" features characterized by inequality of fiber size and structural changes in various muscle fibers. These appearances are considered to be secondary to the sequential regenerative processes that frequently occur in the course of these slowly progressive disorders.

2. Muscle lesions due to primary muscle disease (amyotrophy of myogenic type)

a. General features. *1.* Lack of systematic distribution of the lesions, which is often uneven and disorderly.

2. Inequality of muscle fiber size, with the coexistence, within the same fascicle, of both atrophied and hypertrophied fibers, which usually demonstrate a rounded contour in cross section.

3. Presence of various degenerative lesions, of a scattered and segmental character.

4. Variable involvement of the different fiber types as demonstrated by enzyme histochemistry.

b. Special features. These features permit the recognition of two main types of primary muscle disease: progressive muscular dystrophies (or myopathies) and inflammatory processes (polymyositis).

1. PROGRESSIVE MUSCULAR DYSTROPHIES

Pathological features[1]

The diagnosis is dependent on a number of changes, which include:

The presence of multisegmented hypertrophied fibers (Fig. 225);

The demonstration of lateral sarcoplasmic masses and of striated annulets (Figs. 220 and 221);

---

[1]Note also the normal appearance of the terminal motor nerve fibers, the dystrophic aspect of the motor end-plates, and the classic sparing of neuromuscular spindles.

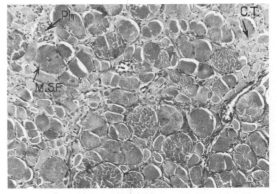

Figure 225. *Muscular dystrophy* (H. and E.). Note the inequality in size of the muscle fibers and the presence of abnormally large fibers, multisegmented fibers (*MSF*), foci of necrosis with phagocytosis (*Ph*), and interstitial infiltration by connective tissue (*CT*).

The very high frequency of centrally displaced sarcoplasmic nuclei;

Conspicuous adipose tissue and interstitial connective tissue proliferation;

The absence or the very great paucity of inflammatory cellular lesions.

None of these changes are, however, specific for, or characteristic of, the various forms of muscular dystrophy or myopathy. The nosological identity of these disorders is primarily contingent on their respective genetic features, on the evolution of their clinical course, and on the distribution of the muscular atrophy, which may or may not be associated with either muscular hypertrophy or myotonia. This caveat applies equally well to the findings of electron microscopy, which has failed to demonstrate any feature that may be regarded as specific for any particular type of myopathy.

Chief etiological forms

Duchenne's pseudohypertrophic muscular dystrophy is a severe form of muscular dystrophy which has a rapid course and is usually fatal around the age of 20 years, with early onset in the muscles of the pelvic girdle associated with a pseudohypertrophic appearance of the calves. It is characteristically recessive and sex-linked, involving males exclusively and being transmitted by a clinically normal maternal carrier.

Lesions are usually severe, with necrotizing features, often of focal distribution.

A more benign variant of later onset and slower evolution is referred to as "dystrophy of the Becker type."

Facioscapulohumeral muscular dystrophy of Landouzy-Dejerine is of slow evolution, compatible with a relatively long life, with its onset in middle childhood or sometimes in the second decade of life. It predominantly involves the facial, neck, and scapular girdle muscles.

Both sexes are affected. The disease is transmitted as an autosomal dominant trait.

Histological lesions are often discrete, and remain so for a considerable time.

The group of the limb-girdle myopathies includes forms of muscular dystrophy that cannot be included in the above-mentioned types. They may have their clinical onset in the second or third decade, predominantly involve the limb girdles (especially the scapular girdle), spare the face, and are not associated with hypertrophy of the calves. Transmission is recessive and is not sex-linked, and the disease is often sporadic.

The structure of the muscle fibers shows dystrophic changes, which are often marked.

This particular group of myopathies, unlike the preceding ones, is not homogeneous, and the diagnosis can be made only after other forms of skeletal muscle involvement have been excluded, especially inflammatory diseases or metabolic disorders, such as glycogen storage disease.

Distal myopathies are much rarer and, with the exception of dominant variants that have been described in Scandinavia, are often difficult to distinguish from certain types of neurogenic atrophy.

Ocular myopathies begin with ptosis and culminate in a picture of total ophthalmoplegia that may resemble certain types of neurogenic disease. They may sometimes be accompanied by involvement of the palato-pharyngeal area and of the limb-girdle musculature.

Some examples of ocular myopathy have shown mitochondrial abnormalities by electron microscopy. In other cases, there is coexistence of retinitis pigmentosa, nervous system manifestations, increased levels of al-bumin in the cerebrospinal fluid, and disorders of cardiac conduction, all of which have been given the name of "ophthalmo-plegia plus."

Myotonic dystrophy is transmitted as an autosomal dominant trait. It presents in young adults as a myopathic disorder with predominantly distal involvement, affecting both the facial and the pharyngeal musculature, and is associated with a myotonic syndrome. Visceral manifestations that may also coexist include baldness, posterior cataracts, endocrine disturbances (involving in particular the sexual organs), and cardiac lesions.

The disease is characterized by the severity and the clear-cut appearance of all the myogenic changes, especially striated annulets (see Fig. 220), lateral sarcoplasmic masses (see Fig. 221), and centrally distributed nuclei arranged in chains (see Fig. 218B).

Enzyme histochemical techniques reveal that the atrophied fibers are mostly of type I, with an overall predominance of muscle fibers belonging to that type (Fig. 226). The extent and frequency of changes in the terminal motor innervation pattern have also been stressed.

Congenital myopathies. Understanding of these diseases is relatively recent. Most of them have been singled out from the group of the childhood hypotonias on the basis of enzyme histochemical and electron microscopic findings.

Many of these cases are characterized by lack of progression in their clinical course and a tendency even to improve with time; this contrasts with the progressive course of hypotonias of neurogenic origin, such as Werdnig-Hoffmann disease.

Central core disease is characterized by the presence of an amorphous central zone devoid of enzymatic activity, involving predominantly type I fibers.

Nemaline myopathy (or rod-body myopathy) may sometimes be identified by means of traditional staining techniques, such as Mallory's trichrome stain, on the basis of the presence of small fuchsinophil rodlets. They are, however, better seen in cryostat-cut sections stained with Gomori's trichrome. They

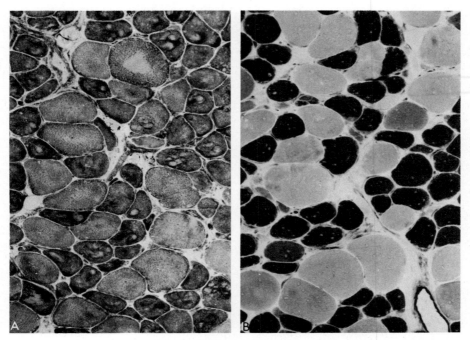

Figure 226. *Myotonic dystrophy.*

A, NADH tetrazolium reductase: numerous atrophied fibers with changes in their sarcoplasm. *B*, ATPase at pH 4.35 (×80): all atrophied fibers are of type I; most type II fibers are hypertrophied.

are situated beneath the sarcolemma. These structures are apparently formed from Z bands.

Megaconial myopathy and *pleoconial myopathy* are identified by the presence of characteristic mitochondrial abnormalities in electron microscopy.

Myotubular myopathy, or centronuclear myopathy, is characterized by the prominence of central nuclei.

Type I fiber hypotrophy may be encountered in single cases as a form of benign congenital hypotonia.

Many of these congenital muscle disorders (to which should be added some that demonstrate lipid storage or inclusions of a fingerprint pattern, etc. as well as other conditions resembling adult myopathy) are still difficult to classify exactly at this stage despite the morphological criteria that have been used for their identification.

2. INFLAMMATORY PROCESSES

Specific myositis

Acute myositis, either viral or infectious (pyogenic, rickettsial, tuberculous, or syphilitic), is rare.

Parasitic myositis (trichinosis, toxoplasmosis, cysticercosis) is less exceptional and fairly common in tropical and subtropical countries.

The diagnosis is based on the identification of the causal agent.

Polymyositis

The diagnostic histological features of polymyositis consist in the association of necrotic lesions involving muscle fibers with an interstitial inflammatory cellular reaction (Fig. 227).

The muscle fiber lesions, which are often segmental, present different degenerative

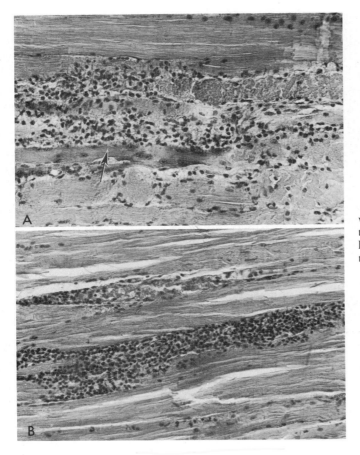

Figure 227. *Polymyositis* (H. and E.). *A*, Necrosis of single muscle fibers, with cellular inflammatory reaction; note the presence of a basophilic fiber with large, pale vesicular nuclei (*arrow*). *B*, Interstitial inflammatory infiltrate.

aspects, which are accompanied by phagocytic features of variable intensity. Muscle involvement shows a disseminated, disorderly distribution, although often with a perifascicular dominance. The presence of coexisting basophilic fibers is generally attributed to a regenerative process.

The inflammatory reaction, which is largely lymphocytic and of variable cellular density, may be distinctly focal or present as interstitial endomysial infiltrates.

Sclerotic lesions and even a few calcifications may be seen in the late stages.

In the *acute form*, the lesions are often edematous and may be associated with mucocutaneous lesions (the picture of dermatomyositis) and with general constitutional signs and symptoms.

In the *chronic form*, the interstitial inflammatory manifestations are often discrete, and the diagnosis is frequently made on the basis of prominent regenerative features (pseudomyopathic form, pseudomyasthenic form, and "late myopathy" of the Nevin type).

Although a precise cause, such as an inflammatory autoimmune reaction or a virus (as suggested) cannot be assigned to most examples of polymyositis, a number of cases (15 to 20 per cent) are associated, in the adult, with visceral cancer, most often bronchopulmonary carcinoma.

Collagenoses

In these disorders the presence of an interstitial nodular myositis may frequently be established microscopically even before muscular disturbances are clinically apparent. When signs and symptoms involving muscle make their clinical appearance, several mechanisms may be brought into play:

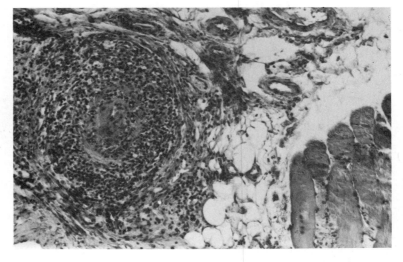

Figure 228. *Polyarteritis no-dosa* (H. and E.). Note the periarteriolar cellular infiltration and the involvement of the vessel wall, with occlusion of the lumen.

Muscle impairment due to a peripheral nerve lesion, especially in polyarteritis nodosa (Fig. 228), in chronic progressive polyarthritis, and less often, in systemic lupus erythematosus;

Peripheral nerve or muscular lesions due to therapy (e.g., corticosteroids, antimalarial drugs);

Muscle lesions allied to those of polymyositis.

Sarcoidosis

The diagnosis of sarcoidosis rests on the observation of interstitial granulomatous foci. Around these foci the parenchymatous lesions are of variable severity and may consist of focal necroses, lymphocytic infiltrates further afield, and replacement by fibroadipose tissue (Fig. 229).

3. Muscle changes occuring in toxic, endocrine, and metabolic disorders. a. Toxic changes. A number of substances, especially drugs (e.g., corticosteroids, chloroquine), may be responsible for the picture of "vacuolar myopathy," in which the vacuoles correspond to disseminated necrotic zones within the muscle fibers.

b. Muscle changes in endocrine disorders. A number of various muscle changes may be encountered in hyperthyroidism, hypothyroidism, corticosteroid over-production, hyperparathyroidism, and hyperinsulinism.

c. Muscle changes in metabolic disorders. Of the many metabolic disorders that are capable of producing muscle lesions, only the chief forms will be mentioned.

1. DYSKALEMIC PARALYSES. These are characterized by abnormalities in the sarcoplasmic reticulum, with the presence of dilatations and vacuoles. Electron microscopy has demonstrated the presence of tubular "pipestem" aggregates.

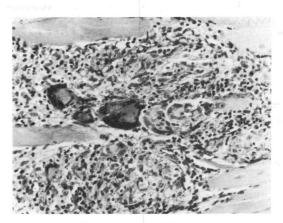

Figure 229. *Sarcoid myositis* (H. and E.). Interstitial granuloma with giant cells.

2. ESSENTIAL PAROXYSMAL MYOGLOBINURIA. During acute episodes a coagulative necrosis of muscle fibers may be seen. This is rapidly followed by phagocytosis of the necrotic zones and, at a later stage, by the onset of a process of muscle fiber regeneration which is virtually complete after a few days.

3. GLYCOGENOSES. A number of glycogenoses are characterized by the presence of glycogen-filled vacuoles within the muscle fibers.

Pompe's disease, or type II glycogenosis, is due to a deficiency of acid maltase; this causes severe hypotonia in the newborn, with cardiac involvement. In the adult it may show the picture of progressive limb-girdle dystrophy.

Forbes' disease, or type III glycogenosis, is due to a deficit of the debranching enzyme amylo-1, 6-glucosidase. It may be the cause of some forms of hypotonia in early childhood and of muscular dystrophy in late childhood.

MacArdle's disease, or type V glycogenosis, is due to a deficiency of phosphorylase. The disease can be diagnosed by histoenzymological techniques.

Type VII glycogenosis is due to a deficiency of phosphofructokinase. It is seen somewhat exceptionally and resembles the picture of MacArdle's disease.

4. AMYLOIDOSIS. The walls of small blood vessels, the small intramuscular nerve fibers, and the interstitial connective tissue are infiltrated by a material which is metachromatic with crystal violet. The lesions in the muscle fibers themselves are essentially those of denervation atrophy.

4. Myasthenia gravis. A special place must be reserved for myasthenia gravis. In addition to the contingent presence of focal interstitial cellular infiltrates known as lymphorrhages (Fig. 230) and to frequent abnormalities in the motor end-plates, one may

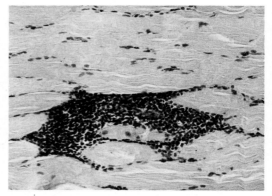

Figure 230. *Myasthenia gravis* (H. and E.). Picture of lymphorrhages.

observe, although very seldom and to a very limited extent, alterations in the size of muscle fibers as well as necrotizing lesions.

C. CONCLUSION

It must be stressed that there is no fundamental lesion diagnostic of a particular etiology. Only the presence of several of these changes taken together may be regarded as characteristic, at least in the majority of cases. For example, striated annulets, lateral sarcoplasmic masses, and an arrangement of sarcoplasmic nuclei in chains, although not diagnostic of myotonic dystrophy, are nevertheless more common and more numerous in this condition than in other forms of muscular dystrophy. The same reservations are applicable to some of the elementary lesions seen by electron microscopy.

Complementary techniques, such as enzyme histochemistry, have provided additional data which have been essential for the diagnosis of certain deceptive forms of denervation atrophy, such as those occurring in slowly progressive neurogenic disease, and for the identification of a number of still poorly defined muscle disorders, such as the limb-girdle myopathies and the "congenital myopathies."

HISTOLOGICAL EXAMINATION OF PERIPHERAL NERVE BIOPSIES

In contrast to muscle biopsy, and despite the use of modern complementary techniques such as teased preparations and electron microscopy, peripheral nerve biopsy does not usually provide data which permit the precise etiology of a particular neuropathy to be determined. This inadequacy is due to two main problems. On the one hand, degenerative lesions of the peripheral nerves do not present any specific well-defined features. On the other, any causative process that may primarily involve either the perikaryon or the axon must perforce escape detection in most cases because of the sampling limitation inherent in the selection of a small distal portion of a nerve which is, moreover, entirely sensory.

A. PRINCIPAL LESIONS

1. Changes in nerve fibers. These changes are rather stereotyped and include three main forms:

a. Wallerian degeneration corresponds to degeneration of the distal end of a nerve fiber secondary to a lesion of the axon or of the nerve cell body. It is characterized by the successive fragmentation and disappearance of axons and myelin sheaths and by secondary proliferation of the Schwann cells. Sprouting of the proximal end is possible in a number of pathological processes (Fig. 231). In traumatic peripheral nerve lesions, which *par excellence* cause wallerian degeneration, perfect restoration of neuritic continuity is necessary in axonal regeneration in order to avoid the development of a post-traumatic neuroma. In the course of so-called axonal neuropathy (which could result from inflammatory, dysmetabolic, or vascular lesions) or following lesions to the perikaryon, the changes observed in peripheral nerves are closely similar to those of wallerian degeneration. Secondary phenomena attributable to regeneration are also important and are characterized by the formation

of clusters of small axons which occupy Büngner's cell bands (resulting from Schwann cell hyperplasia) and undergo more or less complete secondary remyelination. These pathological processes are complex. Their evolution is characteristically progressive: successive and concomitant lesions that are either degenerative or regenerative coexist in both myelinated and unmyelinated axons. They can be analyzed with precision only on the basis of complementing data obtained from traditional light microscopy, from dissociation techniques such as teased preparations, and from electron microscopy. The findings must also be evaluated quantitatively and compared with those obtained in normal control subjects of the same age.

b. Segmental demyelination is characterized by localized scattered destruction of myelin sheaths without axonal lesions and is due to a primary lesion of the Schwann cells (Fig. 232).

Although it is sometimes possible to recognize segmental demyelination with the usual myelin stains (see Fig. 235), this feature can be identified with assurance and studied accurately only through a technique that permits the dissociation of individual nerve fibers, as in teased preparations. Demyelination begins at the node of Ranvier, which becomes widened, and then involves one or more internodes in a variable, irregular manner (Fig. 233).

Potential remission of the neuropathy is explained by the sparing of axons and secondary remyelination. In this process, the involved internodal segment is replaced by shorter internodal segments which result from the multiplication of Schwann cells at that site. The shortening of the internodal distances and the variations in their length permit the segmental process of demyelination followed by remyelination to be recognized in its later stages.

c. Onion-bulb hypertrophy of the Schwann cells is encountered much less fre-

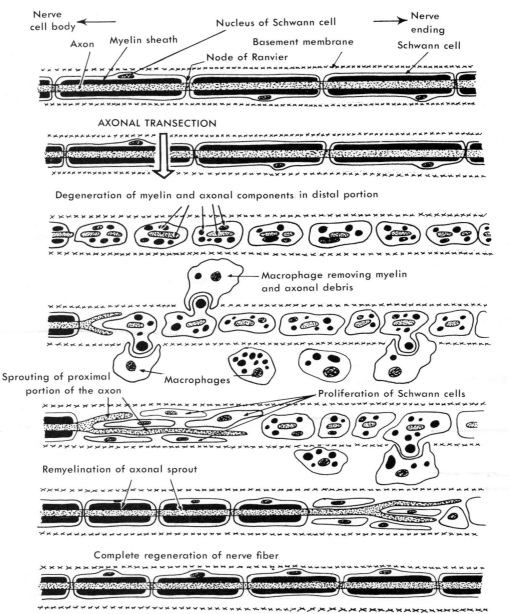

Figure 231. *Diagrammatic representation of the main stages of wallerian degeneration and regeneration of a myelinated peripheral nerve fiber.* (Redrawn and modified after W. G. Bradley, 1974.)

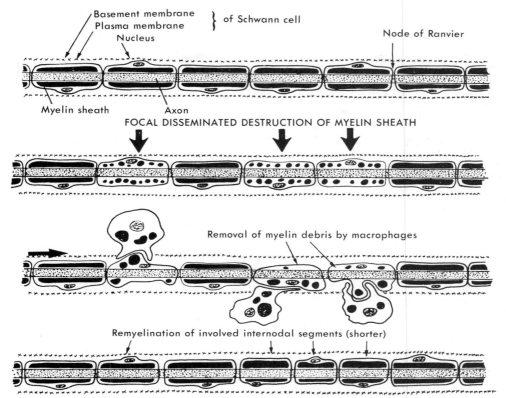

FOCAL DISSEMINATED DESTRUCTION OF MYELIN SHEATH

Figure 232. *Diagrammatic representation of the main stages of segmental demyelination and remyelination of a myelinated peripheral nerve fiber.*

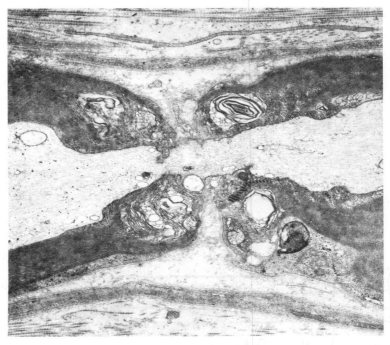

Figure 233. *Electron microscopic appearance of early segmental demyelination at the node of Ranvier.*

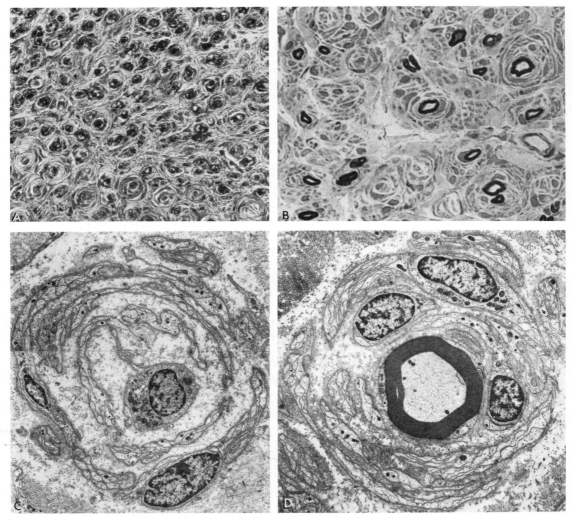

Figure 234.   *Onion-bulb Schwann cell hypertrophy.*

A, Light microscopy (Masson's trichrome).   *B*, Light microscopy of semi-thin section embedded for electron microscopy. *C* and *D*, Electron microscopy.

quently. It is characterized by a whorling proliferation of Schwann cells around axons (Fig. 234). This process was long regarded as specific for Déjerine-Sottas disease (interstitial familial hypertrophic neuropathy) and for certain dysmetabolic neuropathies such as Refsum's disease. However, the lesion is now known to be the terminal phase of various neuropathic processes in which sequential stages of demyelination and remyelination are involved. It may therefore represent only one particular aspect of cer-

tain forms of chronic demyelinating neuropathy.

2. Interstitial changes. As in the case of skeletal muscle, these may include specific alterations (whose recognition will permit an exact diagnosis) and nondiagnostic changes.

a. Diagnostic changes. Chief among these are the lesions of polyarteritis nodosa, sarcoidosis, and amyloidosis (Fig. 237), all three of which are identical with those in muscle; the lesions of lepromatous leprosy (Fig. 236*A*), with the presence of infiltrates of macrophages containing Hansen's bacilli; and those of metachromatic leukodystrophy, characterized by deposits of material that demonstrates brown-red metachromasia with cresyl violet.

b. Nondiagnostic changes. Among these are noted the presence and the extent of edema, connective tissue proliferation, lymphohistiocytic infiltrates (which are often perivascular) and capillary alterations.

B. CHIEF ETIOLOGICAL PROCESSES

Peripheral nervous tissue lesions are, with the exception of traumatic and neoplastic lesions, generally designated as peripheral neuropathies. These may be classified according to the distribution of the lesions—which will account for the clinical picture—or according to the causative histopathological process.

1. Distribution of the lesions. **a. Polyneuritis** affects groups of nerve fibers that have the same biological properties and usually innervate a synergic group of muscle fibers. It gives rise to bilateral and symmetrical functional disturbances which tend in most cases to predominate distally and have a usually progressive clinical evolution.

b. Mononeuritis and **multineuritis** consist respectively in either isolated involvement of a peripheral nerve trunk or successive and disorderly involvement of several nerve trunks. These conditions are clinically distinguishable from polyneuritis by the massive character of the nerve trunk involvement—either sensory or motor—and by the random distribution of the clinical disturbances.

c. Polyradiculoneuritis presents a clinical picture due to a systematic pathological process that involves the nerve roots and to a lesser extent the peripheral nerve trunks, with a usual tendency toward a diffuse and generalized character. Peripheral nerve biopsy does not permit the diagnosis of polyradiculoneuritis to be made,[1] and therefore a clinicopathological evaluation of the findings in peripheral nerve biopsy can be discussed only in regard to polyneuritis, mononeuritis, or multineuritis.

2. Histopathological process. **a. Parenchymatous neuropathies.** These lesions correspond to primary involvement of the nerve fibers. The initial lesion may affect either the nerve cell proper (i.e., the neuronal cell body or the neurite) or the myelin sheath. In a number of cases, both structures are implicated at the same time, albeit unevenly.

1. Peripheral neuropathies resulting from initial involvement of the nerve cell proper. The initial, presumably biochemical, lesion is generally situated in the cell body, but the areas of cytoplasm that are farthest removed from the cell bodies are those which undergo the first changes. Indeed, when the functional integrity of the cytoplasmic organelles in the neuronal cell bodies is disturbed, the integrity of the axodendritic expansions at the periphery is immediately compromised.

Most often, as in alcoholic polyneuritis, the causative process affects equally the cell bodies of the motor neurons in the anterior horns and of the sensory neurons in the spinal root ganglia. Occasionally, in some of the toxic neuropathies, as in lead poisoning, the involvement is virtually selective for motor neurons.

In any event, the first indication of neuronal cell body involvement consists of wallerian degeneration, which makes its appearance at the distal extremity of the neurite and subsequently progresses from the periphery toward the neuronal cell bodies, thus accounting for the initially distal peripheral nerve lesions. This phenomenon has been termed "dying-back neuropathy."

---

[1] In the context of polyradiculoneuritis, Guillain-Barré disease is chiefly characterized by demyelination with edema and lymphocytic inflammatory infiltrates, which may be situated at all levels of the peripheral nervous system. The mechanism of the demyelination is now thought to have an immunoallergic basis.

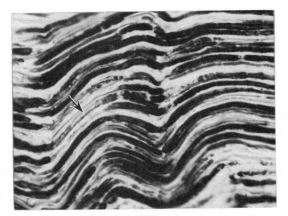

Figure 235. *Diphtheritic polyneuritis* (Loyez stain). Picture of segmental demyelination (*arrow*).

2. Peripheral neuropathies resulting from initial involvement of the myelin sheaths. These lesions typically produce segmental demyelination (Fig. 235), also known as the "segmental periaxial neuritis" of Gombault and Philippe and exemplified in diphtheritic polyneuritis. Since myelin is formed by Schwann cells and since the demyelination is of segmental character, it is probable that the primary mechanism resides in most cases in a disturbance in the metabolic activity of the Schwann cell.

b. Interstitial neuropathies. In contrast to parenchymatous neuropathies the initial lesion in interstitial neuropathies does not lie in the nerve fibers but in the interstitial connective tissue and vascular spaces of the nerve.

Whatever the primary nature of the lesion—whether inflammatory, infectious, metabolic, or otherwise—it is capable of causing secondary lesions of the nerve fibers and therefore wallerian degeneration.

c. Vascular neuropathies. In vascular neuropathy the lesion is primarily situated in the blood vessels supplying the nerve. Whatever the primary cause of the lesion—whether arteritis, atheroma, or vascular compression—it produces ischemia and, consequently, secondary lesions of the nerve fibers characterized by unifocal or multifocal infarcts causing wallerian degeneration.

C. CONCLUSION

Unfortunately, there is no simple and direct correlation between the many etiological factors responsible for peripheral neuropathy and for its three main pathological forms (parenchymatous, interstitial, and vascular), since the same etiological agent may involve the nerve through different pathogenetic mechanisms. As a result, each known etiological factor only seldom corresponds to a diagnostic histopathological picture and most often peripheral nerve biopsy permits simply the recognition of wallerian degeneration and/or segmental demyelination, without providing further information on the etiological diagnosis of peripheral neuropathy.

Thus, in the majority of peripheral neuropathies occurring as the result of deficiency or toxic disorders, or in those of infectious origin, a picture of parenchymatous neuropathy, with initial involvement of the cell body and/or myelin sheath, will be present, but examination of the biopsy specimen will certainly not permit an etiological diagnosis.

On the other hand, there are a few diagnostic conditions which may be established by peripheral nerve biopsy, and in this lies its chief diagnostic value. The main conditions which may be thus diagnosed are the following:

1. In *leprosy,* peripheral nerves may be affected in the lepromatous, tuberculoid, and intermediary forms.

In the *lepromatous form* (Fig. 236*A*), in which the immunological defense reaction is weak, large numbers of Hansen's bacilli may be found in Schwann cells, axons, macrophages, and the perineurium. The demyelinating and axonal lesions undergo a progressive course.

In the *tuberculoid form,* Hansen's bacilli are rare. Focal interstitial histiocytic and lymphocytic cellular infiltrates (Fig. 236*B*) are associated with secondary axonal lesions, but may be missed in a peripheral nerve biopsy.

2. In *collagenoses,* the focal interstitial lesions, which are often limited, are of multineuritic character.

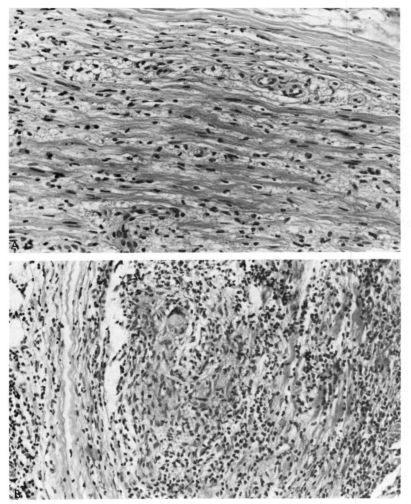

Figure 236. *Leprosy (peripheral nerve lesions)* (H. and E.).
A, Lepromatous form, showing numerous macrophages. *B*, Tuberculoid form, showing nodule composed of histiocytes, lymphocytes and a single giant cell.

In *polyarteritis nodosa*, arteriolar lesions of inflammatory and fibrinoid necrotic nature characteristically coexist with perivascular polymorphonuclear leukocytic infiltrates. In *systemic lupus erythematosus*, peripheral nerve lesions are less frequent. In *chronic progressive polyarthritis*, peripheral nerve lesions are often associated with a picture of nodular interstitial myositis.

3. *Sarcoidosis*, which preferentially affects cranial nerves and especially the facial, may present a multineuritic picture characterized by interstitial granulomas composed of histiocytes, lymphocytes, and giant cells.

4. *Amyloidosis of the nervous system* as a primary disease, either familial or sporadic, is diagnosed by the presence of interstitial deposits that are metachromatic with crystal violet (Fig. 237), congophilic, and birefringent in polarized light. The deposits may be localized to the blood vessel walls or infiltrate the extracellular space as intertwined filaments identifiable by electron microscopy.

Infiltration by amyloid deposits may some-

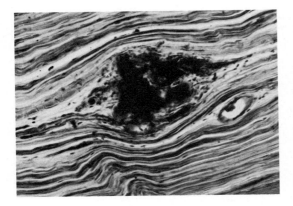

Figure 237. *Amyloidosis of the nervous system* (crystal violet). Nerve fibers dissociated by metachromatic material.

Neuropathies	Histological lesions					Distribution of the lesions			
	Parenchymatous			Interstitial	Vascular	Mono-neuritis	Polyneuropathies		Poly-radiculo-neuritis
	Nerve cell/Axon	Demye-linating	Onion-bulb				Multi-neuritis	Poly-neuritis	
Inflammatory neuropathies									
Collagenoses,* polyarteritis nodosa*	+			⊕	⊕	+	⊕	+	
Leprosy*									
Lepromatous	+	+		+				+	
Tuberculoid	+			⊕		+	+		
Guillain-Barré				+					⊕
Diphtheria								+	
General systemic diseases									
Diabetes	±	+	±		+	+	+	+	
Uremia	+	+						+	
Porphyrias	+							+	
Dysglobulinemias	+				+		+		
Amyloidosis*	+			⊕	+			+	
Metabolic neuropathies									
Metachromatic leukodystrophy*		+		+				+	
Refsum's disease*		+	+					+	
Heredodegenerative diseases									
Déjerine-Sottas disease*		+	⊕					+	
Charcot-Marie-Tooth disease	+	+	±					+	
Avitaminoses									
B_1	⊕	+						+	
B_6	+							+	
B_{12}	+	±						+	
Intoxications									
Ethanol	⊕	+						+	
Lead	+							+	
Malignancies									
Metastases	+			+					+
Paraneoplastic syndromes	+	+						+	
Peripheral nerve compression	+	+				+			

Figure 238. *Histological types and distribution of the lesions in the chief forms of neuropathy.* * = Pathological processes in which the etiology can be elicited from a peripheral nerve biopsy. ⊕ = Chief lesions.

times be encountered in some forms of dys-globulinemia, as in Waldenström's macro-globulinemia and, less often, in multiple myeloma.

5. *Metachromatic leukodystrophy*, or sulfati-dosis, aside from involving the central white matter, often causes prominent peripheral nerve lesions in childhood. The diagnosis is made by demonstrating inclusions that are metachromatic with cresyl violet (brown meta-chromasia). Involvement of myelin sheaths and the presence of typical inclusions within Schwann cells are characteristically revealed by electron microscopy.

6. *Onion-bulb neuropathy* is characteristic of Déjerine-Sottas hypertrophic neuropathy (see Fig. 234), a familial disease that includes pupillary abnormalities and abnormally high levels of albumin in the cerebrospinal fluid.

The picture of onion-bulb neuropathy and the presence of inclusions within Schwann cells demonstrated by electron microscopy are also frequent features of *Refsum's disease*, a neurolipidosis characterized by excessive storage of phytanic acid.

Other neuropathic processes, such as poly-radiculoneuritis, may not be accessible to peripheral nerve biopsy or may demonstrate only nonspecific axonal or demyelinating lesions (Fig. 238).

It will therefore be evident that since the modalities of reaction of peripheral nerves to pathological agents are highly stereotyped (wallerian degeneration and/or segmental demyelination), it is largely the interstitial or vascular peripheral neuropathies that are likely to reveal their etiology through pe-ripheral nerve biopsy.

BRIEF SURVEY OF NEUROPATHOLOGICAL TECHNIQUES

The practice of neuropathology depends on a number of specialized techniques derived from those employed in general pathology and histology.

METHODS OF REMOVAL

I. AUTOPSY

The autopsy of the nervous system cannot be regarded as an isolated procedure and must be part of a complete general autopsy. It must be performed without delay, since the central nervous system is very rapidly altered by postmortem autolysis. It is essential that the prosector adhere to strict technical rules, since central nervous system tissue is delicate and, being enclosed within hard bony structures (skull and spine), is considerably less easily removed than the thoracic and abdominal viscera.

1. Removal of the spinal cord. Removal of the spinal cord should be done at the beginning of the autopsy, as it is technically more difficult when performed after the general postmortem examination. The procedure includes the following steps:

The body is turned face down.

The skin and underlying soft tissues are incised along the spinous processes from the external occipital protuberance to the base of the sacrum.

The soft tissues are freed, first with the knife and then with the scraper, in order to bare the vertebral grooves on either side of the spinous processes.

The vertebral laminae are sectioned on either side of the midline along the entire length of the spine, using a bone cutter or the electric saw.

The spinous processes throughout their entire length, together with their connecting tendinous aponeuroses, are lifted and pulled off.

The cervical enlargement of the spinal cord is sectioned with a scalpel as high up as possible.

The spinal cord is then delivered. This is done by working carefully from above down; the prosector raises the cord with the left hand, using an ordinary forceps clipped onto the dura, while with the right hand the prosector systematically sections the spinal nerve roots down to the cauda equina with a scalpel or scissors.

The dural sheath is opened longitudinally with scissors to permit better penetration by the fixative and thus avoid possible shrinkage and distortion of the underlying cord.

The spinal cord is then immediately immersed in 30 per cent formalin.

2. *Removal of the brain* (Fig. 239). Removal of the brain entails the following steps:

The body is turned face up.

The scalp is incised along a coronal plane from one pinna to the other.

The scalp is freed and reflected forward to the supraorbital ridges and backward to the external occipital protuberance.

The cranial cavity is prized open with the electric saw.

The skull cap thus obtained is lifted by exerting firm traction from front to back, using the wedge of the autopsy hammer inserted in the center of the frontal bone cut. Normally the dura should remain intact.

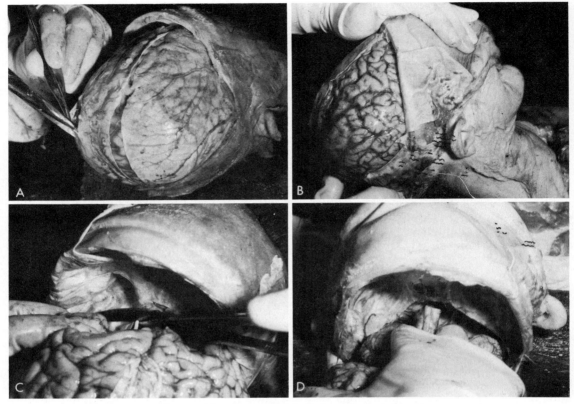

Figure 239.   *Removal of the brain at the time of autopsy.*

A, Parasagittal incision of the dura after removal of the skull cap.

B, Lateral view; the dural flaps have been reflected along the edges of the bony incision.

C, Incision of the tentorium cerebelli along the upper border of the left petrous bone; note that the third cranial nerve has been sectioned.

D, Delivery of the brain; the cut end of the upper cervical cord is lightly held between the right index and middle fingers of the prosector.

The dura is incised first longitudinally, approximately 2 cm on either side of the midline and from front to back, and then in a semicircular fashion, along the edge of the bony cut (Fig. 239*A* and *B*).

The anterior attachment of the falx cerebri is incised down to the crista galli.

The frontal lobes are very gradually raised and freed from front to back by systematically sectioning the anterior connecting structures (optic nerves, internal carotid arteries, pituitary stalk) with scissors.

The tentorium cerebelli is incised along its attached edge to the upper border of the petrous bone (Fig. 239*C*).

The posterior connecting structures (cran-ial nerves, vertebral arteries) are sectioned while, with the left hand, the prosector supports the brain, which will otherwise tend to topple backward.

The brain is then delivered (Fig. 239*D*); with the left hand the prosector continues to support the brain while placing the palm of the right hand on the ventral surface of the pons, inserting the index finger to the left and the middle finger to the right of the medulla.[1] The cut end of the medulla is then

---

[1] If the spinal cord has not been removed beforehand, it will, of course, be necessary to transect the upper cervical cord with a long, thin scalpel.

delivered poised in the air, following which the prosector inserts two fingers under each cerebellar hemisphere. With the left hand the prosector is then able to lift the entire brain, and it only remains for the dura of the posterior fossa to be incised for the brain to be completely freed.

The brain is weighed.

The brain is immediately immersed in 30 per cent formalin, its base facing up, within a receptacle large enough to allow it to float and thus avoid future distortion resulting from possible postmortem compression.

3. Removal of portions of the peripheral nervous system and samples of the skeletal musculature.

The removal of samples of skeletal muscle and of peripheral nerves is both easy and essential, although it is well known that from the histological point of view information derived from autopsy material tends, because of various artifacts, to be less valuable than information obtained from biopsy procedures. In obtaining these samples it is, of course, necessary to avoid multiple skin incisions and disfigurement of the body.

4. Special procedures.

Removal of the spinal cord, the brain, portions of the peripheral nervous system, and samples of the skeletal musculature is part of a complete routine autopsy. However, in some cases this must be supplemented by the examination of certain special areas of the body that are not normally scrutinized in a routine autopsy procedure. This includes, for example, removal of the eyes, examination and sampling of the base and the vault of the skull, and removal *en bloc* of the cervical spine to include the vasculature of the neck. It hardly needs to be pointed out that removal of the pituitary gland is part of any routine autopsy.

II. SURGICAL SPECIMENS

Neurosurgical specimens, which are mostly tumors, must be immediately placed in fixative after their removal by the neurosurgeon. Coagulation by the electrocautery produces artifacts which may render histological interpretation difficult.

Rapid sectioning of a frozen section (preferably cut on the cryostat) may permit a general diagnostic assessment to be made within a few minutes. This may be useful to the surgeon, but the interpretative difficulties of the procedure should not be minimized.

In some centers, brain smears (or the wet film technique) are used by the neuropathologist as a rapid diagnostic method.

III. BIOPSY PROCEDURES

1. Muscle biopsy.

This is a minor surgical procedure, but it is important to stress the strict and meticulous technical care with which it must be performed. Muscle tissue is indeed very delicate, and, if it is not removed with all necessary precautions, the correct interpretation of histological lesions may be considerably impeded by the presence of numerous artifacts.

The operation is performed under local anesthesia, using Xylocaine *and taking care not to inject the local anesthetic beneath the level of the investing aponeurotic fascia.* The incision must be generous enough (at least 3 cm in length) to permit easy dissection of the muscle. After the deep fascia and next the perimysium have been incised, the muscle is dissected by following the plane of cleavage of the muscle bundles in a direction parallel to that of the fibers. A segment of muscle measuring 2 cm in length by 1 cm in thickness is then isolated, *taking care to avoid traction,* and sectioned at either end (Fig. 240). It is placed for approximately 10 minutes in a Petri dish on a piece of surgical gauze soaked in physiological saline. This will obviate artifacts due to shrinkage, and the resulting symmetrical muscle fragment is then later immersed in a specimen jar containing 10 per cent neutral formalin.

From the practical point of view it is important to stress the exact site of removal of the muscle sample. The deltoid or the quadriceps is usually selected in instances of proximal muscle atrophy of myopathic origin. In cases of distal neurogenic atrophy the tibialis anterior or one of the peronei tends to be favored, especially since with the latter a fragment of the superficial musculocutaneous nerve can easily be removed when

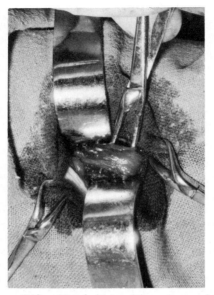

Figure 240. *Muscle biopsy.* Dissection and isolation of muscle fragment.

indicated. It is important to avoid muscles that have undergone the late stages of atrophy, by which time the differential diagnosis may be extremely difficult. It is also preferable to avoid sampling the precise area of previous electromyographic recording, since this may be a source of traumatic artifacts. It is, however, desirable to select a muscle that has been so tested so as to achieve a useful comparison between the electrical and the neuropathological data.

2. Peripheral nerve biopsy.
The indications for peripheral nerve biopsy are more limited than those for muscle biopsy. Sampling of a sensory peripheral nerve is usually done by removing a small fragment of the musculocutaneous nerve of the leg (superficial peroneal nerve).

It is technically easy, in the course of a muscle biopsy of the peroneus brevis, to sample one of the sensory branches of the musculocutaneous nerve at the junction of the middle and inferior thirds of the leg.

A skin incision is made 1 cm anterior to the line that joins the head of the fibula to the external malleolus. This permits easy access to the nerve (Fig. 241). Following longitudinal splitting of the nerve, a frag-

ment measuring 2 cm in length may be removed. Hypoesthesia of the dorsum of the foot will result, but is usually well tolerated. The biopsy fragment is fixed in 10 per cent neutral formalin.

3. Brain biopsy.
Cortical biopsy may be performed in highly specific cases. This is a neurosurgical procedure which does not present any technical difficulty. After administration of the local anesthetic and incision of the scalp, a small disk of bone is drilled with the lobotomy trephine, the dura is incised, and a small fragment of cortex and underlying white matter is removed with the scalpel or, preferably, with a cutting curette. Following this procedure the bone disk is replaced and the scalp is closed. Obviously the biopsy must be performed on a "silent area" (right frontal or occipital lobe). The risk of hemorrhage, infection, reactive edema, or post-traumatic epilepsy is no greater than following ventriculography.

In fact, the indications for brain biopsy raise a problem that is largely ethical. Even if the procedure can be demonstrated to be on the whole innocuous, nevertheless, focal irreparable anatomical damage has been done

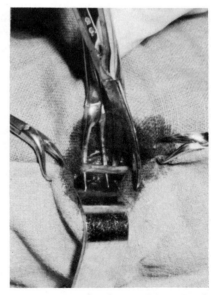

Figure 241. *Peripheral nerve biopsy.* Section of a fragment of the superficial branch of the musculocutaneous nerve of the leg.

to a vital organ incapable of regeneration. For this reason a cortical biopsy must never be a routine procedure and should only be undertaken according to rigorous diagnostic criteria. Most often brain biopsy is envisaged for the diagnosis of some forms of encephalitis, dementia, or neurolipidosis.

4. Other biopsy procedures. In some neurological disorders, largely neurolipidoses, rectal biopsy is sometimes performed in order to examine the ganglion cells of Meissner's plexus. Likewise, it is possible to examine these structures in the appendix.

Skin biopsy may also provide additional information in some cases (e.g., capillary blood vessel walls, terminal nerve endings, cellular inflammatory infiltrates).

FIXATION OF TISSUES

Formalin (formol) is the almost universal fixative used in neuropathology.[1] The most frequently employed formalin solutions are those at 30 per cent, 10 per cent, and 5 per cent. Neutral formalin (calcium formalin) is often recommended and is obtained by pouring powdered calcium carbonate into the fixative container. An alternative method consists in the use of marble chips in the formalin solution.

The amount of fixative to be used depends on the amount of tissues to be fixed and should correspond to approximately 15 to 20 times the volume of tissue. Thus, for the brain as a whole, 5 to 6 liters of a 30 per cent formalin solution is required; the fixative must be changed after 1 to 2 hours, and again after 24 hours.

Good fixation requires a minimum amount of time, depending on the size of the tissue (3 to 6 weeks for a whole brain).

On the other hand, the preservation of tissues in formalin is almost indefinite, provided that the fluid — which turns yellow with age — is changed from time to time and provided that the container is well sealed so as to avoid evaporation. However, fixation that has been prolonged for a considerable period of time will jeopardize some of the staining procedures.

GROSS EXAMINATION OF THE CENTRAL NERVOUS SYSTEM

Gross examination of the central nervous system (brain and spinal cord) must be performed only after 3 to 6 weeks of formalin fixation. In the course of routine neuropathological study the freshly removed brain and spinal cord must be neither handled nor sectioned before their immersion into the fixative. However, as noted below, study of the nervous system by neurochemical and histoenzymological methods requires the sampling of fresh tissues before fixation and their preservation unfixed at low temperature; similarly, sampling and preservation at low temperature of fresh unfixed material are indispensable for virological investigation, and the technical inadequacies of postmortem tissue for electron microscopic study can to some extent be improved by fixing small fragments in buffered glutaraldehyde as soon as possible after death.

The gross examination of the central nervous system is performed in three consecutive steps: (1) inspection of the brain and spinal cord; (2) the cutting of slices and their examination with the naked eye and, if necessary, with the magnifying glass; and (3) the sampling of pieces of tissue for histological examination.

I. INSPECTION OF THE BRAIN AND SPINAL CORD

The brain and spinal cord are carefully examined and any abnormal or interesting features are recorded on schematic diagrams and photographed.

---

[1]There is a frequent and regrettable confusion between formic aldehyde (or formaldehyde) and commercial formalin (or formol). Formaldehyde is an unwieldy gas with which a commercial aqueous 35 or 40 per cent solution is prepared that constitutes the usual formalin. Formalin therefore refers to the commercial formaldehyde solution. Thus, 10 per cent formalin represents a solution prepared by mixing 10 ml of commercial formalin with 90 ml of water.

II. CUTTING OF GROSS SLICES

The usual protocol includes the following steps:

a. Severing the cerebral hemispheres from the brainstem. The arachnoid membrane, which usually obscures the structures of the interpeduncular fossa and the floor of the third ventricle, is first delicately cleared with forceps or fine scissors, the blood vessels of the circle of Willis are then dissected, and the rostral part of the cerebral peduncles is divided with a scalpel along a plane strictly parallel to the base of the brain.

b. Coronal hemispheric slices.[1]   The lower surface of the brain rests on a cork board, with

---

[1] Sectioning of the fixed brain in near-horizontal slices is often performed today in order to obtain better topographic correlation with the findings of computerized tomography (CT scanning) (translator's note).

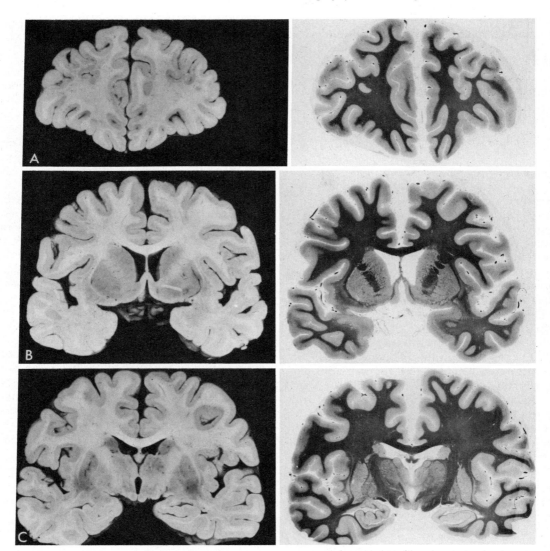

Figure 242.   *Coronal sections through the cerebral hemispheres.*
Left, Gross appearance after fixation; *Right,* myelin stain of corresponding slices after celloidin embedding. *A,* Frontal poles. *B,* Section through the rostral portion of the basal ganglia. *C,* Section through the mamillary bodies.

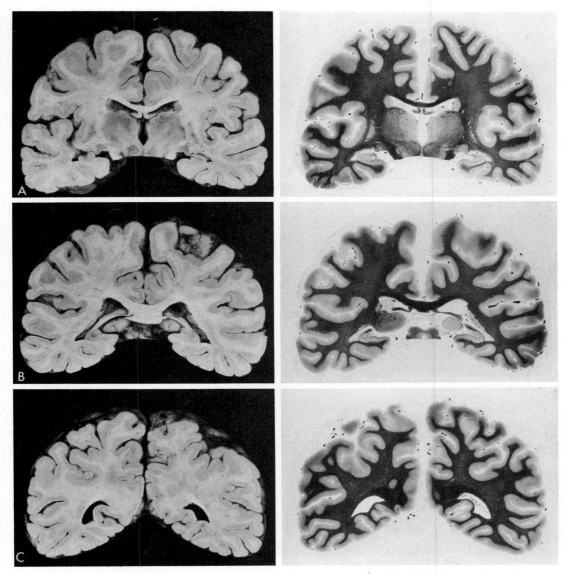

Figure 243.   *Coronal sections through the cerebral hemispheres.*
Left, Gross appearance after fixation; *Right,* myelin stain of corresponding slices after celloidin embedding. *A,* Section through the red nuclei, lateral geniculate bodies, and maximal extent of the optic thalami. *B,* Section through the splenium of the corpus callosum, pulvinars, and trigones. *C,* Posterior section through the occipital horns.

the occipital poles facing the prosector, who holds the brain with the left hand and, with the brain knife in the right, sections the brain in absolutely parallel coronal slices approximately 1 cm thick from the frontal to the occipital poles (Figs. 242 and 243).

c. Coronal sections through the brainstem and

cerebellum. Without separating the cerebellum from the brainstem, coronal sections approximately 1 cm thick are cut from the cerebral peduncles to the medulla (Fig. 244).

d. Transverse sections through the spinal cord. The spinal cord is placed flat on the cork board, and strictly transverse sections, ap-

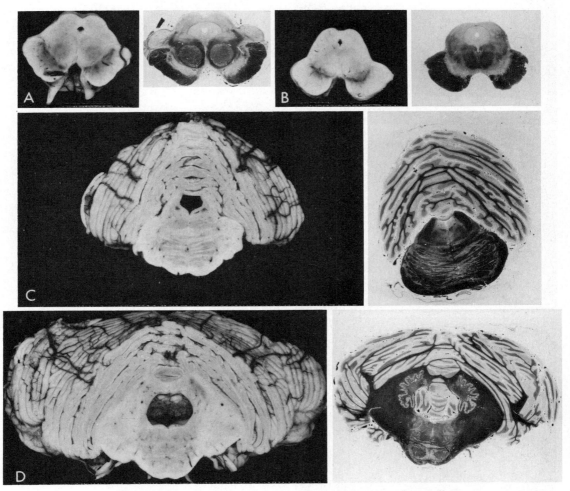

Figure 244. *Coronal sections through the brainstem and cerebellum.*

Left, Gross appearance after fixation; *Right,* myelin stain of corresponding slices after celloidin embedding.

A, Rostral portion of the cerebral peduncles (red nuclei, superior corpora quadrigemina, and exits of third cranial nerves).

B, Caudal portion of the cerebral peduncles (dentatorubral decussation, inferior corpora quadrigemina).

C, Upper pons and superior cerebellar vermis.

D, Midpons and cerebellar hemispheres with dentate nuclei.

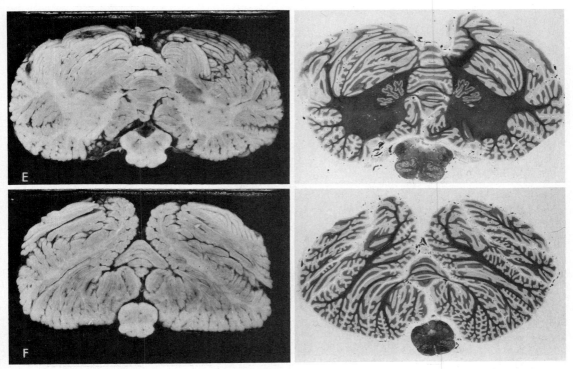

Figure 244. *Continued.*
E, Upper medulla, cerebellar hemispheres with dentate nuclei and inferior vermis.
F, Lower medulla and inferior portion of cerebellar hemispheres.

proximately 1 cm thick, are made using a fresh razor blade held by forceps (Fig. 245).

After the various hemispheric, brainstem, and spinal cord slices have been examined with the naked eye and a magnifying glass, the lesions are recorded on standard stenciled diagrams outlining the main areas of the central nervous system, and gross photographs are taken.

III. HISTOLOGICAL SAMPLING

After the slices have been examined grossly, pieces of tissue are sampled for histological study. In this selection the prosector is guided by the clinical data, the general autopsy findings, the gross study of the slices, and the type of histological technique to be applied to the tissues.

These pieces of tissue must be carefully identified and labeled in order to avoid all possible error.

EMBEDDING, SECTIONING, AND STAINING METHODS

I. EMBEDDING AND SECTIONING PROCEDURES[1]

The neuropathologist most frequently utilizes one or more of the following three techniques:

Paraffin embedding and sectioning with the paraffin microtome;

Celloidin embedding and sectioning with the celloidin microtome;

Frozen sections.

---

[1]For details on embedding and sectioning techniques the reader is referred to general works of reference on histological methods. The indications, advantages, and disadvantages of the various techniques are reviewed here solely within the context of neuropathological practice.

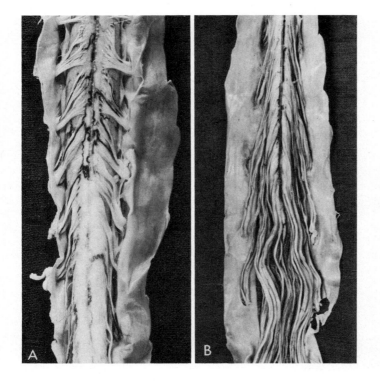

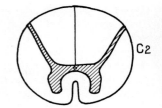

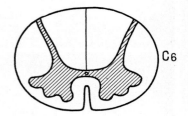

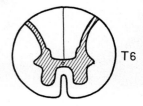

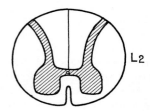

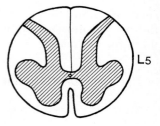

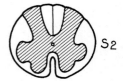

Figure 245.   *Gross appearances of the spinal cord.*

A, Cervicothoracic cord; note the thin thoracic roots (except for T 1), compared to the cervical roots.

B, Lower part of spinal cord; note exits of L 1 roots from the dura at the level of the conus medullaris. At *right,* Diagram of spinal cord sections at various levels.

1. Paraffin embedding. *a. This technique has several disadvantages:*

Paraffin embedding requires preliminary treatment with alcohol and toluene, which are lipid solvents.

Paraffin embedding requires that the tissues be heated during part of the procedure in an oven at a temperature of 56°C (for the paraffin to be melted). Unfortunately, nervous tissue, which is very fragile, tolerates this level of temperature poorly, and this results in numerous artifacts. Nerve cells appear shrunken in the middle of small clear cavities, and the gaping perivascular spaces resemble gaps in the tissue.

Finally, the penetration by paraffin of particularly dense tissues, such as the meninges, may be difficult.

b. However, the advantages of paraffin embedding are considerable:

The embedding method is rapid, much more so than traditional celloidin embedding.

In particular, only paraffin embedding will give very thin sections (5 to 7 μm) as well as easy serial sections. Therefore, in some forms of cytological study this is the method of choice.

Furthermore, certain stains are possible only in paraffin sections.

c. Therefore, paraffin embedding in neuropathology is usually indicated for the study of nervous system tumors, for muscle and peripheral nerve biopsies, and when rapid results are desired (e.g., small fragments of central nervous system tissue may be embedded in paraffin as a preliminary step to subsequent wider sampling for celloidin embedding).

In some laboratories large brain slices are embedded in paraffin, but it is much more difficult to obtain large sections of even quality with this technique.

d. With paraffin embedding the stains listed in Figure 246 can be performed.

2. Celloidin embedding. In contrast to its relatively rare use in general histology, celloidin embedding is often the method of choice in neuropathology. It is done in most laboratories, and many use no other.

a. Its main advantages are:

It permits the embedding and sectioning of very large pieces, such as a cerebral hemisphere or even a whole brain.

The embedding process is very slow and takes place at room temperature so that the highly vulnerable structures of the nervous system are little damaged.

It provides sections that can be handled easily without having to adhere to the slides, a prerequisite without which certain staining methods cannot be utilized.

b. Its main disadvantages are:

The procedure takes several weeks; however, this can now be considerably accelerated by performing the consecutive processing and embedding steps under ultrasonic vibration.

In particular, it is impossible to obtain sections as thin as those acquired with paraffin embedding.

Moreover, as with paraffin embedding, the tissues must be preliminarily processed through fat solvents.

c. In practice, most neuropathology laboratories use celloidin embedding for the routine study of the brain and spinal cord.

d. With celloidin embedding the staining techniques listed in Figure 246 can be used.

3. Frozen sections. *a. This procedure has two main advantages:*

The tissues are not processed through fat solvents, thus permitting the preservation of a number of cell constituents—which disappear after celloidin or paraffin embedding—and the application of special techniques that are impossible in other circumstances.

Frozen sections can be examined under the microscope very soon after fixation (after a few hours); this is of practical importance when rapid histological diagnosis is important (e.g., in biopsies).

b. Naturally these sections are not as thin as those obtained with paraffin embedding.

c. In practice, frozen sections are utilized to permit a number of special stains and also in histochemistry; however, in some laboratories they are often used for routine purposes.

d. The staining procedures possible with frozen sections are listed in Figure 246.

			Paraffin	Celloidin	Frozen section
General histological stains		Hematoxylin-eosin	++	++	++
		Masson's trichrome	+	−	−
		Van Gieson stain	+	+	+
Nerve cell stains	Nissl bodies	Thionin (Nissl variant)	±	++	−
		Cresyl violet	++	+	++
	Neurofibrils	Bielschowsky	±	−	++
	Axons	Bodian	++	±	−
		Gros	−	−	++
Myelin stains		Loyez	±	++	+
		Woelcke	+	++	++
		Luxol fast blue	++	+	+
Glial cell stains	Astrocytes	Hortega's lithium carbonate	−	−	++
		Holzer	+	−	++
		Mallory's P.T.A.H.	+	+	+
	Microglia	Silver carbonate	−	−	+
Connective and vascular tissue stains	Collagen fibers	Masson's trichrome	+	−	−
		Van Gieson	+	+	+
	Reticulin fibers	Perdrau; Wilder; Gordon-Sweets; Gomori; Laidlaw; Foot	++	±	−
	Elastic fibers	Orcein; Weigert-Hart; Verhoeff; resorcin-fuchsin	++	+	+

Figure 246. *Principal stains in common use according to the embedding procedure.*

II. STAINING PROCEDURES

It is not possible to give here a detailed account of the many staining procedures employed in neuropathology. Figure 247 lists those most frequently utilized.

SPECIAL TECHNIQUES

A number of special morphological techniques, such as enzyme histochemistry and electron microscopy, as well as neurochemical and virological methods are often employed today in human neuropathology. They are usually research techniques, essentially performed on biopsy fragments.[1] Their

---

[1] Whereas the utilization of some of these techniques on autopsy material presents serious interpretative limitations due to the development of postmortem autolysis, they nevertheless may be valuable in certain instances, as follows:

Electron microscopy may be used to search for, and to identify, viral particles.

Neurochemical studies may be performed on freshly removed, unfixed material that may be spared from neuropathological examination, such as an occipital or a frontal pole; such tissues must be frozen without delay.

Virological studies, particularly in tissue culture, may be undertaken, but sampling has to be performed in a sterile manner on the brain *in situ*, after aseptic removal of the skull cap.

	Central nervous system	Peripheral nerves	Muscles	Tumors
General histological stains (hematoxylin-eosin, trichomes)	+ +	+ +	+ +	+ +
Stains for Nissl bodies (thionin, cresyl violet)	+ +			
Myelin sheath stains (Loyez, Woelcke, luxol fast blue)	+ +	+ +		±
Neurofibrillar stains (Bielschowsky)	±			
Axon stains (Bodian, Gros)	±	+ +		±
Astrocytic stains (Hortega's lithium carbonate; Holzer; Mallory's P.T.A.H.)	±			±
Microglial stains (silver carbonate)	±			±
Collagen fiber stains (trichomes, van Gieson)	±	±	±	±
Elastic fiber stains (Orcein; Weigert-Hart; Verhoeff)	±	±	±	±
Reticulin stains (Perdrau; Wilder; Gordon-Sweets; Gomori; etc.)	±	±	±	±

Figure 247. *Utilization of the various stains according to the material studied.*

success depends on the adherence to certain technical rules of removal and subsequent processing.

1. **Muscle biopsy** may, in addition to the

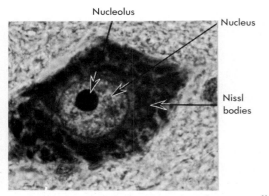

Figure 248. *Cell body of a normal nerve cell stained with the Nissl method.*

usual histological study of paraffin-embedded material, require supplementary methods of investigation in some cases.

Enzyme histochemistry permits the study of the distribution of various histochemical types of muscle fibers. For this purpose it is necessary to freeze without delay the muscle biopsy fragment in isopentane cooled to $-160°C$ in liquid nitrogen. The specimen is stored at $-35°C$ for subsequent serial sectioning in the cryostat at $10 \mu m$.

Study of the motor nerve endings necessitates removal of the sample from the area of motor innervation. This is followed by identification of the nerve fibers after dissection under the dissecting microscope, and by subsequent silver impregnation. The study of the terminal motor nerve ending is performed conjointly with that of the subneural apparatus, which is based on a histoenzymological method in which acetylthiocholine is employed as a substrate (cholinesterase preparation).

Electron microscopic examination requires *in situ* fixation, performed at the time of removal, in 2.5 per cent phosphate-buffered (ph 7.4) glutaraldehyde, followed by fixation for 4 to 6 hours at 0°C and by postfixation in 1 per cent osmium tetroxide for 1 hour at room temperature.

2. Peripheral nerve biopsies often require, in addition to the usual histological procedures performed on frozen section and on paraffin-embedded tissue, and in addition to immunofluorescence study that may sometimes be needed:

Electron microscopy after fixation in glutaraldehyde;

Quantitative assessment of nonmyelinated and myelinated fibers in order to determine their respective caliber, complemented by histograms drawn on the basis of transversely sectioned semi-thin sections;

Examination of dissociated fibers in teased preparations.

The latter is done by dissociating nerve fascicles measuring 2 cm in length under the dissecting microscope, using a needle. This permits some of the nerve fiber elements, such as the axons and myelin sheaths, to be studied in longitudinal section. The internodal distance and any lesions due to segmental demyelination may also be evaluated. The fragment removed at biopsy is im-

mersed in 1 per cent osmic acid for several hours. then in 60 per cent glycerol for 48 hours. The dissociation procedure itself is performed in 100 per cent glycerol. The nerve fibers are subsequently immersed in creosote, aligned on glass slides, dehydrated, and mounted in Canada balsam for microscopic examination.

3. The investigation of brain biopsies must include, in addition to traditional light microscopic study, the use of various other techniques.

For electron microscopy, it is necessary for a brain biopsy fragment to be immediately fixed for 1 hour in 4 per cent glutaraldehyde buffered in Millonig solution, followed by rinsing in the buffer, postfixation in 1 per cent osmic acid, progressive dehydration in 70, 96, 100 per cent alcohol and propylene oxide, and embedding in Epon 812.

Neurochemical studies must be performed on fragments that have been frozen without delay. Catecholamines may be demonstrated by specific histofluorescence on cerebral biopsy fragments fixed by immersion in 2 per cent glyoxylic acid, followed by sectioning with a vibratome.

Virological investigations, such as animal inoculation and culture on appropriate nutrient media, must be planned on a fragment that has been kept sterile. Such a fragment may also be stored at −80°C for further studies.

BIBLIOGRAPHY

In view of the elementary didactic nature of this manual, a full bibliography has not been provided. For further details the reader is referred to the following textbooks and treatises.

Neuropathological techniques

Adams (C. W. M.). *Neurohistochemistry.* Elsevier, Amsterdam, 1965, 753 pp.

Gasser (G.). *Basic neuropathological technique.* Blackwell Scientific Publications, Oxford, 1961, 77 pp.

Ráliš (H. M.), Beesley (R. A.) and Ráliš (Z. A.). *Techniques in neurohistology.* Butterworths, London, 1973, 162 pp.

Tedeschi (C. G.). *Neuropathology. Methods and diagnosis.* Little, Brown and Co., Boston, 1970, 874 pp.

Pathology of the central nervous system

Adams (R. D.) and Sidman (R. L.). *Introduction to neuropathology.* McGraw-Hill Book Co., New York, 1968, 629 pp.

Biggart (J. H.). *Pathology of the nervous system.* 3rd ed. Livingstone, Edinburgh and London, 1961, 368 pp.

Blackwood (W.), and Corsellis (J. A. N.). *Greenfield's neuropathology.* 3rd ed. Edward Arnold, London, 1976, 946 pp.

Blackwood (W.), Dodds (T. C.) and Sommerville (J. C.). *Atlas of neuropathology.* 2nd ed. Livingstone, Edinburgh and London, 1964, 234 pp.

Burger (P. C.) and Vogel (F. S.). *Surgical pathology of the nervous system and its coverings.* J. Wiley and Sons, New York, 1976, 623 pp.

Crome (L.) and Stern (J.). *Pathology of mental retardation.* 2nd ed. Williams & Wilkins, Baltimore, 1972, 544 pp.

Friede (R. L.). *Developmental neuropathology.* Springer-Verlag, New York, 1975, 524 pp.

Hughes (J. T.). *Pathology of the spinal cord.* Lloyd Luke, London, 1966, 196 pp.

Lewis (A. J.). *Mechanisms of neurological disease.* Little, Brown and Co., Boston, 1976, 540 pp.

Malamud (N.) and Hirano (A.). *Atlas of neuropathology.* 2nd ed. University of California Press, Berkeley, 1974, 462 pp.

Minckler (J.). *Pathology of the nervous system.* McGraw-Hill Book Co., New York, 3 vols., 1968–1972, 3088 pp.

Slager (U. T.). *Basic neuropathology.* Williams & Wilkins, Baltimore, 1970, 311 pp.

Smith, (J. F.). *Pediatric neuropathology.* McGraw-Hill Book Co., New York, 1974, 265 pp.

Vinken (P. J.) and Bruyn (G. W.). *Handbook of clinical neurology.* North Holland Publishing Co., Amsterdam. Volumes 6 (1968, 889 pp.), 7 and 8 (1970, 680 and 556 pp.), 9 (1970, 706 pp.), 10 (1970, 699 pp.), 11 and 12 (1972, 719 and 696 pp.), 13 (1973, 493 pp.), 15 (1974, 860 pp.), 21, 22 and 23 (1975, 636, 586 and 742 pp.), 24, 25 and 26 (1976, 860, 522 and 550 pp.).

Zacks (S. I.). *Atlas of neuropathology.* Harper & Row, New York, 1971, 394 pp.

Zimmerman (H. M.). *Progress in neuropathology.* Grune and Stratton, New York, Vol. I (1971, 316 pp.), Vol. II (1973, 460 pp.), Vol. III (1976, 495 pp.).

Tumor pathology

Barnard (R. O.), Logue (V.) and Reaves (P. S.). *An atlas of tumours involving the central nervous system.* Baillière-Tindall, London, 1976, 158 pp.

Harkin (J. C.) and Reed (R. J.). *Tumors of the peripheral nervous system.* Armed Forces Institute of Pathology, Washington, D.C., Atlas of Tumor Pathology, Second series, fasc. 3, 1969, 174 pp.

Kernohan (J. W.) and Sayre (G. P.). *Tumors of the central nervous system.* Armed Forces Institute of Pathology, Washington, D.C., Atlas of Tumor Pathology, First series, Section X, fasc. 35 and 37, 1952, 128 pp.

Rubinstein (L. J.). *Tumors of the central nervous system.* Armed Forces Institute of Pathology, Washington, D.C., Atlas of Tumor Pathology, Second series, fasc. 6, 1972, 400 pp.

Russell (D. S.) and Rubinstein (L. J.). *Pathology of tumours of the nervous system.* 4th ed. Edward Arnold, London, 1977, 448 pp.

Stout (A. P.). *Tumors of the peripheral nervous system.* Armed Forces Institute of Pathology, Washington, D.C., Atlas of Tumor Pathology, First series, Section II, fasc. 6, 1949, 57 pp.

Vinken (P. J.) and Bruyn (G. W.). *Handbook of clinical neurology.* North-Holland Publishing Co., Amsterdam. Volumes 14 (1972, 821 pp.), 16 and 17 (1974, 748 and 746 pp.), 18 and 19 (1975, 582 and 393 pp.), 20 (1976, 859 pp.).

Zülch (K. J.). *Brain tumors. Their biology and pathology.* 2nd ed. Translated by J. Olszewski and A. B. Rothballer. Springer, New York, 1965, 326 pp.

Zülch (K. J.). *Atlas of gross neurosurgical pathology.* Springer-Verlag, Berlin, Heidelberg and New York, 1975, 228 pp.

Neuromuscular pathology

Adams (R. D.). *Diseases of muscles.* 3rd ed. Hoeber Medical Books, Harper & Row, New York, 1975, 588 pp.

Bethlem (J.). *Muscle pathology. Introduction and atlas.* North-Holland Publishing Co., Amsterdam and London, 1970, 132 pp.

Coërs (C.) and Woolf (A. L.). *The innervation of muscle. A biopsy study.* Blackwell Scientific Publications, Oxford, 1959, 149 pp.

Dubowitz (V.) and Brooke (M. H.). *Muscle biopsy. A modern approach.* W. B. Saunders Co., Philadelphia, 1973, 475 pp.

Dyck (P. J.), Thomas (P. K.) and Lambert (E. H.). *Peripheral neuropathy.* W. B. Saunders Co., Philadelphia, 2 vols., 1975, 1438 pp.

Greenfield (J. G.), Shy (G. M.), Alvord (E. C.) and Berg (L.). *An atlas of muscle pathology in neuromuscular diseases.* Livingstone, Edinburgh and London, 1957, 104 pp.

Mair (W. G. P.) and Tomé (F. M. S.). *Atlas of the ultrastructure of diseased human muscle.* Churchill Livingstone, Edinburgh and London, 1972, 249 pp.

Walton (J. N.). *Disorders of voluntary muscles.* 3rd ed., Churchill Livingstone, Edinburgh and London, 1974, 1149 pp.

INDEX

Note: Numbers set in **boldface** type are Figure numbers, not page numbers.

Abscess, amebic, **139**
  cerebral, 64, 105, **133, 134**
  epidural, 105
  epidural tuberculous, 107
  mycotic, 111
  subdural, 105
  subdural tuberculous, 108
Acanthocytosis, 172, **192**
Acidosis, lactic, congenital, 174
Acromegaly, 44
Acropathia, ulcero-mutilans, 146
Adenomas, pituitary, 44, **30, 31, 32, 59**
Adenoviruses, 113
Adrenoleukodystrophy, 129
Afibrinogenemia, **86**
Agammaglobulinemia, 162
Agenesis, of cerebellum, 181, 184, **212**
  of cerebrum, 180
  of corpus callsoum, 49, 180, **204**
  of olfactory bulbs, 180, **205, 206**
  of septum lucidum, 180, **202**
Agyria, 181, **207**
Alcoholic cerebellar atrophy, 140, 160, **189**
Alcoholism, chronic, 158
Alexander's disease, 131, **158**
Alzheimer's ameboid glia, 9
Alzheimer's disease, 6, 135, **162**
Alzheimer's glia, type I, 9
  type II, 9, 157, 175, **16**
Alzheimer's neurofibrillary degeneration, 4, 134, **9, 161**
Amaurotic idiocies, 166, 167
Amebiasis, **139**
Ameboid glia of Alzheimer, 9
Amenorrhea-galactorrhea syndrome, 44
Aminoacidurias, 131, 175
Ammon's horn, sclerosis, 190
Amyloid, 134
Amyloidosis, 164, 202, 206, 209, **237, 238**
Amyotrophic lateral sclerosis, 3, 16, 149, **172, 173, 174**
  Guam form, 6, 149
Amyotrophy, myogenic, 197
  neurogenic, 185, 195, **222, 223, 224**
  spinal hereditary, 146, **174**
Anemia, sickle-cell, **86**
Anencephaly, 178, **200**
Aneurysms, arterial congenital, 72, **86, 94, 95, 96, 97, 98**
  arteriovenous, 77, **86, 101, 102**
  atherosclerotic, 77, **99**
  infectious, 77, **100**
  miliary (see *Microaneurysms*)
  mycotic, 77, **100**
  of vein of Galen, 79, **103**
  post-traumatic, 77

Aneurysms (*Continued*)
  spinal arteriovenous, 79, **101, 102**
  vestigial, 73, **94**
Angioblastic meningiomas, 44, 51
Angiokeratosis, diffuse, 172
Angiomas, cavernous, 79, 80, **86**
  cerebral (see *Aneurysms, arteriovenous*)
Angiomatosis, encephalotrigeminal (see *Sturge-Weber disease*)
  retinocerebellar (see *von Hippel–Lindau disease*)
Angiopathy, congophilic, 134
  dyshoric, 134
Angioreticuloma (see *Hemangioblastoma*)
Angle, pontocerebellar, tumors of, 33, 46, **27, 31, 47**
Anisomorphous gliosis, 9
Annulets, striated, 193, 198, 202, **220**
Anoxia, cerebral, 14, 150, **22, 175, 176, 177, 178, 179**
Anterior poliomyelitis, acute, 115
  chronic, 147, **174**
Anticoagulant therapy, 81, **86**
Antigens, tissue-type, in multiple sclerosis, 126
Aplasia paleocerebellar, 181
Apparatus, subneural, 225
Aqueductal stenosis, 15, 183, 187
Arachnoidal cysts, 182, **211**
Arachnoiditis, 14, 183, **135**
Arbovirus, 113, 115
Arbovirus encephalitis, 115
Argyrophilic (argentophilic) neuronal inclusions, 6, 136, **10**
Arhinencephaly, 180, **205, 206**
Arnold-Chiari malformation, 176, 184
Arrest, cardiac, 150, 152, **177**
Arsenic intoxication, 158
Arterial hypertension, 67, 69, 71, 73, 101, **86, 89**
Arteriolar hyalinosis, 72, 101, 135, **92**
Arteriolosclerosis, 72, 101, **92**
Arteriopathic dementia, 102, 103
Arteriovenous malformations, 77, **86, 101, 102**
Arteritis, 90, 108, **136**
  syphilitic, 90, 110
Artery, anterior cerebral, infarct of territory of, 91, **117, 118**
  anterior choroidal, infarct of territory of, 94, **117, 118**
  middle cerebral, infarct of territory of, 92, 95, **117, 118**
  posterior cerebral, infarct of territory of, 96, **117, 120**
Arthrogryposis, 147
Artifacts, freezing, 15, **25**
  gross, 15
  microscopic, 15, 223, **25**
  muscle, 192, 215
Arylsulfatase, 169, 170, 171, **192**

Ascariasis, **139**
Aspergillosis, 112
Astrocytes, basic lesions of, 7, **14, 15, 16**
   gemistocytic, 8, **15, 107**
   giant, 9, 120, **146**
   pilocytic, 25
Astrocytomas, 23, **30, 31, 32, 33, 34, 35, 36**
   cerebellar, 25, **31, 32**
   fibrillary, 23, 25
   gemistocytic, 23, **35**
   microcystic, 23, **35**
   of brainstem, 25
   of cerebral hemispheres, 23, **31, 32, 34, 35**
   of optic nerves and chiasm, 25
   of spinal cord, 25, **33, 36**
   of third ventricle, 25
   pilocytic, 25
   protoplasmic, 23, 25
Ataxia, Friedreich's, 3, 16, 143, 144, **171, 174**
   hereditary cerebellar, 144
Atherosclerosis, 87, 102, 135, **109, 111, 112, 113**
Atherosclerotic emboli, 90
Atrophy, cerebellar, 139, 141, 160, **167, 168, 170, 189**
    alcoholic, 140, 160, **189**
     crossed, 141
     (Holmes), 3, 140
     paraneoplastic, 140, 162, **170, 191**
   cerebello-olivary, 3, 139, **167, 170**
   cerebral, 12, 135, **162**
   congenital, of granular layer, 140, **170**
   denervation, 195, **218, 222, 223, 224**
   dentatorubral (see *Ramsay Hunt syndrome*)
   fascicular, 193, 195, **222**
   granular, of cerebral cortex, 102, **128**
   infantile spinal muscular (see *Werdnig-Hoffmann disease*)
   lobar and hemispheric, 135
   muscular, denervation, 195, **218, 222, 223, 224**
    myogenic, 197
    neurogenic, 195, **218, 222, 223, 224**
   of Gudden, 3
   of subthalamic nuclei (corpora Luysii), 138
   olivopontocerebellar, 3, 141, **168, 169, 170**
   optic, 144
   pallidal (pure), 138
   pigment (of neurons), 2
   simple neuronal, 2, 3, 7
   striatonigral, 138
Austin's disease, 171, **192**
Autopsy of the nervous system, 213, **239**
Avitaminosis B_1, 153, 159, **238**
Avitaminosis B_6, **238**
Avitaminosis B_{12}, 156, **185, 238**
Avitaminosis E, 7
Avitaminosis PP factor (see *Encephalopathy, pellagra*)
Axonal changes, 6
Axonal neuropathy, 203
Axonal reaction (see *Chromatolysis, central*)
Axonal swellings, 7, **13**

Baló's concentric sclerosis, 129
Basophilic fibers, 193, 200, **227**
Bassen-Kornzweig's disease, 172, **192**
Batten-Mayou disease, 168
Behçet's disease, 120

Bergmann glia, 140
Beriberi (see *Avitaminosis B_1*)
Bilharziasis, **139**
Binswanger, subcortical encephalopathy of, 103, **129**
Biopsy, cerebral, technique of, 216, 226
   cortical, 216, 226
   muscle, histological examination of, 191
    technique of, 215, 225, **240**
   peripheral nerve, histological examination of, 203
    technique of, 216, 226, **241**
   rectal, 217
   skin, 217
Bismuth salts, 158
Blastomatous dysplasias, 187
Blepharoplasts, 28
Blood dyscrasias, 67, 81, **86, 104**
Brain, biopsy, 216, 226
   removal of, 213, **239**
   "Swiss-cheese," 15, **24**
Brain smears, 215
Brainstem, hemorrhages of, primary, 71, **91**
    secondary, 56, **75, 83, 86**
   infarcts of, 96, **121**
Brucellosis, 111
Buerger's disease, 103
Bullae of putrefaction, 15, **24**
Büngner's cell bands, 203

Calcifications, intracranial, 118, 188
Calcium metabolism, 157
Canavan's disease, 13, 131, 167
Candidiasis, 111
Capillary endothelial proliferation, 26, **38**
Capillary telangiectases, 79, **86**
Capsulolenticular hemorrhage, 69, **87**
Carbon monoxide poisoning, 14, 123, 138, 152, **178, 179**
Carcinoma, metastatic, 51, **67, 68, 69, 70**
Carcinomatous meningitis, 14, 51, **23, 69, 70**
Cardiac arrest, 150, 152, **177**
Cardiac emboli, 90, **114**
Cardiopathies, congenital, 107
Caroticocavernous fistulae, 79
Catecholamines, demonstration of, 226
Cauda equina, tumors of, 28, 33, **48, 68**
Cavernomas, 80
Cavernous angiomas, 79, 80
Cavum vergae, 180
Cell loss, neuronal, 1, 150
Celloidin embedding, 223
Cellular lesions, basic, 1
Central chromatolysis, 2, 136, 155, 159, **2, 3, 4, 184**
Central core disease, 198
Central pontine myelinolysis, 123, 159, **188**
Centrilobar sclerosis (Foix-Marie), 189
Ceramide, 166, 172, **192**
Cerebello-olivary atrophy, 3, 139, **167, 170**
Cerebellum, agenesis of, 181, 184, **212**
   atrophy of, 139, 141, 160, **167, 168, 170, 189**
    alcoholic, 140, 160, **189**
    crossed, 141
    paraneoplastic, 140, 162, **170, 191**
   hematoma of, 71, **90**
   infarcts of, 98, **122**

Note: Numbers set in **boldface** type are Figure numbers, not page numbers.

Cerebral atrophy, 12, 135, **162**
Cerebral biopsy, technique of, 216, 226
Cerebral diplegia, infantile, 188
Cerebral emboli, 85, 87, 89, 90, 96, 103, **113, 114, 115**
Cerebral hemiplegia, infantile, 188
Cerebral hemorrhage, 67, **85, 86, 87, 88, 90, 91, 104**
Cerebromeningeal hemorrhage, 67, **85**
Cerebrosides, 168, **192**
Cerebrum, agenesis of, 180
    atrophy of, 12, 135, **162**
Ceroid-lipofuscinoses, 168, **194**
Ceruloplasmin, 175
Cestodiasis, **139**
Chagas' disease, **139**
Charcot-Marie-Tooth disease, 144, 146, 197, **174, 238**
Charcot's disease (see *Amyotrophic lateral sclerosis*)
Chemodectomas, 44
Chickenpox, 113
Chloroquine myopathy, 201
Cholesteatomas, 32, 45, **30, 62, 63**
Cholesterol storage diseases, 172, **192**
Cholinesterase preparations, 226
Chondroitin sulfate, 173
Chondrosarcomas, 44
    mesenchymal, 44
Chordomas, 48, **30**
Chorea, chronic (see *Huntington's chorea*)
Choriomeningitis, lymphocytic, 113
Choroid plexus papillomas, 29, 183, **30, 42**
Chromatolysis, central, 2, 136, 155, 159, **2, 3, 4, 184**
    peripheral, 3, **4**
Cirrhosis, hepatic, 9, 157, 158
Clasmatodendrosis, 9
Coccidioidomycosis, 112
Coenurosis, **139**
Collagenoses (collagen diseases), 164, 200, 208, **238**
Colloid cysts of third ventricle, 30, **30, 43**
Coma, hepatic, 9
    hypoglycemic, 157
    prolonged, 64
Commotio cerebri, 64, **83**
Commotio cordae, 66
Compound granular corpuscles, 10, 83, **18, 19, 107**
Concentric sclerosis, Baló, 129
Congophilic angiopathy, 134
Connective tissue and vascular changes, 14
Contusions, cerebral, 63, 64, **82, 83**
    spinal cord, 66
Cord, spinal (see *Spinal cord*)
Cornea verticillata, 172
Corpora amylacea, 9
Corpus callosum, agenesis of, 49, 180, **204**
    necrosis of (see *Marchiafava-Bignami disease*)
Corpuscles, compound granular, 10, 83, **18, 19, 107**
Cortical biopsy, 216, 226
Coxsackie virus, 113, 115
Craniopharyngiomas, 45, **30, 31, 60, 61**
Craniorachischisis, 178
Cranium, fractures of, 60, **78, 83**
Creutzfeldt-Jakob disease, 120, 132, 149, **147**
Criggler-Najjar syndrome, 175
Crocker's form of Niemann-Pick disease, 171
Crossed cerebellar atrophy, 141
Cryptococcosis, 111, **138**
Curvilinear bodies, 168, **194**
Cushing's disease, 45
Cyanide poisoning, 150, 152

Cyclocephaly, 178
Cystathionine synthetase, 175
Cysticercosis, 199, **139, 140**
Cysts, arachnoidal, 182, **211**
    colloid, of third ventricle, 30, **30, 43**
    dermoid, 46, **63**
    epidermoid, 45, 46, **62**
    of septum lucidum, 180, **203**
Cytoid bodies, 131
Cytomegalovirus, 118

Dandy-Walker syndrome, 183, **212**
Dawson's inclusion body encephalitis, 116
Deficiency diseases, 153
Degeneration, acute neuronal (of Nissl), 1
    granular, of Spielmeyer, 1
    granulovacuolar, 4, 134, 135, **9**
    hepatolenticular (see *Wilson's disease*)
    mucoid, of oligodendrocytes, 10
    neurofibrillary, of Alzheimer, 4, 134, **9, 161**
    of muscle fibers, 193, **217**
    of nerve cell, chronic (see *Neuronal atrophy, simple*)
    opticocochleodentate, 143
    pallidonigral, 138
    retrograde (see *Central chromatolysis*)
    spongy, of neuraxis, 131, 167
        of white matter, 13
    striatonigral, 138
    subacute combined, of spinal cord, 13, 156, **185**
    trans-synaptic, 3
    wallerian, 7, 123, 203, 207, 208, 211, **149, 231**
Déjerine and Thomas' type of olivopontocerebellar atrophy, 141
Déjerine-Sottas familial hypertrophic neuropathy, 206, 211, **234, 238**
Dementia(s), arteriopathic, 102, 103
    mixed, 135
    organic, 132
    senile, 6, 132, 135, **159**
Demyelinating diseases, 121, 123, **150**
Demyelination, 13, 121
    segmental, 203, 208, 211, 226, **232, 233, 235**
Denervation atrophy, 195, **218, 222, 223, 224**
Denny-Brown, hereditary sensory neuropathy, 146, **174**
Dentatorubral atrophy, 143
Depopulation, neuronal, 1
Dermal sinus, congenital, 177, **199**
Dermatomyositis, 161, 200
Dermoid cysts, 46, **63**
Derry's disease, 167, **192**
Diabetes mellitus, nervous system lesions in, 164, **238**
Diffuse sclerosis (see *Schilder's disease*)
Dilatation, ventricular, 12, 132, 138, 179, 183, **42, 73, 77, 135, 201, 212**
Diphtheritic polyneuritis, 208, **235, 238**
Diplegia, cerebral infantile, 188
Disseminated sclerosis (see *Multiple sclerosis*)
Dissociation, myelin-axonal, 121, 125, **152**
DNA viruses, 117
Down syndrome, 176, 182
Duchenne's pseudohypertrophic muscular dystrophy, 197
Dying-back neuropathy, 207

Note: Numbers set in **boldface** type are Figure numbers, not page numbers.

Dysglobulinemias, 162, 211, **238**
Dyshoric angiopathy, 134
Dyskalemias, 201
Dysmyelinating diseases, 130
Dysplasias, blastomatous, 187
Dysraphic states, 176
Dyssynergia, myoclonic cerebellar (see *Ramsay Hunt syndrome*)
Dystasia, hereditary areflexic (see *Roussy-Lévy syndrome*)
Dystrophy(ies), muscular, 197, **225, 226**
    myotonic, 197, 202, **218, 220, 221, 226**
    neuroaxonal, 7, 139

Echinococcus, **139**
Echovirus, 113, 115
Economo, von, encephalitis of, 120
Ectopias (see *Heterotopias*)
"Ectopic pinealoma," 32
Edema, cerebral, 13, 54, 64, 82, **21, 77, 83, 105**
Electron microscopy techniques, 224, 226
Embedding, celloidin, 223
    paraffin, 223
Emboli, atherosclerotic, 90
    cardiac, 90, **114**
    cerebral, 85, 87, 89, 90, 96, 103, **113, 114, 115**
    fibrin, 89
    platelet, 89
Empyema, subdural, 105
    ventricular, 107
Encephalitides, 11, 12, 14, 113, 114, **141**
    arbovirus, 115
    Central European, 115
    cytomegalovirus, 118
    Dawson's inclusion body, 116
    DNA viruses, 117
    Eastern and Western equine, 115
    granulomatous, 42
    hemorrhagic, 114
    herpesvirus, 117, **144, 145**
    Japanese B, 115
    limbic, 162
    mosquito-borne, 115
    Murray Valley, 115
    necrotizing, 6, 118, 162, **144**
    papovavirus, 120, **146**
    paramyxovirus, 116, **143**
    perivenous, 113
    postinfectious, 113
    primary, 114
    RNA viruses, 115
    Russian spring-summer, 115
    St. Louis, 115
    tick-borne, 115
    viral, 114
Encephalitis lethargica, 120
Encephalo-araphia, 178
Encephaloceles, 178
Encephalomalacia (see *Infarcts*)
Encephalomyelitis, 114
    acute disseminated, 113
    experimental allergic, 114, 128
Encephalo-myelo-araphia, 178
Encephalomyocarditis, 113

Encephalopathy, bismuth, 158
    hemorrhagic, 114
    hepatic, 9, 157, 158, 160, **16**
    infantile, 188
    lead, 158
    metabolic, 157
    pancreatic, 157
    paraneoplastic, 162
    pellagra, 3, 155, **184**
    perinatal vascular, 190
    portocaval, 157
    postepileptic, 190
    pseudopellagra, 156
    respiratory, 157
    subacute necrotizing, 174
    subcortical, of Binswanger, 103, **129**
    toxic, 157
    Wernicke's, 3, 153, 159, **180, 181, 182, 183**
Encephalotrigeminal angiomatosis (see *Sturge-Weber disease*)
Endocarditis, infective, 77, 90
    nonbacterial thrombotic, 90, 162
    subacute bacterial, 77
Entamoeba histolytica, **139**
Enteroviruses, 113, 115
Enzyme histochemistry techniques, 191, 194, 195, 197, 198, 202, 225, **224, 226**
Ependymal changes, 14
Ependymal tubules, 28, **41**
Ependymitis (see *Granulations, ependymal*)
Ependymoblastomas, 29
Ependymomas, 28, **30, 31, 32, 33, 40, 41**
    malignant, 29
    myxopapillary, 29
    papillary, 29,
Epidermoid cysts, 45, 46, **62**
Epidural abscess, 105
Epidural neoplasms, 51, **33, 68**
Epilepsy (see also *Encephalopathy, postepileptic*)
    congenital, 188
    myoclonic, 6, 174, **12**
    post-traumatic, 64
"État criblé," 102
"État glacé," 16, 140
"État lacunaire," 102
"État marbré," 189
External granular layer, 31
Extracranial metastases, 26, 59
Extradural hematoma, 61, 66, **79, 83, 85**

Fabry's disease, 172, **192**
Facioscapulohumeral dystrophy, 198
Fahr's disease, 157
Fallot's tetrad, 107
Farber's lipogranulomatosis, 172, **192**
Fascicular atrophy of muscle fibers, 193, 195, **222**
Fat emboli, 90
Fenestrated neurons, 3, **5**
Ferrugination, 4, **6**
Fetal external granular layer, 31
Fibers, basophilic, 193, 200, **227**
    ring, 193, 198, 202, **220**
    Rosenthal, 25, 131, **158**
    target, 193, 195, **219**

Note: Numbers set in **boldface** type are Figure numbers, not page numbers.

Fibers (*Continued*)
  vacuolated, 193
Fibrillary gliosis, 7, 8, **15**
Fibrin emboli, 89
Fibrosarcoma, 42
Fibrous xanthoma, 42
Fifth ventricle, 180, **203**
Filariasis, **139**
Filum terminale, ependymomas of, 28
Fingerprint pattern, 168, 199
Fistulae, caroticocavernous, 79
Fixation procedures, 217
  for demonstration of catecholamines, 226
  for electron microscopy, 226
  for teased preparations, 226
Flukes, **139**
Foam cells, 10, **18**
Foix and Alajouanine, "subacute necrotic myelitis," 79, **102**
Foix and Marie's centrilobar sclerosis, 189
Foramen magnum, tumors of, 18, **26, 27**
Forbes' disease, 202
Fractures, of skull, 60, **78, 83**
  of spine, 66, **84**
Freezing artifacts, 15, **25**
Friedreich's ataxia, 3, 16, 143, 144, **171, 174**
Frozen sections, 223
Fucosidosis, 174
Fungal infections, 111, **138**

Galactosemia, 174
Galactosidase, 167, 169, 172, **192**
Gangliogliomas, 31, **30**
Ganglioneuromas, 31, **30**
Gangliosidoses, 166, **192**
Gargoylism, 166, 173
Gaucher's disease, 168, **192**
Gemistocytic astrocytes, 8, **15, 107**
General paralysis of the insane, 12, 111, **20**
Germinomas, pineal, 32, **30, 46**
Glia, Alzheimer, type I, 9
    type II, 9, 157, 175, **16**
  ameboid, of Alzheimer, 9
  Bergmann, 140
  subependymal, proliferation of, 15
Glial changes, 7
Glial necrosis, 9
Glioblastomas, 25, **30, 31, 32, 33, 37, 38**
  giant-cell, 26, 42
Gliomas, **30, 31**
  brainstem, 25, 187, **31**
  multifocal, 25
  of chiasm, 25, 187
  of spinal cord, 25, 186, **36**
  subependymal, 29
"Gliosarcoma," 26
Gliosis, 7, **14, 15**
  anisomorphous, 9
  fibrillary, 7, 8, **15**
  isomorphous, 8
  naked nuclei, 9, 157
  protoplasmic, 7, 8, **15**
Globoid body leukodystrophy (see *Krabbe's disease*)
Glomus jugulare tumors, 44, **30**

Glucosidase, 169, **192**
Glucuronyltransferase, 175
Glycogenoses, 174
  muscular, 202
Glycosaminoglycans, 173
Glycosphingolipids, 166, **192**
Granular atrophy of cerebral cortex, 102, **128**
Granular degeneration of Spielmeyer, 1
Granular layer, congenital atrophy, 140, **170**
Granulations, ependymal, 14
Granulovacuolar degeneration, 4, 134, 135, **9**
Grinker's myelopathy, 123, 152, **179**
Grouping (enzyme histochemistry) of muscle fibers, 194, 195, **224**
Guam, amyotrophic lateral sclerosis, 6, 149
  Parkinsonian dementia syndrome, 149
Gudden's atrophy, 3
Guillain-Barré's disease, 207, **238**
Gumma, syphilitic, 110

Hallervorden-Spatz disease, 139
Hand-Schüller-Christian disease, 172
Hartnup's disease, 175
Hemangioblastomas, 44, 49, 187, **30, 31, 64, 65, 66**
Hemangioblastomatosis, 49, **66**
Hemangiopericytoma, 43, 44, 51
Hematoma, extradural, 61, 66, **79, 83, 85**
  intracerebral, 67, 77, **85, 96, 97, 98**
    traumatic, 63, **83**
  of cerebellum, 71, **90**
  subarachnoid, 73, **97, 98**
  subdural, 61, 62, 66, **80, 81, 83, 85**
    of newborn, 188
Hematomyelia, 66
Hemiballismus, 138
Hemiplegia, cerebral infantile, 188
Hemochromatosis, 157
Hemoglobinuria, paroxysmal, 162
Hemophilia, **86**
Hemorrhages, 12, 67, **85, 86**
  basal ganglia, 69, **87**
  brainstem, primary, 71, **91**
    secondary, 56, **75, 83, 86**
  capsulolenticular, 69, **87**
  cerebral, hemispheric, 67, **85, 86, 87, 88, 90, 91, 104**
    white matter, 69, **88**
  cerebromeningeal, 67, **85**
  hypertensive, 67, 69, 71, **86, 89**
  intracerebellar, 69, **90**
  intracerebral (see *Hemorrhages, cerebral*)
    of newborn, 188
  intracranial, 67, **83, 85**
  meningeal, nontraumatic, 67, 73, 79, **85, 86, 97, 98**
    of newborn, 188
  meningocerebral, 67, 77, **85, 96, 97**
  slit, 69, **89**
  subarachnoid, nontraumatic, 67, 73, 79, 81, **85, 86, 97, 98**
    of newborn, 188
  thalamic, 69, **87**
  traumatic, 61, 63, 66, **79, 80, 82, 83**
Hemorrhagic encephalopathy, 114
Hemosiderosis, marginal, 73

Note: Numbers set in **boldface** type are Figure numbers, not page numbers.

Heparin sulfate, 173
Hepatic cirrhosis, 9, 157, 158
Hepatic coma, 9
Hepatic encephalopathy, 9, 157, 158, 160, **16**
Hepatic insufficiency, 9, 157, 160
Hepatitis, viral, 113, 157
Hepatolenticular degeneration (see *Wilson's disease*)
Hereditary areflexic dystasia (see *Roussy-Lévy syndrome*)
Hereditary cerebellar ataxia, 144
Hereditary degenerative spinocerebellar disease, 144, **171, 174**
Hereditary sensory neuropathy (Denny-Brown), 146, **174**
Hereditary spasmodic paraplegia, 144, **174**
Herniations, cerebellar, 58, **76**
  cerebral, 55, 64, **74, 75, 77, 81, 83**
  external, 56, **74**
  hippocampal, 56, **74, 75**
  tonsillar, 58, **76**
Herpes simplex, 9, 117
Herpesvirus, 6, 113, 117, **145**
Herpes zoster-varicella, 118
Heterotopias, 179, 181, 187, **209**
Hexosaminidase, 166, 167, **192**
Hippocampal herniation, 56, **74, 75**
Hirano bodies, 136
Histochemistry, enzyme (techniques of), 191, 194, 195, 197, 198, 202, 225, **224, 226**
Histofluorescence for catecholamines, 226
Histological stains of the nervous system, **246, 247**
Hodgkin's disease, 120, 162
Holmes' familial cerebello-olivary atrophy, 3, 140
Holoprosencephaly, 180, **206**
Homocystinuria, 175
Hunter's disease, 173
Huntington's chorea, 138, **166**
Hurler's disease, 173, **198**
Hurst's acute hemorrhagic leukoencephalitis, 114
Hyalinosis, arteriolar, 72, 101, 135, **92**
Hydatid disease, **139**
Hydranencephaly, 179, **201**
Hydrocephalus, 15, 30, 55, 183, **42, 73, 135, 201**
  acute, 30, 64
  "normal-pressure," 64
Hydromyelia, 187
Hygromas, subdural, 61, 183
Hyperbilirubinemia, congenital familial, 175
Hypercapnea, 157
Hypercholesterolemia, familial, 172
Hyperlipemia, familial, 172
Hypertension, arterial, 67, 69, 71, 73, 101, **86, 89**
  intracranial, 55, **77**
  malignant, 164
Hypertensive hemorrhage, 67, 69, 71, **86, 89**
Hypertrophy, olivary, 4, **5**
  schwannian, onion-bulb, 203, 211, **234, 238**
Hypoglycemia, 157
Hypoparathyroidism, 157
Hypophyseal adenomas, 44, **30, 31, 32, 59**
Hypoplasia, pontoneocerebellar, 181
Hypotension, orthostatic, 139
Hypotrophy, type I muscle fibers, 199

Idiocies, amaurotic, 166
  congenital, 167
  late infantile, 167
Inclusion body encephalitis, Dawson's, 116
Inclusion disease, cytomegalic, 118
Inclusions, argyrophilic, (argentophilic) neuronal, 6, 136, **10**
  intracytoplasmic, 6, 115, 116, 136, 137, **10, 11, 12**
  intranuclear, 6, 10, 115, 116, 118, 120, **143, 145, 146**
    oligodendroglial, 10, 120, **143, 146**
  viral, 6, 10, 115, 116, 118, 120, **143, 145, 146**
Incrustated neurons, 4, **6**
Incrustations, capillary, 14, 137, 152
Infantile cerebral diplegia, 188
Infantile cerebral hemiplegia, 188
Infantile neuroaxonal dystrophy, 139
Infantile spinal muscular atrophy (see *Werdnig-Hoffmann disease*)
Infarcts, anemic, 82, **105**
  boundary zone, 87, 95, 98, **110, 119**
  brainstem, 96, **121**
  carotid territory, 91, **118, 119**
  cerebellar, 98, **122**
  cerebral, 82, **105, 106, 107, 108, 109, 110, 118, 119, 120**
  edematous, 82, **105**
  etiological factors, 87, **109**
  hemodynamic factors, 85, **109, 110**
  hemorrhagic, 83, **108**
  myocardial, 90
  of spinal cord, 66, 98, **125, 126**
  pale, 82, **105**
  venous, 104, **130**
  vertebrobasilar territory, 95, **120, 121, 122**
  watershed, 87, 95, 98, **110, 119**
Infections, bacterial, 105, **131, 132, 133, 134, 135, 136, 137**
  brucellosis, 111
  fungal, 111, **138**
  listeria, 105
  parasitic, 112, **139, 140**
  pyogenic, 105, **131, 132, 133, 134**
  rickettsial, 113
  slow-virus, 113, 120, **147**
  syphilitic, 12, 90, 110, **20**
  tuberculous, 90, 107, **135, 136, 137**
  viral, 113, **141, 142, 143, 144, 145, 146**
Inflammatory cellular lesions, 13, 114, 115, 123, 124, 126, 128, **141, 152, 155**
Influenza, 116
Injuries, craniocerebral, 60, **78, 79, 80, 81, 82, 83**
  spinal and radicular, 66, **84**
Innervation, terminal motor (study of), 225
Insufficiency, hepatic, 9, 157, 160
Intoxications, 150, 157, 158
Intracerebral hematoma, 67, 77, **85, 96, 97, 98**
  traumatic, 63, **83**
Intracerebral hemorrhages, 67, 69, 71, **85, 86, 87, 88, 89, 90, 91, 104**
  of newborn, 188
Intracranial hypertension, 55, **77**
Intraspinal hemorrhages, 66
Iodoquinoline, 158
Iron metabolism, 157

Note: Numbers set in **boldface** type are Figure numbers, not page numbers.

Ischemic nerve cell change, 2, 150, **1**
Isomorphous gliosis, 8
Isoniazid, 158

Jakob-Creutzfeldt disease, 120, 132, 149, **147**
Jansky-Bielschowsky disease, 168
Jaundice, nuclear, 175, 190

Kahler's disease, 162
Kernicterus, 175
Kernohan's notch, 56, **75**
Kinky-hair disease, 175
Korsakoff's syndrome, 159, **186**
Krabbe's disease, 169, **150, 192, 195**
Kufs' disease, 168
Kuru, 120

Lactic acidosis, congenital, 174
Lacunae, 101, **127**
Lafora bodies, 6, 174, **12**
Laminar sclerosis (Morel), 160
Landouzy and Déjerine's facioscapulohumeral dys-
    trophy, 198
Layer, fetal external granular, 31
Lead poisoning, 158, 207, **238**
Leigh-Feigin disease, 174
Leprosy, 207, 208, **236, 238**
Lesions, basic cellular, 1
Leucinosis, 175
Leukemia, acute, 81, 162, **104**
    chronic lymphatic, 120, 162
    chronic myeloid, 81
    hemorrhages in, 81, 162, **104**
Leukodystrophy, 121, 123, 124, 129, 169, 170, 211,
    150, 156, 157, 192, 195, 196, 238
    globoid cell (see *Krabbe's disease*)
    metachromatic, 121, 170, 211, **150, 192, 196, 238**
    of Löwenberg and Hill, 131
    sudanophilic, 130, **150, 156, 157**
Leukoencephalitis, acute disseminated, 113
    hemorrhagic, of Weston Hurst, 114
    subacute sclerosing, 116
Leukoencephalopathy, progressive multifocal, 9, 10,
    120, **146**
Lewy bodies, 6, 137, 139, **11**
Limb-girdle myopathy, 198
Limbic encephalitis, 162
Lindau's disease, 49, 187, **66**
Lipid neuronal storage, 4, 166, 167, 168, 170, 171,
    173, **7, 8, 192, 193**
Lipid phagocytes, 11, **18**
Lipidoses, 4, 165, **8, 192**
    infantile, 140, 167
    generalized neurovisceral (Norman-Landing), 167
    late, 132
    late neurovisceral, juvenile or adult, 169
Lipofuscin, 4, 9, 134, 137, **7, 161**
Lipogranulomatosis of Farber, 172, **192**

Lipohyalinosis, arterial, 72
Lipomas, 49, 180
Lipomucopolysaccharidosis (Spranger), 174
Lipopigment (see *Lipofuscin*)
Lipoproteinoses, 172, **192**
Lissencephaly, 181, **208**
Listeria infection, 105
Little's disease, 188
Liver cirrhosis, 9, 157, 158
Loss of neuronal cells, 1, 150
Löwenberg and Hill, leukodystrophy of, 131
Lupus erythematosus, systemic, 164, 201, 209
Lymphocytic meningitis 113
Lymphomas, malignant, nervous system lesions in, 162
Lymphorrhages, 202, **230**

MacArdle's disease, 202
Macroglobulinemia, 162, 164, 211
Macrophages (see *Compound granular corpuscles*)
Malaria, **139**
Malformations, arteriovenous, 77, **86, 101, 102**
    vascular, 67, 72, 77, 79, 90, **86, 101, 102, 103**
Malta fever, 111
Manganese poisoning, 138
Mannosidosis, 174
Maple syrup urine disease, 175
Marchiafava-Bignami disease, 123, 159, 160, **187**
Masses, sarcoplasmic, 193, 198, 202, **221**
Measles, 113, 116, 117, **143**
Measles infection, and multiple sclerosis, 126
Measles virus, 117, **143**
Medulloblastomas, 31, 59, **44**
Megaconial myopathy, 199
Megalencephaly, 131, 178
Meissner's plexus, 217
Melanomas, 41, **70**
Melanomatosis, meningeal, 14
Membranous cytoplasmic bodies, 166, 173, **193**
Meningeal changes, 14
Meningeal hemorrhages, nontraumatic, 67, 73, 79, **85,
    86, 97, 98**
    of newborn, 188
Meningiomas, 36, 187, **53, 54, 55, 56, 57**
    angioblastic, 44, 51
    sarcomatous, 44
Meningiomatosis, 187
Meningitis, acute viral lymphocytic, 113
    carcinomatous, 14, 51, **23, 69, 70**
    fungal, 111, 112, **138**
    listeria, 105
    lymphocytic, 113
    purulent, 105, **131, 132**
    sequelae and complications of, 14, 108, **135**
    serous, 61, 183
    syphilitic, secondary, 110
    tertiary, 110
    tuberculous, 14, 90, 108, **135, 136**
Meningocele, 117, **199**
Meningoencephalitis, 114
    amebic, **139**
Meningoencephalomyelitis, 114
Meningoencephaloradiculitis, 114

Note: Numbers set in **boldface** type are Figure numbers, not page numbers.

Menkes' disease, 175
Menzel's type of olivopontocerebellar atrophy, 141
Metabolic encephalopathy, 157
Metachromatic leukodystrophy, 121, 170, 211, **192, 196, 238**
Metastases, extracranial, 59
  from glioma, 59
  from medulloblastoma, 31
Metastatic carcinoma, 51, **67, 68, 70**
Metazoa, **139**
Microaneurysms, 71, 101, **93**
Microangiopathy, thrombotic, 162
Microcephaly, 178
Microencephaly, 178
Microglia, lesions of, 10, 42
  rod-shaped, 11, 111, 115, **20, 141**
Microglial nodules, 12, 115, **141**
Microgliomas, 42, **58**
Microgyria, 179, 181, **210**
Mineralization of neurons, 4, **6**
Mink encephalopathy, 120
Mitochondria, abnormalities of, 198, 199
Mixed glioma and sarcoma, 26
Mongolism, 176, 182
Monocytes, 11, **19**
Mononeuritis, 207, **238**
Mononucleosis, infectious, 113
Morel's laminar sclerosis, 160
Moschowitz disease, 162
Motor nerve endings, study of, 225
Mucoid degeneration of oligodendrocytes, 10
Mucolipidoses, 174
Mucopolysaccharidoses, 9, 171, 173, **198**
Mucormycosis, 112
Mucosulfatidosis, 171, **192**
Multiceps multiceps, **139**
Multineuritis, 207, **238**
Multiple myeloma, 162, 211
Multiple sclerosis, 9, 10, 16, 121, 123, 124, **150, 151, 152, 153**
  acute, 126
Mumps, 113, 116
Muscle biopsy, histological examination of, 191
  technique of, 215, 225
Muscle fiber atrophy, 195, 197, **218, 222, 223, 224**
Muscle fiber degeneration, 193, **217**
Muscle fiber regeneration, 193, 200, **227**
Muscle fibers, typing, 194, 195, 197, 198, 199, 225, **224, 226**
Muscle nuclei, abnormalities of, 193, **218, 223**
Muscular dystrophies, 197, **225, 226**
Muscular glycogenoses, 202
Myasthenia gravis, 202, **230**
Mycoses, cerebral, 111, **138**
Mycotic aneurysms, 77, **100**
Myelin sheath, 121, **148**
Myelin-axonal dissociation, 121, 125, **152**
Myelinolysis, central pontine, 123, 159, **188**
Myelitis, subacute necrotic, of Foix and Alajouanine, 79, **102**
Myelo-araphia, 176
Myeloma, multiple, 162, 211
Myelomalacia, 66
Myelomeningocele, 176, 185, **199**
Myelopathy, acute necrotizing, 126, 161
  Grinker's, 123, 152, **179**
  necrotizing, paraneoplastic, 161

Myoclonic cerebellar dyssynergia (Ramsay Hunt), 143, **170**
Myoclonic epilepsy, 6, 174, **12**
Myoglobinuria, paroxysmal, 202
Myopathy, centronuclear, 199
  chloroquine, 201
  congenital, 198, 202
  distal, 198
  facioscapulohumeral, of Landouzy and Déjerine, 198
  late (Nevin), 200
  limb-girdle, 198, 202
  megaconial, 199
  myotubular, 199
  nemaline, 198
  ocular, 198
  pleoconial, 199
  rod-body, 198
  steroid, 201
  vacuolar, 201
Myositis, 161, 199
Myotonic dystrophy, 198, 202, **218, 220, 221, 226**
Myotubular myopathy, 199
Myxedema, 45
Myxosarcoma, 44
Myxovirus, 6, 116, **143**

Naegleria, **139**
"Naked nuclei" gliosis, 9, 157
Necrosis, glial, 9
  laminar, of cerebral cortex, 152, **177**
  of nerve cell, acute (see *Ischemic nerve cell change*)
  of neural tissue, 12
  of neurons, 2, **1**
Necrotizing encephalitis, 6, 118, 162, **144**
Necrotizing myelopathy, 126, 161
Negri bodies, 6, 116
Nemaline myopathy, 198
Nematodes, **139**
Nerve, peripheral, biopsy, histological examination of, 203
  technique of, 216, 226
Nerve cell, acute necrosis (see *Ischemic nerve cell change*)
Nerve cell change, ischemic, 2, 150, **1**
Nerve cell degeneration, chronic (see *Neuronal atrophy, simple*)
Nerve endings, motor, study of, 225
Neural tube, closure defects of, 176, **199**
Neurilemmomas (see *Schwannomas*)
Neurinomas (see *Schwannomas*)
Neuroanemic syndromes, 156
Neuroaxonal dystrophy, 7, 139
Neuroblastoma, 31
Neurobrucellosis, 111
Neurochemical investigations, 224, 226
Neurofibrillary degeneration, 4, 134, **9, 161**
Neurofibromas, 35, 187, **51, 52**
Neurofibromatosis of von Recklinghausen, 33, 35, 187, **48**
Neurolipidoses, 4, 9, 166, 168, 172, **8, 192, 193, 194, 196, 197, 198**
  juvenile atypical, 168
Neuromyelitis optica acuta, 126
Neuronal atrophy, simple, 2, 3, 7
Neuronal cell disease of Nissl, acute, 1
Neuronal cell loss, 1, 150

Note: Numbers set in **boldface** type are Figure numbers, not page numbers.

Neuronal changes, 1
Neuronophagia, 2, 12, 115, **141**
Neurons, basic lesions of, 1
  binucleated, 4
  dark, 16
  distended, 4, **8**
  fenestrated, 3, **5**
  ferrugination of, 4, **6**
  incrustated, 4, **6**
  mineralized, 4, **6**
  pale, 16
  vacuolated, 3, **5**
Neuropathy, amyloid, 209, **237, 238**
  axonal, 203
  dying-back, 207
  hypertrophic, of Déjerine-Sottas, 206, 211, **234, 238**
  interstitial, 208, **238**
  mixed sensorimotor, 161
  motor, 161
  onion-bulb, 206, 211, **234, 238**
  paraneoplastic sensory, 161, **190, 238**
  parenchymatous, 207, **238**
  sensory, of Denny-Brown type, 146, **174**
  vascular, 208, **238**
Niemann-Pick disease, 171, **192, 194**
Nissl's acute neuronal cell disease, 1
Nissl's severe cell disease, 1
Nitrofurantoin, 158
Nodules, microglial, 12, 115, **141**
Norman-Landing disease, 167, **192**
Nova Scotia variant of Niemann-Pick disease, 171
Nuclear bodies, 8
Nuclear jaundice, 175, 190
Nuclei, muscle fiber, abnormalities of, 193, **218, 223**

Occlusion, arterial, 85, 87, 90, **109, 110, 111, 113, 114, 115**
Ocular myopathy, 198
Olfactory bulbs, agenesis of, 180, **205**
Oligoastrocytoma, 27
Oligodendrocytes, basic lesions, 10
  mucoid degeneration of, 10
Oligodendroglial swelling, 10
Oligodendrogliomas, 26, **30, 39**
Olivary hypertrophy, 4, **5**
Olivopontocerebellar atrophy, 3, 141, **168, 169, 170**
Onion-bulb schwannian hypertrophy, 203, 211, **234, 238**
Opalski cells, 175
Ophthalmoplegia plus, 198
Opticocochleodentate degeneration, 143
Orthostatic hypotension, 139

Pachygyria, 181, **207, 208**
Pachymeningitis, hemorrhagic, 63
Paleocerebellar aplasia, 181
Pallidonigral degeneration, 138
Pallidum, atrophy of, 138
Palsy, supranuclear progressive, of Steele-Richardson-Olszewski, 6, 139
Panencephalitis, of Pette and Döring, 116
  subacute sclerosing, 6, 9, 10, 116, 128, **142, 143**
Papillomas of choroid plexus, 29, 183, **30, 42**

Papovavirus, 120, **146**
Paraffin embedding, 223
Paragonimiasis, **139**
Paralysis, general, of the insane, 12, 111, **20**
  labioglossopharyngeal, 149
Paramyxovirus, 116, **143**
Paraneoplastic cerebellar atrophy, 140, 162, **170, 191**
Paraneoplastic syndromes, 161, **190**
Paraplegia, hereditary spasmodic, 144, **174**
Parasitic diseases, 112, 199, **139, 140**
Parkinsonian dementia syndrome of Guam, 149
Parkinsonian syndromes, 137
Parkinson's disease, 6, 137, 139, **11, 165**
Paroxysmal hemoglobinuria, 162
Paroxysmal myoglobinuria, 202
Pearly tumors, 45
Pelizaeus-Merzbacher's disease, 130
Pellagra encephalopathy, 3, 155, **184**
Perinatal vascular encephalopathy, 190
Peripheral chromatolysis, 3, **4**
Peripheral nerves, biopsy technique, 216, 226
  histological examination of, 203
  removal at autopsy, 215
Perithelial sarcoma, 42
Perivascular space of Virchow-Robin, 14, **23**
Perivenous encephalitis, 113
Phagocytes, lipid, 11, **18**
Phakomatoses, 187
Phenylketonuria, 175
Phlebitis, cerebral, 103, 104, 162
Phycomycosis, 112
Physaliphorous cells, 48
Phytanic acid storage, 172, 211, **192**
Pick bodies, 136
Pick's disease, 6, 135, 149, **10, 163, 164**
Pigment atrophy, 2
"Pinealoma," 31, **45, 46**
"Pinealoma, ectopic," 32
Pineoblastoma, 32, **30**
Pineocytoma, 32, **30**
Pituitary adenoma, 44, **30, 31, 32, 59**
Plaques, senile, 133, 135, 164, **159, 160**
  shadow, 125, **152**
Plasmodium falciparum, **139**
Platelet emboli, 89
Platybasia, 184
Pleoconial myopathy, 199
Poisoning, bismuth, 158
  carbon monixide, 14, 123, 138, 152, **178, 179**
  cyanide, 150, 152
  lead, 158, 207, **238**
  manganese, 138
  tetraethyl tin, **21**
  tin salts, 131, 158
Polioencephalitides, 113
Polioencephalitis, acute superior hemorrhagic, 153
Poliomyelitis, acute anterior, 115
  chronic anterior, 147, **174**
Poliovirus, 115
Polyarteritis nodosa, 90, 164, 201, 206, 209, **228, 238**
Polyarthritis, chronic progressive, 164, 201, 209
Polycythemia, 162
Polymicrogyria, 181, **210**
Polymyositis, 161, 199, **227**
Polyneuritis, 207, **238**
  alcoholic, 207, **238**
  diphtheritic, 208, **235, 238**

Note: Numbers set in **boldface** type are Figure numbers, not page numbers.

Polyradiculoneuritis, 207, 211, **238**
Pompe's disease, 174, 202
Pontocerebellar angle, tumors of, 33, 46, **27, 31, 47**
Pontoneocerebellar hypoplasia, 181
Porencephaly, 179, **201, 202**
Porphyria, 175, **238**
Portocaval encephalopathy, 157
Postepileptic encephalopathy, 190
Postinfectious encephalitis, 113
Post-traumatic epilepsy, 64
Pott's disease, 107
Presbyophrenia, 134
Progressive multifocal leukoencephalopathy, 9, 10, 120, **146**
Progressive supranuclear palsy of Steele-Richardson-Olszewski, 6, 139
Proliferation, capillary endothelial, 26, **38**
Protoplasmic gliosis, 7, 8, **15**
Protozoa, **139**
Psammoma bodies, 37, 40, **56**
Pseudocalcium, 137, 152, 157
Pseudohypertrophic muscular dystrophy (Duchenne), 197
Pseudopalisades, 26, **38**
Pseudopellagra encephalopathy, 156, 159
Pseudopolydystrophy, 174
Pseudoporencephaly, 189, **201, 216**
Pseudorosettes, 28, **38, 41**
Pseudosyringomyelia, 186
Purpura, thrombocytopenic, 162, **86**
Purulent meningitis, 105, **131, 132**
Putrefaction, bullae of, 15, **24**
Pyocephalus, 105
Pyogenic infections, 105

Rabies, 6, 115
Ramsay Hunt syndrome, 143, 144, **170**
Rathke's pouch, 45
Rectal biopsy, 217
Recurrence, tumor, 58
Refsum's disease, 172, 206, 211, **192, 238**
Reticulum-cell sarcomas, 42, **58**
Retinocerebellar angiomatosis (see *von Hippel–Lindau's disease*)
Retrograde degeneration (see *Central chromatolysis*)
Rhabdomyosarcoma, 44
Rhabdovirus, 115
Rickettsial infections, 113
Ringbinden (ringfibers), 193, **220** (see also *Annulets, striated*)
RNA virus, 115
Rocky Mountain spotted fever, 113
Rod-body myopathy, 198
Rod-shaped microglia, 11, 115, **20, 141**
Rosenthal fibers, 25
  electron microscopy, 131, **158**
Roussy-Lévy syndrome, 144
Rubella, 113, 176
Rupture, ventricular, 67, 71, 77, 107, **85, 96**

Sandhoff disease, 166, **192**
Sanfilippo's disease, 173
Sarcoidosis, 195, 201, 206, 209, **229**

Sarcomas, "arachnoidal," 42
  "circumscribed cerebellar," 31, 42
  fibrosarcomas, 42
  "monstrocellular" (see *Glioblastoma, giant cell*)
  perithelial, 42
  reticulum-cell, 42, **58**
Sarcomatosis, meningeal, 42
Sarcoplasmic masses, 193, 198, 202, **221**
Satellitosis, 10, **17**
Scars, traumatic, 64, 65
Schilder's disease, 9, 10, 123, 128, **15, 150, 154, 155**
Schistosomiasis, **139**
Schizencephaly, 179
Schwannian onion-bulb hypertrophy, 203, 211, **234, 238**
Schwannomas, 33, 187, **30, 47, 48, 49, 50, 52**
  acoustic, 33, **31, 32, 47**
    bilateral, 187
  intracranial, 33, **31, 32, 47**
  intraspinal, 33, **33, 48**
Sclerosis, acute multiple, 126
  Ammon's horn, 190
  amyotrophic lateral, 3, 16, 149, **172, 173, 174**
  Guam form, 6, 149
  centrilobar, of Foix and Marie, 189
  concentric, of Baló, 129
  diffuse (see *Schilder's disease*)
  disseminated (see *Sclerosis, multiple*)
  laminar, of Morel, 160
  multiple, 9, 10, 16, 121, 123, 124, **150, 151, 152, 153**
    acute, 126
  transitional, 129
  tuberose, of Bourneville, 4, 178, 187
Scrapie, 120
Segmental demyelination, 203, 208, 211, 226, **232, 233, 235**
Seitelberger's disease, 131
Senile dementia, 6, 132, 135, **159**
Senile plaques, 133, 135, 164, **159, 160**
Septum lucidum, agenesis of, 180, **202**
Shadow plaques, 125, **152**
Shingles, 118
Shy-Drager's disease, 139
Sickle-cell anemia, **86**
Siderosis, subpial cerebral, 73
Sinus, congenital dermal, 177, **199**
  superior sagittal, thrombosis of, 104
Skin biopsy, 217
Skull, fractures of, 60, **78, 83**
Slit hemorrhages, 69, **89**
Slow-virus infections, 113, 120
Smallpox, 113
Space, extracellular, 13, **21**
  perivascular, 14, **23**
  Virchow-Robin, 14, **23**
Spasm, arterial, 77, 85
Sphingolipidoses, 166, **192**
Sphingomyelin, 171, **192**
Spielmeyer's acute swelling, 1
Spielmeyer's granular degeneration, 1
Spielmeyer-Vogt disease, 168
Spina bifida, 176, 177, 185, **199**
Spinal cord, degenerative disorders of, 144, **174**
  infarcts of, 98, **125, 126**
  injuries of, 66, **84**
  removal of, 213
  subacute combined degeneration of, 13, 156, **185**

Note: Numbers set in **boldface** type are Figure numbers, not page numbers.

Spinal cord (*Continued*)
  tumors of, 18, 25, 26, 28, 49, **29, 33, 36, 66**
Spinal hereditary amyotrophy, 146, **174**
Spine, fractures, 66, **84**
Spongiosis, 13, 120, 131, 156, **147, 185**
Spongy degeneration, of neuraxis, 131, 167
  of white matter, 13
Stains, histological, of nervous system, **246, 247**
Status cribratus, 102, 137
Status lacunatus, 102
Status marmoratus, 189
Status spongiosus (see *Spongiosis*)
Steele-Richardson-Olszewski disease, 6, 139
Stenosis, aqueductal, 15, 183, 187
  arterial, 85, 88, **109, 111, 112, 113**
Steroid myopathy, 201
Storage, lipid neuronal, 4, 166, 167, 168, 170, 171,
  173, **7, 8, 192, 193**
Striated annulets, 193, 198, 202, **220**
Striatonigral degeneration, 138
Strumpell-Lorrain disease, 144, **174**
Sturge-Weber's disease, 188
Subacute bacterial endocarditis, 77
Subacute combined degeneration, of cord, 13, 156, **185**
"Subacute necrotic myelitis" of Foix and Alajouanine,
  79, **102**
Subacute sclerosing leukoencephalitis, 116
Subacute sclerosing panencephalitis, 6, 9, 10, 116, 128,
  142, 143
Subarachnoid hemorrhage, nontraumatic, 67, 73, 79,
  81, **85, 86, 97, 98**
  of newborn, 188
Subclavian steal syndrome, 89
Subcortical encephalopathy of Binswanger, 103, **129**
Subdural abscess, 105
Subdural empyema, 105
Subdural hematoma, 61, 62, 66, **80, 81, 83, 85**
  of newborn, 188
Subdural hygromas, 61, 183
Subependymal glia, proliferation of, 15
Subependymoma, 29
Subneural apparatus, demonstration of, 225
Subpial cerebral siderosis, 73
Subthalamic nuclei (corpora Luysii), atrophy of, 138
Sudanophilic leukodystrophy, 130, **150, 156, 157**
Sulfatide lipidosis (see *Sulfatidoses*)
Sulfatidoses, 169, 211, **192, 196, 238**
Sulfotransferase, 169
Supranuclear progressive palsy of Steele-Richardson-
  Olszewski, 6, 139
SV40 virus, 120
Swellings, axonal, 7, **13**
  oligodendroglial, 10
"Swiss-cheese brain," 15, **24**
Syphilis of the central nervous system, 12, 90, 110, **20**
Syphilitic gumma, 110
Syringobulbia, **214**
Syringomyelia, 185, 187, **213**
Syringomyelobulbia, 185
Systemic lupus erythematosus, 164, 201, 209

Tabes dorsalis, 111
Taenia echinococcus, **139**
Taenia solium, **139, 140**
Tangier's disease, 172, **192**

Tapeworms, **139**
Target fibers, 193, 195, **219**
Tay-Sachs disease, 9, 166, **192, 193**
Teased preparations, 203, 226
Telangiectases, 79, **86**
Tentorial notch tumors, 18, **26, 27**
Teratomas, 49, **30**
  atypical, 32
Tetraethyl lead poisoning, 158
Tetraethyl tin poisoning, **21**
Thalamus, hemorrhage in, 69, **87**
  infarct of, 96, **120**
Thesaurismosis, 165
Third ventricle, colloid cysts of, 30, **30, 43**
Thrombocytopenic purpura, 162, **86**
Thrombosis, arterial, 85, 87, 89, **109, 112, 113, 115**
  of basilar artery, 89, 96, **115**
  of internal carotid artery, 89, 92, 95, **112, 113, 115**
  of middle cerebral artery, 89, **115**
  of posterior cerebral artery, 89, **115**
  of subclavian artery, 89
  of superior sagittal sinus, 104
  of vein of Galen, 104
  of vertebral artery, 89, 96, **115**
  venous superficial, 104, **130**
Thrombotic microangiopathy, 162
Tin poisoning, 131, 158
Tissue-type antigens, and multiple sclerosis, 126
Tonsillar herniation, 58, **76**
Torpedoes, 7, **13**
Torulosis, 111, **138**
Toxoplasmosis, 176, 199, **139**
"Tramcar" nuclei, 193, **218**
Transitional sclerosis, 129
Trans-synaptic degeneration, 3
Trauma, craniocerebral, 60, 65, **83**
  obstetric, 188
  to spinal cord and nerve roots, 66, **84**
Traumatic scars, 64, 65
Trematodes, **139**
Treponema pallidum, 111
Trichinosis, 199, **139**
Trichopoliodystrophy, 175
Trihexosylceramide, 172, **192**
Trisomy 13–15, 176, 180, **205**
Trisomy 21, 176, 182
Trypanosomiasis, **139**
Tryptophan, 175
Tube, neural, closure defects of, 176, **199**
Tuberculoma, 110, **137**
Tuberculosis, spinal, 107
Tuberculous meningitis, 14, 90, 108, **135, 136**
Tuberose sclerosis, 4, 178, 187
Tubules, ependymal, 28, **41**
Tumors, age incidence and type, 18, 20, **32**
  bone, 54
  causing radiculospinal compression, 18, **29, 33**
  classification, histological, 18, **30**
    topographical, 18, **26, 27**
  extramedullary spinal, 18, **29, 33**
  infratentorial, 18, **26, 27, 28, 31**
  intramedullary spinal, 18, **29, 33**
  intraspinal, 18, **29, 33**
  metastatic, 51, **67, 68, 69, 70**
  of foramen magnum, 18, **26, 27**
  of posterior fossa, 18, **28, 32**
  of tentorial notch, 18, **26, 27**

Note: Numbers set in **boldface** type are Figure numbers, not page numbers.

Tumors (*Continued*)
  primary, 23, **30, 31**
  secondary, 51, **70**
  supratentorial, 18, **26, 27, 31**
Type I fiber hypotrophy, 199
Typhus, 113
Typing, muscle fibers, 194, 195, 197, 198, 199, 225, **224, 226**
Tyrosinosis, 175

Ulegyria, 188, **215**
Unverricht-Lundborg myoclonic epilepsy, 174
Uremia, **238**
Uveo-meningoencephalitides, 120

Vaccination, against rabies, 116, 128
  against smallpox, 113
Vacuolar myopathy, 201
van Bogaert and Bertrand's disease (see *Canavan's disease*)
Varicella, 118
"Varix" of vein of Galen, 79, **103**
Vascular malformations, 67, 72, 77, 79, 90, **86, 101, 102, 103**
Vein of Galen, thrombosis of, 104
Ventricles, dilatation of, 12, 132, 138, 179, 183, **42, 73, 77, 135, 201, 212**
  fifth, 180, **203**
  third, colloid cysts of, 30, **30, 43**
Ventricular rupture, 67, 71, 77, 107, **85, 96**
Vertebral fractures, 66, **84**
Vincristine, 158

Viral diseases, 112
Virchow-Robin space, 14, **23**
Virological investigations, 224, 226
Viruses, DNA, 117
  RNA, 115
  slow, 113, 120
von Economo's encephalitis lethargica, 120
von Hippel–Lindau disease, 49, 187, **66**
von Recklinghausen's disease, 33, 35, 187, **48**

Waldenström's macroglobulinemia, 162, 164, 211
Wallenberg's syndrome, 96, **121**
Wallerian degeneration, 7, 123, 203, 207, 208, 211, **149, 231**
Werdnig-Hoffmann's disease, 146, 198, **174**
Wernicke's encephalopathy, 3, 14, 153, 159, **180, 181, 182, 183**
Wet film technique, 215
Whorls, 40, **56**
Wilson's disease, 9, 157, 175, **16**
Wolman's disease, 172, **192**
Wounds, cerebral, 65

Xanthogranuloma, juvenile, 172
Xanthoma, fibrous, 42
Xanthomatoses, 172
Xanthosarcoma, 42

Zebra bodies, 173, **198**
Zona, 118

Note: Numbers set in **boldface** type are Figure numbers, not page numbers.